Progress in Oncology 2002

Edited by

Vincent T. DeVita, Jr.
Yale Cancer Center
New Haven, Connecticut

Samuel Hellman
Department of Radiation Oncology
University of Chicago
Chicago, Illinois

Steven A. Rosenberg
National Cancer Institute
National Institutes of Health
Bethesda, Maryland

JONES AND BARTLETT PUBLISHERS
Sudbury, Massachusetts
BOSTON TORONTO LONDON SINGAPORE

World Headquarters
Jones and Bartlett Publishers
40 Tall Pine Drive
Sudbury, MA 01776
info@jbpub.com
www.jbpub.com

Jones and Bartlett Publishers Canada
2406 Nikanna Road
Mississauga, ON L5C 2W6
CANADA

Jones and Bartlett Publishers International
Barb House, Barb Mews
London W6 7PA
UK

ISBN 0-7637-2063-1

ISSN 1535-9980

Acquisitions Editor: Christopher Davis
Production Editor: Elizabeth Platt
Cover and Interior Design: Anne Spencer
Cover Image: © Nancy Kedersha/Science Photo/Custom Medical Stock Photo
Manufacturing Buyer: Amy Bacus
Composition: Modern Graphics, Inc.
Printing and Binding: Malloy Lithographing
Cover Printer: Malloy Lithographing

The authors, editor, and publisher have made every effort to provide accurate information. However, they are not responsible for errors, omissions, or for any outcomes related to the use of the contents of this book and take no responsibility for the use of the products described. Treatments and side effects described in this book may not be applicable to all patients; likewise, some patients may require a dose or experience a side effect that is not described herein. Drugs and medical devices are discussed that may have limited availability controlled by the Food and Drug Administration (FDA) for use only in a research study or clinical trial. The drug information presented has been derived from reference sources, recently published data and pharmaceutical tests. Research, clinical practice, and government regulations often change the accepted standard in this field. When consideration is being given to use of any drug in the clinical setting, the health care provider or reader is responsible for determining FDA status of the drug, reading the package insert, reviewing prescribing information for the most up-to-date recommendations on dose, precautions, and contraindications, and determining the appropriate usage for the product. This is especially important in the case of drugs or therapies that are new or seldom used.

Printed in the United States of America
06 05 04 03 10 9 8 7 6 5 4 3 2

Contents

Current Controversies in Oncology

List of Contributors

Hakan Akbulut, MD
Ankara University Faculty of Medicine, Department of Medical Oncology, Ankara, Turkey

Sunil J. Advani, PhD
The Marjorie B. Kovler Viral Oncology Laboratories and The Department of Radiation and Cellular Oncology, The University of Chicago, Chicago, Illinois

James P. Allison, PhD
Cancer Research Laboratory, University of California at Berkeley, Berkeley, California

Dario C. Altieri, MD
Department of Pathology, Boyer Center for Molecular Medicine, Yale University School of Medicine, New Haven, Connecticut

Charles M. Balch, MD
The Johns Hopkins Medical Institutions, Baltimore, Maryland, and the American Society of Clinical Oncology, Alexandria, Virginia

Donald A. Berry, PhD
Department of Biostatistics, The University of Texas M. D. Anderson Cancer Center, Houston, Texas

Smita Bhatia, MD, MPH
City of Hope National Medical Center, Duarte, California

Renier Brentjens, MD, PhD
Gastrointestinal Oncology Service, Department of Medicine, Memorial Sloan Kettering Cancer Center, New York, New York

Antonio Buzaid, MD
Hospital Sirio Libanes, San Paulo, Brazil

Shu-Hsia Chen, PhD
Gene Therapy and Molecular Medicine, Derald H. Ruttenberg Cancer Center, New York, New York

Albert Deisseroth, MD, PhD
Sidney Kimmel Cancer Center, San Diego, California

George D. Demetri, MD
Center for Sarcoma and Bone Oncology, Dana-Farber Cancer Institute, and Harvard Medical School, Boston, Massachusetts

Deborah Dillon, MD
Yale University School of Medicine, New Haven, Connecticut

Raymond N. DuBois, MD, PhD
Departments of Medicine and Cell Biology, Vanderbilt University Medical Center and Department of Veterans Affairs Medical Center, Nashville, Tennessee

Isaiah J. Fidler, MD
Department of Cancer Biology, The University of Texas M. D. Anderson Cancer Center, Houston, Texas

Patricia L. Fiero, PhD
Medical University of South Carolina, Charleston, South Carolina

Rajnish A. Gupta, MD
Departments of Medicine and Cell Biology, Vanderbilt University Medical Center and Department of Veterans Affairs Medical Center, Nashville, Tennessee

Claudia I. Henschke, MD, PhD
Department of Radiology, Joan and Stanford I. Weill Medical College of Cornell University, New York, New York

Daniel B. Kopans, MD
Harvard Medical School and Massachusetts General Hospital, Boston, Massachusetts.

Wendy Landier, RN, MSN, CPNP
City of Hope National Medical Center, Duarte, California

Scott Leischow, PhD
Tobacco Control Research Branch, Division of Cancer Control and Population Sciences, National Cancer Institute, Bethesda, Maryland

Douglas R. Lowy, MD
Laboratory of Cellular Oncology, National Cancer Institute, Bethesda, Maryland

Eva Matthews, MPH
Health Promotion Sciences, University of Arizona, Tucson, Arizona

Olli S. Miettinen, MD, PhD
Department of Medicine, Weill Medical College of Cornell University, New York, New York, and the Departments of Epidemiology and Biostatistics and of Medicine, Faculty of Medicine, McGill University, Montreal, Canada.

Glen Morgan, PhD
Tobacco Control Research Branch, Division of Cancer Control and Population Sciences, National Cancer Institute, Bethesda, Maryland

Michael S. O'Reilly, MD
Departments of Cancer Biology and Radiation Oncology, The University of Texas M. D. Anderson Cancer Center, Houston, Texas

James O. Prochaska, MD
Cancer Prevention Research Center, University of Rhode Island, Kingston, Rhode Island.

Leslie L. Robison, PhD
Division of Pediatric Epidemiology and Clinical Research, University of Minnesota, Minneapolis, Minnesota

Leonard Saltz, MD
Department of Medicine, Joan and Stanford I. Weill Medical College of Cornell University, New York, New York

John T. Schiller, PhD
Laboratory of Cellular Oncology, National Cancer Institute, Bethesda, Maryland

James P. Smith, MD
Department of Medicine, Joan and Stanford I. Weill Medical College of Cornell University, New York, New York

Seng-Jaw Soong, PhD
University of Alabama at Birmingham, Birmingham, Alabama

Kathryn Stone, MD
HHMI Biopolymer/W.M. Keck Foundation, Biotechnology Resource Laboratory at Yale University, New Haven, Connecticut

Max W. Sung, MD
Department of Medicine, Medical Oncology Division, Derald H. Ruttenberg Cancer Center, New York, New York

John F. Thompson, MD
Sydney Melanoma Unit, Royal Prince Alfred Hospital and University of Sydney, Sydney, Australia

Ralph R. Weichselbaum, MD
Department of Radiation and Cellular Oncology, The University of Chicago, Chicago, Illinois

Robert M. Weiss, MD
Department of Surgery (Urology), Yale University School of Medicine, New Haven, Connecticut

Kenneth Williams, PhD
HHMI Biopolymer/W.M. Keck Foundation, Biotechnology Resource Laboratory at Yale University, New Haven, Connecticut

Savio L. C. Woo, PhD
Carl C. Icahn Institute for Gene Therapy and Molecular Medicine, New York, New York

David F. Yankelevitz, MD
Department of Radiology, Joan and Stanford I. Weill Medical College of Cornell University, New York, New York

Chapter 1

Potential Application for Proteomics in Oncology

Deborah Dillon

Kathryn Stone

Kenneth Williams

With recent advances in our knowledge of the sequence of the human genome has come a renewed interest in the structure, function, and interactions of the encoded proteins. The term *proteome* was first used in 1995 to refer to all of the proteins expressed by a given genome.[1] *Proteomics* has since come to refer to the global analysis of cellular proteins (reviewed in Refs. 2–7). Recent interest in this new field of study pays tribute to a growing awareness within the scientific community that the genomic sequence is, by itself, of only limited utility in understanding cellular functions and disease pathogenesis.

There are a number of reasons why the global analysis of proteins is expected to provide a more accurate reflection of disease processes than are global mRNA expression analyses. Several studies have provided evidence that mRNA expression levels are correlated only moderately with protein abundance.[8–10] Furthermore, genomic information does not reflect posttranscriptional regulation or posttranslational modifications, such as glycosylation or phosphorylation, which have a major impact on protein function. Gene sequence and mRNA expression data also fail to reflect protein-protein interactions and pathways within the cell, critical to higher-level organizational function.[11] Thus, although global protein analysis is inherently more complex and more difficult to study, it also promises to be more informative.

The analysis of cellular proteins has typically been performed using two-dimensional polyacrylamide gel electrophoresis (2D-PAGE) for separation and visualization of proteins, followed by mass spectrometry for identification (Fig. 1.1). These studies are labor-intensive and, due to the requirement for large amounts of protein, have mostly been performed using cell lines and bulk tissue samples. Fueling the new "postgenomic" era of proteomic research are advances in complementary fields leading to the development of high-throughput technologies, improved cell separation techniques, and better image analysis and database software. These advances offer the hope of resolving and identifying large numbers of cellular proteins more efficiently and accurately than ever before, and they make it possible to begin contemplating clinical applications for these technologies.

The ultimate hope is that the ability to perform global expressed protein comparisons between well-defined groups of cells (e.g., different stages of tumor development, different recognized prognostic categories, or different drug susceptibilities) will lead to new insights into the mechanisms of tumor progression,

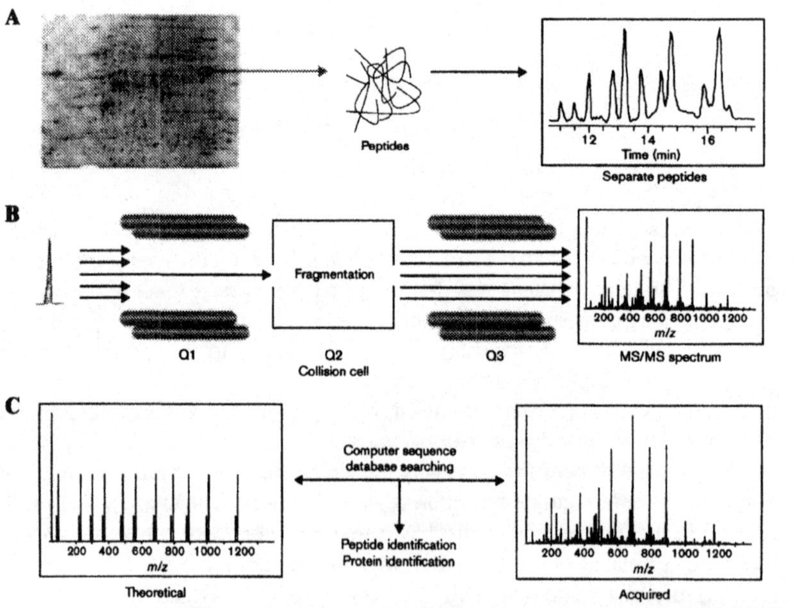

FIGURE 1.1. Standard proteomic analysis by two-dimensional polyacrylamide gel electrophoresis and mass spectrometry. Proteins are first separated by two-dimensional polyacrylamide gel electrophoresis and are excised from the gel (A); peptides are ionized by electrospray and fragmented (B); and the acquired tandem mass spectrometry spectrum is compared to predicted spectra from a sequence database (C). (Gygi SP et al. Curr Opin Biotechnol 2000; 11:396–401. Reprinted with permission.)

new protein markers for early detection, new prognostic and predictive markers, new therapeutic targets, and new endpoints for measuring therapeutic efficacy and toxicity. Here, we review the technologies used in these efforts, their strengths and limitations, and preliminary results of proteomic studies in areas of critical interest in cancer diagnosis, prognosis, and therapeutics.

TECHNOLOGY FOR PROTEOMIC ANALYSIS

Cell Enrichment Techniques

Many proteomic studies of cancer have used tumor cell lines or whole-tumor tissues. The effects of tissue culture on protein profiles or dilution of the signal of interest in the background of a mixed cell population must be kept in mind in interpreting results of these studies. Considerable interest exists in facilitating the study of patient samples within their native tissue environment, as opposed to cultured or transplanted cells, the expressed proteins of which may be very different. However, tissues are complex heterogeneous mixtures of cells, and the presence of contaminating cells within a tissue sample will dilute any specific signal generated from the cell population of interest. Thus, for the most informative results, it is critical to achieve significant enrichment prior to proteomic analysis. This enrichment for the cell population of interest may be achieved using any of a number of cell separation techniques, including flow cytometry, antibody purification (when appropriate antibodies are available), and microdissection.

Laser microdissection is particularly well suited to the analysis of tissues. Using laser microdissection, one can effectively separate and collect specific cell populations under direct morphologic guidance.[12] Proteins solubilized from laser-captured tissues retain their expected electrophoretic mobility on two-dimensional gels as compared with bulk samples of the tissue.[13–15] Mass spectrometry profiles also appear to be unaffected by laser capture. Efforts to couple laser capture microdissection with proteomic analysis have shown promising results and are beginning to yield proteins of potential clinical utility.[13,14]

Sample Preparation for Protein Identification

The completion of draft versions of the human and many other genomes has quickly redirected most protein chemistry and mass spectrometry core laboratories from trying to obtain just enough peptide sequence to enable oligonucleotide primers and probes to be synthesized to identifying proteins—which invariably have been separated by one-dimensional or two-dimensional sodium dodecyl sulfate (SDS) PAGE. No other current technology rivals the ability of SDS PAGE to resolve complex protein mixtures in amounts sufficient for subsequent protein identification. Currently, 2D-PAGE remains the method of choice for protein profiling of large numbers of proteins—albeit from small numbers of samples—because it is difficult to achieve high throughput with 2D-PAGE. In this regard, Gygi and colleagues[16] visualized > 1,500 silver-stained yeast protein spots using a 1.0-pH-unit isoelectric focusing range in the first dimension. By extrapolation, they estimate that a full complement of 7 × 1.0 pH-unit gels might be able to resolve 10,500 features.

Assuming that 2D gels have been run to compare the proteome of a control versus an experimental sample and that several spots have been shown to differ substantially in level of expression between these two samples, the next goal is to identify the proteins in these selected spots. Because 80%–90% of proteins from higher eukaryotes appear to have "blocked" N-terminals,[17] with the blocking most often resulting from in vivo protein acetylation, proteins usually cannot be identified by direct amino acid sequencing via Edman degradation. Rather, they usually must first be proteolytically digested with trypsin (which cleaves after lysine or arginine) or endopeptidase Lys-C (which cleaves after lysine). In this instance, the normal Coomassie blue staining and destaining procedure removes the buffers, salts, SDS, and other reagents present during SDS PAGE, leaving behind a denatured protein eminently susceptible to proteolysis and transiently trapped in the gel slice. After the destaining solution is removed and the gel band is dried, it can be rehydrated in the volatile buffer used for trypsin digestion, and the relatively low molecular weight enzyme then can be diffused into the gel to digest the protein.

Protein Identification and Database Searching

After trypsin digestion, the resulting peptides are extracted from the polyacrylamide gel with volatile solvents, which puts them in an ideal format to be subjected to one or more of the protein identification strategies summarized in Table 1.1. The three strategies are arranged in order of their general reliability and the amount of protein required, with usable peptide mass data often being obtained from matrix-assisted laser desorption ionization mass spectrometry (MALDI-MS) studies carried out on as little as 10–25 fmol of protein digests. Figure 1.2 shows a typical strategy that might be used to identify "unknown" proteins submitted to a large biotechnology core laboratory. Because of its relative ease of use and very high sensitivity, MALDI-MS analysis of aliquots of nonfractionated tryptic digests followed by peptide mass database searching is probably the protein identification approach that is used most widely. A further advantage of this approach is that it is amenable to high-throughput analysis. Instrumentation is available to automate virtually all required steps (in-gel digestion, extraction-spotting onto MALDI-MS targets, MALDI-MS, and database searching) in this process with consequent large savings in cost and turnaround time.

Several factors can be brought into play either to confirm or to weaken an identification based on peptide mass database searching. First, the identified

TABLE 1.1 Protein Identification Approaches Often Available in Biotechnology Core Laboratories

Type of Peptide Data Acquired	Minimum Recommended Amount of Polyacrylamide Gel-Separated Protein	Type of Analysis Usually Carried Out	Representative Database Search Algorithm
MALDI-MS masses (with high accuracy)	100 fmol	MALDI	ProFound,[1] PepSea[2]
Uninterpreted peptide MS/MS fragmentation data	0.1–1.0 pmol	MS/MS via nanospray or LC/MS/MS	Sequest[3]
Edman sequencing	5 pmol	Preparative capillary HPLC followed by Edman sequencing	NCBI nr[4]

HPLC, high-pressure liquid chromatography; LC, liquid chromatography; MALDI-MS, matrix-assisted laser desorption ionization mass spectrometry; MS/MS, tandem mass spectrometry.

[1] *http://129.85.19.192/profound_bin/WebProFound.exe*

[2] *http://195.41.108.38/PA_PepSeaForm.html*

[3] Sequest is distributed by Finnigan Corporation, a division of ThermoQuest Corporation.

[4] *http://www.ncbi.nlm.nih.gov/BLAST/*

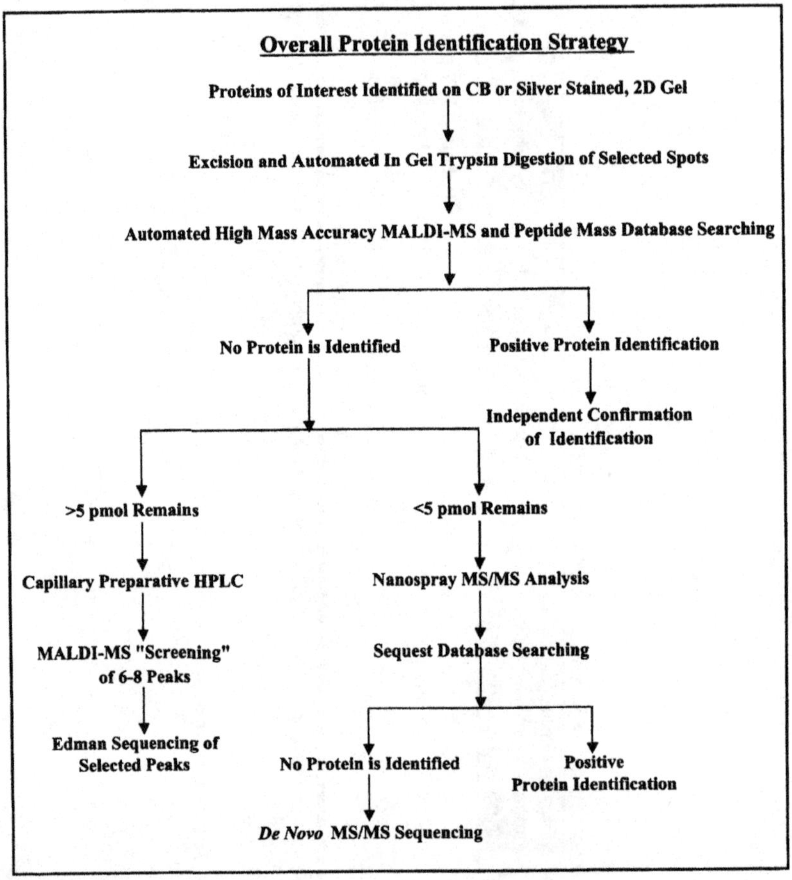

FIGURE 1.2 Typical strategy for identification of proteins submitted to a large biotechnology core laboratory.

protein should be from the correct species. If the organism from which the protein was isolated has not been sequenced in its entirety (i.e., the gene encoding the protein of interest has not yet been sequenced), it is possible that the best match may be to a protein that is structurally homologous and having a gene that has been sequenced already from a different organism. Second, the molecular weight observed by SDS PAGE generally should be within a 0.5- to 1.5-fold "window" around the predicted molecular weight or there should be a good explanation for its falling outside this window. Third, if the sample was isolated by 2D-PAGE, the observed versus predicted pI will provide an additional criterion. Fourth, the functional properties or activities (e.g., affinity for nucleic acids, adenosine triphosphatase activity) of the identified protein should be consistent with the known or presumed properties of the isolated protein (e.g., ability to bind nucleic acids). Although any part and all of these data may be used to quickly bolster or cast doubt on an identification based on peptide mass searching, it is strongly recommended that additional studies (Western blotting/antibody detection, tandem mass spectrometry [MS/MS], or Edman sequencing of one or more tryptic peptides) be carried out prior to drawing firm conclusions. Finally, it must be kept in mind always that if the sample has not been purified sufficiently, the major protein in the Coomassie blue or silver-stained band may not be the protein responsible for the activity being followed. In this regard, it is interesting that Gygi et al.[16] detected as many as six proteins comigrating to the same faintly silver-stained spot on a 2D gel.

An alternative mass spectrometric approach to protein identification is MS/MS. In this instance, the mass spectrometer is used both to isolate a specific peptide ion from a digest mixture and then to fragment it. In contrast to MALDI-MS-based protein identification, MS/MS protein identification uses both peptide mass and peptide fragmentation data. The MS/MS data usually are acquired either via liquid chromatography–MS, as described by Stone et al,[18] or by nanospray analysis of the unfractionated in-gel tryptic digest.[19] During this approximately 30-minute analysis, it is generally possible to manually select and fragment 6–15 peptide ions that generate the MS/MS spectra. These are then individually searched against the National Center for Biotechnology Information (NCBI) nonredundant database using the Sequest algorithm.[20] For each MS/MS spectrum selected, the corresponding peptide mass is first searched by Sequest against a database for every peptide with an equivalent mass. Using the tandem mass correlation algorithm developed by Yates et al,[21] the MS/MS spectra of the mass-matched peptides are then compared to the observed MS/MS spectra and are ranked. The final ranking of peptide sequences by Sequest is based on a correlation score (C) that provides a quantitative description of how well the observed MS/MS peptide fragmentation spectrum correlates with the theoretical MS/MS spectrum of the candidate peptide. It is important to mention that Sequest database searching is carried out with uninterpreted MS/MS spectra, bringing this technology within reach of investigators and staff who may have relatively little training in mass spectrometry.

Finally, it is also possible to fractionate in-gel tryptic digests of proteins via reverse-phase high-pressure liquid chromatography (HPLC), to collect the resulting fractions, and then to subject one or more of the isolated peptides to amino acid sequencing via Edman degradation. The resulting peptide sequence can then be searched against the NCBI nonredundant database. In many instances, a single tryptic peptide sequence spanning 10–15 residues is sufficient to identify the parent protein unambiguously. Because of the expertise and time required to carry out "internal" Edman sequencing on low picomole amounts of SDS PAGE–separated proteins, most biotechnology core laboratories first "screen" samples submitted for identification via MALDI-MS or MS/MS analysis for known proteins prior to embarking on the more involved preparative liquid chromatography and internal Edman sequencing of selected peptides.

Glimpses of the Future: Quantitative Analysis of Genome Level Protein Expression

Although two-dimensional gel electrophoresis followed by mass spectrometry–based protein identification has been the most common way to assess relative protein expression and remains the gold standard for protein discovery, this methodology has a number of limitations. Two-dimensional gel electrophoresis does not adequately separate hydrophobic proteins[22] and does not allow visualization of low-abundance proteins (10–1,000 copies per cell), which can often be obscured by highly expressed proteins, such as the structural proteins (> 10,000 copies per cell).[16,23,24] In addition, in terms of assessing the potential for the application of proteomic studies to routine clinical use, two-dimensional gels are laborious and time-consuming and, thus, are likely to be of limited practical use. In response to this need, several new platforms have been developed for high-throughput proteomic analysis.

Two related technologies already in use are biomolecular interaction analysis mass spectrometry and surface-enhanced laser desorption ionization (SELDI) spectrometry either to simplify the ensemble of proteins analyzed or to direct the analysis toward a specific target protein or proteins. In both technologies, the surface of the MALDI-MS sample plate is derivatized so that it either has a defined chromatography-like characteristic (e.g., cationic, hydrophilic, hydrophobic) or has a covalently bound ligand (e.g., protein, oligonucleotide, antibody, enzyme substrate) that binds to the target protein with high affinity. Hence, a crude extract might be passed over a SELDI chip containing bound DNA to specifically enrich for a transcription factor of interest. After a brief washing to remove noninteracting proteins, the SELDI chip is subjected to MALDI-MS so that a mass spectrum can be produced and will provide the mass profile for the noncovalently bound proteins. In the case of biomolecular interaction analysis mass spectrometry, a phenomenon called *surface plasmon resonance* can be used to detect the presence of noncovalently bound proteins prior to subjecting the chip to MALDI-MS.[25] Attractive features of biomolecular interaction analysis mass spectrometry and SELDI include the ability to direct the analysis toward the class or individual protein of interest and, in the case of SELDI, the relative ease of automating the technology to permit high-throughput analysis of the same protein from numerous samples. Both approaches suffer from the limitations inherent in MALDI-MS analysis of intact proteins, which provide substantially decreased response and resolution (due to their higher molecular weight) as compared to tryptic peptides that, because of their small size and relatively uniform net positive charge, are ideally suited for MALDI-MS analysis. Hence, SELDI analysis of epithelial cells detected only about three proteins in the 20,000- to 60,000-Da range and only one protein beyond this range with poor resolution.[26] SELDI may, however, provide a reasonable approach for high-throughput expression analysis of small subsets of proteins.

Perhaps the most promising approach to quantitative, "genome-wide" protein profiling is the isotope-coded affinity tag (ICAT) methodology devised by Gygi et al.[27] The ICAT reagent contains two crucial functional groups: a thiol-specific reactive group that covalently and specifically links the ICAT reagent to cysteine residues in proteins and a biotinyl tag that allows rapid separation and isolation of the modified peptides. The key to this technology is the availability of two forms of the ICAT reagents—heavy and light—that differ in mass by 8 Da due to the incorporation of 8 deuteriums in the heavy reagent in place of 8 hydrogens in the light reagent. These two reagents are thus analogous to the Cy3 and Cy5 dyes used in DNA microarray analysis and permit the two samples being compared to be mixed together prior to mass spectrometric analysis.

A typical experiment might begin by modifying a whole-cell protein isolate from a sample of interest (e.g., tumor tissue) with the heavy ICAT reagent while a control protein sample isolate (e.g., normal tissue) is modified with the light ICAT reagent. At this point, the two samples are mixed and subjected to trypsin digestion. After fractionating this extremely complex peptide mixture via cation exchange chromatography, each of the resulting fractions is subjected to an avidin affinity step to isolate cysteine-containing tryptic peptides and then to liquid chromatography-MS/MS, with the liquid chromatography being carried out on a reverse phase column, providing exceptionally good resolution of tryptic peptides. During this analysis, each modified tryptic peptide will produce a signal for both its heavy and light forms. The ratio of the areas of these two peaks provides an accurate estimation of the relative abundance of this particular tryptic peptide in each digest, which in turn provides the relative abundance of the parent protein in the two samples being compared. It is estimated that > 80% of human proteins contain cysteine. Hence, slightly different approaches, perhaps based on modification of histidine, methionine, or another amino acid, eventually may be needed to monitor expression of proteins that do not contain cysteine. Both the cation exchange and avidin chromatography steps are important, as they substantially reduce the complexity of the resulting digest and thus enable more isotopic peptide pairs to be resolved and more of their parent proteins to be quantified. Han et al[28] used this overall approach to identify and determine the ratios of abundance (within ± 20%) of 491 proteins contained in the microsomal fractions of naive and in vitro differentiated human myeloid leukemia (HL-60) cells.

Detection and Identification of Posttranslational Modifications

Because protein function is often modulated by posttranslational events, there is intense interest in identifying and quantifying the relative level of phosphorylation and other protein modifications. One general approach for detecting and identifying the locations in proteins of many modifications is to carry out comparative analysis (e.g., MALDI, liquid chromatography–MS, comparative tryptic peptide HPLC mapping) of an experimental sample of protein isolated from its normal biological host versus the same protein that has been cloned and expressed in *Escherichia coli,* which lacks many of the enzymes that add posttranslational modifications to proteins from humans and other higher organisms. Hence, comparative HPLC tryptic peptide mapping of the human heterogeneous nuclear ribonucleoprotein A1 versus the same protein that was expressed in *E. coli* quickly identified several HPLC peaks that did not co-elute. Amino acid sequencing and mass spectrometric analysis of the nonaligning human A1 peptide peaks demonstrated that they contained a total of four arginine residues that had been posttranslationally methylated.[29] Another similar approach is to carry out the comparative HPLC or mass spectrometric studies before and after removing the posttranslational modification of interest (e.g., by enzymatic or chemical removal of carbohydrate modifications).

A major challenge that confounds the analysis of protein posttranslational modifications, such as phosphorylation (often involved in modulating protein function), is that the stoichiometry of the modification may be very low. Hence, only 5% or fewer of the total number of molecules of a certain protein may actually be phosphorylated, which makes it extremely difficult to use such conventional approaches as mass spectrometry to identify their location within the protein structure. Although radiochemical labeling may be used in this instance to help bring about an identification, often it is not feasible to carry out radiochemical labeling studies in higher organisms. In this instance, the modified ICAT approach devised by Goshe et al[30] not only allows the enrichment and isolation of phosphorylated tryptic peptides but permits their relative quantitation, thus providing for the intriguing possibility of carrying out comparative, quantitative analysis of phosphoproteomes.

APPLICATION OF PROTEOMICS IN ONCOLOGY

Two broad categories of proteomics research, essentially different in their approach, have been distinguished: (1) the determination of global protein profiles that characterize cell and tissue types, with determination of the profile changes that occur with disease, drug action, or other biological stimuli (so-called expression proteomics), and (2) determination of the subcellular localization of proteins and protein-protein interactions by purification of cellular organelles or complexes and subsequent identification of components by mass spectrometry, or "cell-map proteomics."[3] Both approaches have potential utility in identifying proteins involved in tumor development and progression. The proteins characteristic of different types of tumors at different stages of development may then be used as biomarkers in the early detection of cancer, in refining prognostic and therapeutic categories, in molecular staging, and as potential drug targets and markers of drug efficacy and toxicity. Preliminary studies have been performed in many of these areas; in addition to demonstrating proof of principle, they also highlight the particular challenges that lie ahead.

Elucidation of Tumor Development and Progression

The histologic changes that accompany the progression from normal epithelium to in situ carcinoma and invasive carcinoma are generally well-characterized in each organ and, in the setting of a well-oriented, well-preserved tissue section of adequate size, rarely present diagnostic difficulty. However, diagnostic challenges for the pathologist occur in the setting of small, nonoriented biopsy specimens; artifacts that due to handling result in obscured architecture and cytology; small numbers of atypical cells; and metastatic tumors of unknown origin. Immunohistochemical stains are currently available to provide additional information about the origin and nature of cells observed under the microscope and can be a significant diagnostic aid in challenging cases. Examples are the use of leukocyte-common antigen and cytokeratins to help to distinguish lymphoma from poorly differentiated carcinoma and the use of keratin 903 for basal cells to help in the evaluation of atypical glands in the prostate for the possibility of invasive adenocarcinoma.

Although these immunostains have been extremely helpful in addressing important diagnostic questions, access to a global scan of protein differences might extend diagnostic decision-making capabilities even further. The ability of proteomic profiles to address diagnostic questions will require first the establishment of large, reliable databases from which one can extract the subset of proteins that best distinguish two diagnostic entities (e.g., reactive atypia vs. in situ carcinoma; atypical hyperplasia vs. in situ carcinoma; in situ vs. invasive carcinoma; or primary ovarian carcinoma vs. metastatic breast carcinoma). The initial characterizations of distinctive protein profile subsets will require microdissection, so that salient differences in the cell populations of interest can best be appreciated. For proteomic profiles to be diagnostically useful, they also must be highly sensitive, so that small samples will be able to yield the necessary distinctions. Finally, high-throughput assays will be required, so that the cost of analysis will be reasonable and information will be available within a clinically useful time frame.

Preliminary studies in prostate cancer progression by Paweletz and colleagues[26] have coupled the use of laser-capture microdissection and proteomic analysis by SELDI spectrometry. Patient-matched tissues showing normal epithelium, prostatic intraepithelial neoplasia, invasive carcinoma, and endothelial cells were laser-microdissected and analyzed by SELDI-time-of-flight (TOF) mass spectrometry. Results of these studies showed that a specific and reproducible protein phenotype was obtained for each individual cell type. Interestingly, and highly compatible with our biological conception of tumor progression, the spectra for microdissected premalignant cells demonstrated a profile intermediate between the normal and tumor protein fingerprints.

Although still very preliminary, this work addresses two important issues. First, it demonstrates that a relatively small number of cells (as few as 1,500) may be required to obtain distinctive protein profiles, as compared with the 50,000 cells required for the performance of a typical two-dimensional gel analysis. As many morphologically significant findings are much smaller than 50,000 cells, it is important that differential protein profiles were obtained by SELDI for small lesions that one might want to assay clinically. Second, the short time required for performance of the assay (approximately 10 minutes) supports the notion that the newer proteomic technologies will be able to meet the high-throughput and rapid turnaround times required for clinically relevant testing.

Identification of New Diagnostic and Prognostic Markers

Once characteristic proteomic profiles have been generated on the basis of careful microdissection studies, the subsets of proteins that best distinguish clinically important diagnostic entities will have to be validated as biomarkers for screening and clinical monitoring (reviewed in Ref. 31). It will be most useful if the major tumor types have distinctive profiles, so that, for instance, the proteomic profile of a needle biopsy of a tumor mass will be able to complement the histologic evaluation in determining the tissue origin of the tumor. Indeed, proteomic studies in a number of different organ systems are beginning to result in the identification of proteins that are distinctive of the tissue of origin and that appear to play important roles in carcinogenesis in that organ.

One further hopes that more subtle differences will also be reflected: proteins responsible for the differences in nuclear and histologic grades, long recognized to be prognostically important in a number of cancers, might help us to refine and improve currently used histologic prognostic indicators. Such prognostic proteomic profiles would then have the potential to refine preoperative treatment planning by providing better information about tumor type and about invasive and metastatic potential. Ongoing studies are starting to reveal proteins that might serve as biomarkers in a number of common epithelial cancers; examples of these are briefly reviewed.

Colon Cancer In an effort to understand better the complex biological events underlying the process of colorectal carcinogenesis, Stulik and colleagues[32] examined normal and colon tumor pairs by 1D-PAGE and 2D-PAGE followed by Western blotting or mass spectrometry to look for proteins altered in this process. Proteins found to be down-regulated in colorectal carcinoma were liver fatty acid–binding protein, actin-binding protein–smooth muscle protein 22-alpha and cyclooxygenase 2. Upregulated proteins included a novel variant of heat shock protein 70 and several members of the S100 protein family of calcium-binding proteins.

Using two-dimensional gel electrophoresis of colorectal carcinomas and normal colonic epithelium, Jungblut et al[33] identified another low-molecular-weight protein, calgranulin B, which appears to be expressed only in dysplasia and tumor tissues. Additional testing is required to determine whether detection of calgranulin B and of other proteins expressed or up-regulated in colorectal carcinoma might be useful in noninvasive screening prior to colonoscopy or in monitoring patients with a prior history of colonic polyps or colorectal carcinoma.

Protein profiles that were obtained by Paweletz and colleagues[34] combined laser-microdissected patient-matched colon tissues and SELDI. In addition to the demonstration of a distinct protein profile for colon tumor compared with normal colonic epithelium, a similar profile was found in the colon tumor metastasis to liver, fairly distinct from the profile of normal liver (Fig. 1.3). These investigators

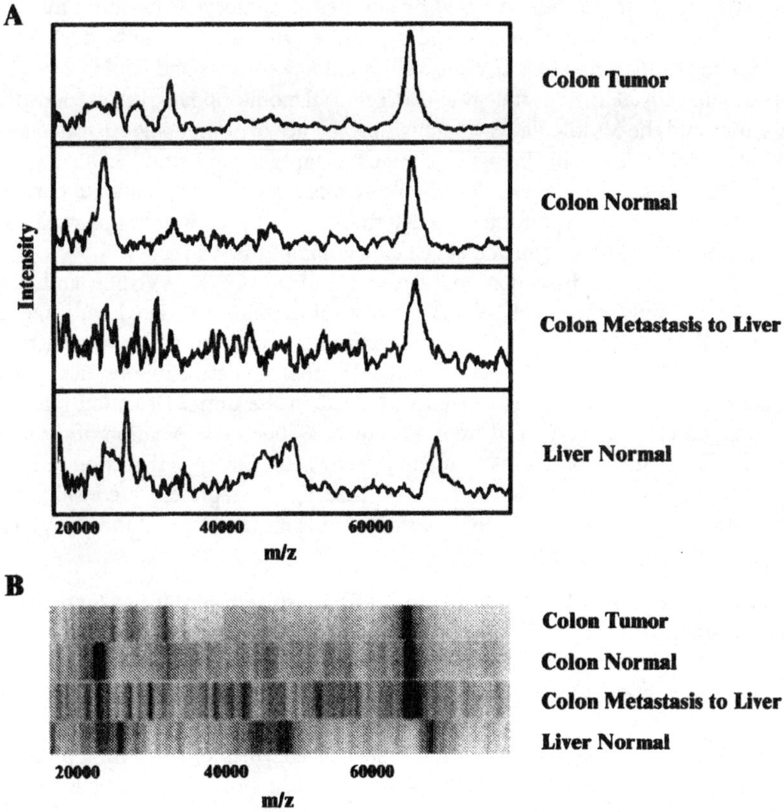

FIGURE 1.3 Surface-enhanced laser desorption ionization analysis of microdissected colon tumor and colon tumor metastasis to liver. Distinct protein profiles are seen for normal colonic epithelium and colon tumor. The colon-specific peak is clearly present in the liver metastasis, creating a profile that is distinct from that of normal liver. (From Paweletz CP et al. Drug Dev Res 2000;49:34–42. Reprinted with permission.)

also described reproducible protein expression changes that were discriminatory for a number of different tumor types, including esophagus, prostate, breast, and ovary. If these alterations remain consistent over a large number of cases, distinct protein profiles may be helpful in identifying tumors of unknown origin and for distinguishing metastatic from new primary tumors.

Bladder Cancer Celis et al[35] developed a comprehensive database of expressed proteins from two-dimensional gel analysis of bulk bladder tumor tissues and urine of bladder cancer patients. This database includes profiles of both transitional and squamous cell carcinomas. So far, only one candidate marker—psoriasin, a putative marker for squamous cell carcinomas of the bladder—has emerged from these studies, perhaps reflecting the fact that bulk tissues rather than microdissected tissues were used. Psoriasin is a low-molecular-weight calcium-binding protein that is also excreted by cultured keratinocytes. Psoriasin may be useful as a diagnostic marker for squamous cell carcinoma of the bladder, as it is excreted in the urine of squamous cell carcinoma patients and could be developed as an early detection strategy and as a clinical monitoring marker in countries in Africa and the Middle East with a high prevalence of *Schistosoma haematobium*. However, some reversible benign squamous metaplasias and stratified squamous epithelium in the female trigone may also express psoriasin. Additional clinical studies will have to be performed to determine the clinical utility of psoriasin as a diagnostic marker for squamous cell carcinoma of the bladder.

Using laser microdissection coupled with SELDI-TOF-MS, Vlahou and colleagues[36] recently screened 94 urine samples for proteins associated with transitional-cell carcinoma (TCC). These investigators uncovered five potential new TCC biomarkers. One has been identified further as defensin. Another seven protein clusters were also associated with TCC in the urine. Detection rates of the individual markers ranged from 43% to 70%, but a combination of the five markers and the seven clusters resulted in an 87% sensitivity of detection of TCC in the urine, with a specificity of 66%. These figures represent a considerable improvement over cytology alone, particularly for the detection of the low-grade transitional cell carcinomas.

Breast Cancer Protein expression profiles have also been established for purified normal breast epithelial cells and myoepithelial cells using double antibody magnetic affinity cell sorting. In two-dimensional gel electrophoresis, Page et al[37] found 170 protein spots differentially expressed at least two-fold between the two populations. Subsequent characterization of 51 of these by MS/MS revealed the myoepithelial cells to contain muscle-specific enzymes and structural proteins consistent with their contractile muscle–related functions. As one hallmark of early breast cancer progression from in situ to invasive carcinoma is the loss of myoepithelial cells, it has been suggested that one or more of the proteins identified by these investigators may have a cancer-suppressing function.[38] If loss of these proteins correlates with invasive carcinoma, assessment of the status of these proteins will then have potential diagnostic applications in the evaluation of small biopsy or cytology samples.

A potential marker for noncancerous breast epithelial cells was recently identified using 2D-PAGE and MALDI-TOF. In contrast to other isoforms, the sigma form of the molecular chaperone 14-3-3 protein appears to be strongly down-regulated in primary breast carcinomas.[39] Additional evidence that the gene encoding this protein is silenced by hypermethylation in breast cancer[40] suggests that this protein is a tumor suppressor. Breast cancer cells transfected with 14-3-3σ show inhibition of cyclin-dependent kinase activity and cell-cycle progression, further implicating this protein in the development of breast cancer.[41] Thus, detection of 14-3-3σ, as one component of a protein profile, may prove to be a marker of benignity.

Esophageal Carcinoma Emmert-Buck and colleagues[14] used two cases of esophageal carcinoma in their recent demonstration of a strategy for combined laser-capture microdissection with subsequent analysis by two-dimensional gel electrophoresis and MS/MS microsequencing. In these studies, 50,000 cells were captured from frozen sections of esophageal carcinoma, with an additional 50,000 cells separately captured from the normal squamous esophageal epithelium. Two-dimensional gels revealed 675 distinct proteins (or isoforms) with 98% identity between normal and tumor cells. Subject to very strict criteria, 17 proteins still showed tumor-specific alterations, with 10 proteins present only in the tumors and 7 only in the normal epithelium. Two of the altered proteins were subsequently characterized by mass spectrometry and immunoblot analysis; cytokeratin 1 was identified only in the tumors, and annexin I was identified only in the normal epithelium. In addition to demonstrating the power of microdissection to highlight differences between the normal and diseased epithelium, this study also identified several potential new markers of esophageal cancer.

Renal Cell Carcinoma A two-dimensional gel database for normal and cancerous human kidney proteins has been created by Sarto et al.[42] These studies have shown that four polypeptides synthesized in normal kidney tissues are not found in renal cell carcinoma. Two of these proteins have been identified as ubiquinol cytochrome *c* reductase and mitochondrial nicotinamide adenine dinucleotide-ubiquinone oxidoreductase complex I. The loss of expression of these two proteins in carcinoma may be due to unknown deletions or to changes in gene transcription or translation, because neither protein has a gene locus in a region known to be deleted in renal cell carcinoma. Using MALDI-TOF-MS, Sarto and colleagues[43] further identified multimeric isoforms of manganese superoxide dismutase only in renal cell carcinomas and isomeric forms of glutathione peroxidase only in normal kidneys, supporting a potential diagnostic role for these two proteins. Von Eggeling et al[44] also analyzed renal cell carcinoma, with patient-matched normal, peripheral, and central tumor tissue using SELDI-TOF-MS, also noting differentially expressed protein profiles.

Lung Cancer Two-dimensional gel electrophoresis studies have identified different protein profiles associated with different histologic subtypes of lung cancer. In particular, high expression of β-tubulin, heat shock proteins 73 and 90, lamin B, and proliferating cell nuclear antigen constituted a profile specific for small-cell lung carcinomas.[45] Two polypeptide markers, TAO1 and TAO2, have been identified by 2D-PAGE as being highly expressed in 80%–90% of lung adenocarcinomas, compared with metastatic carcinoma of colon or breast.[46] Mass spectrometry of tryptic peptides has more recently shown that TAO1/TAO2 is identical to napsin A, a member of the aspartic protease family.[47] Potential utility for these proteins in distinguishing primary from metastatic carcinomas in the lung is apparent.

Brichory and colleagues[48] used a proteomic approach to identify proteins that induce a humoral response in lung cancer. Using 2D-PAGE followed by Western blotting with more than 50 patient sera and more than 100 controls, they found that 60% of patients with lung adenocarcinoma and 33% of patients with squamous cell lung carcinoma (but none of the noncancer controls) made antibodies against glycosylated annexin I or glycosylated annexin II (or both). Clearly, serum-based screening and clinical follow-up assays may use both a combination of proteins shed or secreted by tumors and the humoral response to these proteins.

Prostate Carcinoma Studies in the prostate by Alaiya et al[9] used 2D-PAGE to examine six cases of hyperplasia and six cases of carcinoma. Malignant tumors showed increased expression of proliferating cell nuclear antigen; calreticulin; HSP 90 and pHSP 60; oncoprotein 18(v); elongation factor-2; glutathione S-transferase π; superoxide dismutase; and triose phosphate isomerase and decreased expression of cytokeratin 18 and tropomyosin-1 and -2. If these differences are maintained in larger studies, they have potential for development as markers for prostate cancer in early detection strategies, in molecular staging, or in clinical screening for tumor recurrence.

Using laser capture microdissection and 2D-PAGE, Ornstein and colleagues[49] examined normal and malignant prostate epithelium from prostatectomy specimens. In both cases examined, the same six proteins were seen only in malignant cells, whereas two others were seen only in benign epithelium. These eight proteins were not seen in the microdissected stromal cells but were present in the profiles from the whole-tissue sections. The profiles generated from the microdissected patient tissue sections were also compared with protein profiles from a patient-matched in-vitro cell line and from two metastatic prostate cancer cell lines (LnCaP and PC3); fewer than 20% of proteins identified on 2D-PAGE were identical to those seen in the cell lines. That study highlights the importance both of using patient tissue samples and tissue microdissection. Microdissected prostate tissue specimens exhibiting carcinoma, prostatic intraepithelial neoplasia, and normal epithelium also showed a number of differentially expressed proteins when analyzed by SELDI-MS.[50]

Proteomics in Screening and Molecular Staging

Of particular interest is the possibility of detection of tumor-specific protein alterations in body fluids, such as blood, urine, cerebrospinal fluid, or sputum, because these might then serve as tumor markers for noninvasive screening or monitoring of disease treatment. It will be important in these studies to rely on already established protein profiles characteristic of normal and tumor tissues. Such cytologic applications as these will benefit from some type of cell separation performed prior to proteomic analysis to enrich for the cell population of interest; antibody methods are likely to be of use in this regard.

Serum samples from breast cancer patients have been examined by two-dimensional gel electrophoresis after depletion of abundant serum proteins (albumin, immunoglobulin heavy and light chains, transferrin, and haptoglobin) to determine breast cancer–associated serum protein profiles. These studies have resulted in the identification of previously unknown associations of several serum proteins in patients with breast cancer.[51] In a similar approach to search for surrogate serum protein markers of primary hepatocellular carcinoma, 10 differentially expressed proteins that were identified might represent possible markers; these included haptoglobin 1 and 2, four complement factors, and two novel proteins. Studies are ongoing to compare these markers to α-fetoprotein and to determine their relationship to tumor burden.[51] The detection of disease-specific protein marker profiles in serum and other body fluids has a large number of potential applications in screening, molecular staging, and monitoring of therapeutic efficacy.

Characterization of Intracellular Events and Elucidation of Disease Mechanisms

Both expression proteomics and cell-map proteomics will be useful in the elucidation of disease mechanisms and the characterization of intracellular events. The integration of both global genomic and proteomic analyses is likely to be particularly powerful in elucidating cellular pathways and their regulation and interconnection with other cellular pathways. This was demonstrated recently by Ideker and colleagues.[10] Using the yeast galactose utilization pathway as a model, these investigators measured global mRNA and protein responses to various perturbations to critical pathway components and developed a complex integrated physical-interaction network. Such an integrated approach to the study of cell signaling pathways, cell-cycle control pathways, and other pathways deregulated in cancer will surely deepen our understanding of these processes, suggesting new hypotheses and new therapeutic targets.

In another example integrating gene expression data and proteomic data, Nelson et al[52] investigated the androgen receptor and the androgen-response pathway, both critically important in the development and progression of prostate cancer and in the treatment of patients with advanced disease. By cDNA microarray, androgen was found to induce the expression of 20 genes in prostate cancer cells, including such known androgen-regulated genes as prostate-specific antigen, and several novel cDNAs. Interestingly, the protein expression profiles of these cells by two-dimensional gel electrophoresis and mass spectrometry identified the metastasis-suppressor gene *nm23*. This finding is compatible with the reduced metastatic potential observed when these cells express a functional androgen receptor pathway.

Improved cell fractionation and protein identification techniques will continue to facilitate our understanding of functional intracellular protein complexes. Rout and colleagues[53] recently applied proteomic analysis to a characterization of the individual protein components of the yeast nuclear pore complex. Forty proteins associated with the nuclear pore complex were identified. A subset of these were also localized within the nuclear pore complex, resulting in a map of its molecular architecture and contributing significantly to further work in understanding nucleocytoplasmic exchange.

Identification of New Predictive Markers, Therapeutic Targets and Patient-Specific Therapies

The comparative study of protein expression profiles in tumor cells before, during, and after treatment should elucidate the mechanisms of action and efficacy of existing and investigational drugs and should suggest new drug targets, better ways to monitor for drug toxicity, and better predictors of therapeutic response. In an effort to speed the identification of new protein targets for drug development in cancer, the National Cancer Institute recently established a Tissue Proteomics Initiative in collaboration with the U.S. Food and Drug Administration. Preliminary results from these and other investigators are beginning to point to suitable targets for further study.

Functional proteomic screening for proteases important in colon cancer progression recently was carried out by McKerrow et al[54] in an attempt to identify proteases suitable for drug targeting. Using an automated microtiter plate enzymatic assay, these investigators analyzed 15 sets of matched colorectal carcinoma tumor and normal biopsies and liver metastases for protease activity. A number of proteases were detected, including the matrix metalloproteases, cathepsin B, and cathepsin D, that might prove to be suitable targets for low-molecular-weight protease inhibitors.

The first genome-wide proteomics attempt to analyze protein kinase function recently was reported by Zhu and colleagues,[55] who used a protein kinase chip to test almost the entire set of yeast protein kinase homologs to determine the catalytic efficiency of each one with 17 different substrates. This protein chip technology is of great interest because of its potential automatability and potential for adaptation to identify potent and selective inhibitors of protein kinases in a high-throughput fashion. In spite of the recognized limitations of this technology (including a possibly deleterious effect of chemical linking to the substrate and possible lack of cofactors or activators in the reaction), the potential for large-scale screening efforts is exciting and will likely reveal physiologically relevant enzyme-substrate combinations and uncover new kinase inhibitors.[56]

CONCLUSION

Proteomic studies hold much promise for the development of a comprehensive understanding of cellular events that occur during the course of disease. Advances in two broad areas are fueling the current excitement surrounding protein analysis in this "postgenomic" era: first, the rapid growth of protein databases and improved software analysis tools for mining these databases; second, newer, highly sensitive, automatable protein analysis platforms that will be able to process large numbers of cellular proteins efficiently. In oncology, it is reasonable to expect that these advances will lead to the delineation of protein profiles characteristic of different tumor types at different stages of progression, profiles characteristic of therapeutic responsiveness and resistance, and identification of new candidate drug and vaccine targets. Ultimately, these studies may also lead to rapid, high-throughput, integrated genomic-proteomic analysis of a patient's individual tumor and patient-tailored therapies.

A number of alternate global protein analysis strategies are also in development. These include the production of ordered protein microarrays, using purified proteins, recombinant proteins, or antibodies on a coated microscope slide. Binding events of proteins in a complex solution can then be measured by the relative intensity of different fluorescent dyes, allowing for the automated evaluation of potentially hundreds of thousands of proteins in parallel.[57] Other MALDI-TOF-based assays have been proposed, including polymerase chain reaction amplification of a gene of interest, with subsequent in vitro transcription-translation for high-throughput detection of mutations in genes of interest in cancer. Garvin and colleagues[58] used this approach to detect mutations in BRCA1 in patients with breast cancer. Other proteomic approaches have been explored, including automated quantitative immunoassay for prostate-specific antigen from laser-microdissected prostate tissues.[59]

The success of these approaches will depend on the sensitivity of detection of significant differences (likely in low-abundance proteins) against a background of high-abundance proteins that show no difference between neoplastic and nonneoplastic cells. Robust cell separation techniques, such as magnetic bead separation, may be able to compensate for limitations in sensitivity by increasing the cell population of interest prior to protein analysis (e.g., separation of small numbers of tumor cells in lymph nodes, bone marrow, or blood) in molecular staging assays. Thus far, only a small number of cases of each tumor type have been examined, and results are fairly preliminary. However, within the next few years, we are likely to have large numbers of proteins of potential diagnostic, prognostic, and therapeutic utility. Then will come the arduous task of validation, before any of these proteins reaches routine clinical use. Progress will be accelerated by the concomitant development of sophisticated data analysis tools, comprehensive databases of the protein profile differences correlating with clinically important decision-making points and, finally, the commitment of resources and energy to large, carefully conducted clinical validation trials.

REFERENCES

1. Wasinger VC, Cordwell SJ, Cerpa-Poljak A et al. Progress with gene-product mapping of the Mollicutes: *Mycoplasma genitalium*. Electrophoresis 1995;16:1090–1094.
2. Wilkins MR, Williams KL, Appel RD, Hochstrasser DF, eds. Proteome Research: New Frontiers in Functional Genomics. Berlin: Springer-Verlag, 1997.
3. Blackstock WP, Weir MP. Proteomics: quantitative and physical mapping of cellular proteins. Trends Biotechnol 1999;17:121–127.
4. Chambers G, Lawrie L, Cash P, Murray GI. Proteomics: a new approach to the study of disease. J Pathol 2000;192:280–288.
5. Williams KL. Genomes and proteomes: towards a multidimensional view of biology. Electrophoresis 1999;20:678–688.
6. Harry JL, Wilkins MR, Herbert BR, et al. Proteomics: capacity versus utility. Electrophoresis 2000; 21:1071–1081.
7. Bichsel VE, Liotta LA, Petricoin EF. Cancer proteomics: from biomarker discovery to signal pathway profiling. Cancer J 2001;7:69–78.
8. Anderson L, Seilhamer J. A comparison of selected mRNA and protein abundances in human liver. Electrophoresis 1997;18:533–537.
9. Alaiya AA, Franzen B, Auer G, Linder S. Cancer proteomics: from identification of novel markers to creation of artificial learning models for tumor classification. Electrophoresis 2000;21:1210–1217.
10. Ideker T, Thorsson V, Ranish JA et al. Integrated genomic and proteomic analyses of a systematically perturbed metabolic network. Science 2001;292:929–934.
11. Humphrey-Smith I, Cordwell SJ, Blackstock WP. Proteome research: complementarity and limitations with respect to the RNA and DNA worlds. Electrophoresis 1997;18:1217–1242.
12. Emmert-Buck MR, Bonner RF, Smith PD et al. Laser capture microdissection. Science 1996;274: 998–1001.
13. Banks RE, Dunn MJ, Forbes MA et al. The potential use of laser capture microdissection to selectively obtain distinct populations of cells for proteomic analysis—preliminary findings. Electrophoresis 1999;20:689–700.
14. Emmert-Buck MR, Gillespie JW, Paweletz CP et al. An approach to proteomic analysis of human tumors. Mol Carcinog 2000;27:158–165.
15. Lawrie LC, Curran S, McLeod HL, et al. Application of laser capture microdissection and proteomics in colon cancer. J Clin Pathol Mol Pathol 2001;54:253–258.
16. Gygi SP, Corthals GL, Zhang Y, et al. Evaluation of two-dimensional gel electrophoresis–based proteome analysis technology. Proc Natl Acad Sci USA 2000;97:9390–9395.
17. Driessen HP, de Jong WW, Tesser GI, Bloemendal H. The mechanism of N-terminal acetylation of proteins. CRC Crit Rev Biochem 1985;18:281–325.
18. Stone KL, DeAngelis R, LoPresti M, et al. Use of liquid chromatography-electrospray ionization tandem mass spectrometry (LC-ESI-MS/MS) for routine identification of enzymatically digested

proteins separated by sodium dodecyl sulfate-polyacrylamide gel electrophoresis. Electrophoresis 1998;19:1046–1052.

19. Wilm M, Shevchenco A, Houthaeve T et al. Femtomole sequencing of proteins from polyacrylamide gels by nano-electrospray mass spectrometry. Nature 1996;379:466–469.

20. Eng JK, McCormack AL, Yates JR. An approach to correlate tandem mass spectral data of peptides with amino acid sequences in a protein database. J Am Soc Mass Spectrom 1994;5:976–989.

21. Yates JR, Eng JK, McCormack AL. Mining genomes: correlating tandem mass spectra of modified and unmodified peptides to sequences in nucleotide databases. Anal Chem 1995;67: 3202–3210.

22. Wilkins MR, Gasteiger E, Sanchez JC, et al. Two-dimensional gel electrophoresis for proteome projects: the effects of protein hydrophobicity and copy number. Electrophoresis 1998;19: 1501–1505.

23. Celis JE, Rasmussen HH, Gromov P et al. The human keratinocyte two-dimensional gel protein database (update 1995); mapping components of signal transduction pathways. Electrophoresis 1995;16:2177–2240.

24. Gygi SP, Rist B, Aebersold R. Measuring gene expression by quantitative proteome analysis. Curr Opin Biotechnol 2000;11:396–401.

25. Nedelkov D, Nelson R. Biomolecular interaction analysis mass spectrometry: a multiplexed proteomics approach. Bio Pharm 2001;8:28–33.

26. Paweletz CP, Liotta LA, Petricoin EF. New technologies for biomarker analysis of prostate cancer progression: laser capture microdissection and tissue proteomics. Urology 2001;57:160–163.

27. Gygi S, Rist B, Gerber S, et al. Quantitative analysis of complex protein mixtures using isotope-coded affinity tags. Nat Biotechnol 1999;17: 994–999.

28. Han DK, Eng J, Zhou H, Aebersold R. Quantitative profiling of differentiation-induced microsomal proteins using isotope-coded affinity tags and mass spectrometry. Nat Biotechnol 2001;19: 946–951.

29. Kim S, Merrill BM, Rajppurohit R et al. Identification of N^G-methylarginine residues in human heterogeneous RNP protein A1: Phe/Gly-Gly-Gly-Arg-Gly-Gly-Gly/Phe is a preferred recognition motif. Biochemistry 1997;36:5185–5192.

30. Goshe MB, Conrads TP, Panisko EA, et al. Phosphoprotein isotope-coded affinity tag approach for isolating and quantitating phosphopeptides in proteome-wide analyses. Anal Chem 2001;73: 2578–2586.

31. Srinivas PR, Srivastava S, Hanash S, Wright GL Jr. Proteomics in early detection of cancer. Clin Chem 2001;47:1901–1911.

32. Stulik J, Koupilova K, Osterreicher J et al. Protein abundance alterations in matched sets of macroscopically normal colon mucosa and colorectal carcinoma. Electrophoresis 1999;20: 3638–3646.

33. Jungblut PR, Zimmy-Arndt U, Stulik J et al. Proteomics in human disease: cancer, heart and infectious diseases. Electrophoresis 1999;20:2100–2110.

34. Paweletz CP, Gillespie JW, Ornstein DK et al. Rapid protein display profiling of cancer progression directly from human tissue using a protein biochip. Drug Dev Res 2000;49:34–42.

35. Celis JE, Ostergaard M, Rasmussen HH et al. A comprehensive protein resource for the study of bladder cancer: *http://biobase.dk/cgi-bin/celis*. Electrophoresis 1999;20:300–309.

36. Vlahou A, Schellhammer PF, Mendrinos S et al. Development of a novel proteomic approach for the detection of transitional cell carcinoma of the bladder in urine. Am J Pathol 201;158: 1491–1502.

37. Page MJ, Amess B, Townsend RR et al. Proteomic definition of normal human luminal and myoepithelial breast cells purified from reduction mammoplasties. Proc Natl Acad Sci USA 1999; 96:12589–12594.

38. Liotta LA, Petricoin EF. Beyond the genome to tissue proteomics. Breast Cancer Res 2000;2: 13–14.
39. Vercoutter-Edouart A-S, Lemoine J, Bourhis XL et al. Proteomic analysis reveals that 14-3-3σ is down-regulated in human breast cancer cells. Cancer Res 2001;61:7680.
40. Ferguson AT, Evron E, Umbricht C et al. High frequency of hypermethylation at the 14-3-3σ locus leads to gene silencing in breast cancer. Proc Natl Acad Sci USA 2000;97:6049–6054.
41. Laronga C, Yang HY, Neal, Lee MH. Association of the cyclin-dependent kinases and 14-3-3σ negatively regulates cell cycle progression. J Biol Chem 2000;275:23106–23112.
42. Sarto C, Marocchi A, Sanchez JC et al. Renal cell carcinoma and normal kidney protein expression. Electrophoresis 1997;18:599–604.
43. Sarto C, Frutiger S, Cappellano F et al. Modified expression of plasma glutathione peroxidase and manganese superoxide dismutase in human renal cell carcinoma. Electrophoresis 1999;20: 3458–3466.
44. von Eggeling F, Junker K, Fiedle W et al. Mass spectrometry meets chip technology: a new proteomic tool in cancer research? Electrophoresis 2001;22:2898–2902.
45. Okuzawa K, Franzen B, Lindholm J et al. Characterization of gene expression in clinical lung cancer materials by two-dimensional polyacrylamide gel electrophoresis. Electrophoresis 1994; 15:382–390.
46. Hirano T, Fujioka K, Franzen B et al. Relationship between TAO1 and TAO2 polypeptides associated with lung adenocarcinoma and histocytological features. Br J Cancer 1997;75:978–985.
47. Chuman Y, Bergman A, Ueno T et al. Napsin A, a member of the aspartic protease family, is abundantly expressed in normal lung and kidney tissue and is expressed in lung adenocarcinomas. FEBS Lett 1999;462:129–134.
48. Brichory FM, Misek DE, Yim AM et al. An immune response manifested by the common occurrence of annexins I and II autoantibodies and high circulating levels of IL-6 in lung cancer. Proc Natl Acad Sci USA. 2001;98:9824–9829.
49. Ornstein DK, Gillespie JW, Paweletz CP et al. Proteomic analysis of laser capture microdissected human prostate cancer and in vitro prostate cell lines. Electrophoresis 2000;21:2235–2242.
50. Wright GL, Cazares LH, Leung S-M et al. ProteinChip surface enhanced laser desorption/ionization (SELDI) mass spectrometry: a novel protein biochip technology for detection of prostate cancer biomarkers in complex protein mixtures. Prostate Cancer Prostate Dis 1999;2:264–276.
51. Kennedy S. Proteomic profiling from human samples: the body fluid alternative. Toxicol Lett 2001;120:379–384.
52. Nelson PS, Han D, Rochon Yet al. Comprehensive analyses of prostate gene expression: convergence of expressed sequence tag databases, transcript profiling and proteomics. Electrophoresis 2000; 21:1823–1831.
53. Rout MP, Aitchison JD, Suprapto A, et al. The yeast nuclear pore complex: composition, architecture, and transport mechanism. J Cell Biol 2000;148:635–652.
54. McKerrow JH, Bhargava V, Hansell E et al. A functional proteomics screen of proteases in colorectal carcinoma. Mol Med 2000;6:450–460.
55. Zhu H, Klemic JF, Chang S et al. Analysis of yeast protein kinases using protein chips. Nat Genet 2000;26:283–289.
56. Williams DM, Cole PA. Kinase chips hit the proteomics era. Trends Biochem Sci 2001;26:271–273.
57. Haab BB, Dunham MJ, Brown PO. Protein microarrays for highly parallel detection and quantitation of specific proteins and antibodies in complex solutions. Genome Biol 2001;2:1–13.
58. Garvin AM, Parker KC and, Haff L. MALDI-TOF based mutation detection using tagged in vitro synthesized peptides. Nat Biotechnol 2000;18:95–97.
59. Simone NL, Remaley AT, Charboneau L et al. Sensitive immunoassay of tissue cell proteins procured by laser capture microdissection. Am J Pathol 2000;156:445–452.

Chapter 2

Modulation of the Inhibitory Effects of CTLA-4 in the Enhancement of Immunologic Responses Against Cancer

James P. Allison

One of the main goals of tumor immunotherapy is the development of strategies for the induction of anti-tumor T-cell responses of sufficient potency to obtain tumor rejection and immunity to reoccurrence. Recent advances in basic immunology are leading to novel and rational approaches towards this goal. Of particular interest are recent insights into the regulation of the early stages of T-cell activation. The fact that T-cell activation is regulated not only by antigen-specific signals, but also by positive and negative costimulatory signals, has offered the possibility of new targets for manipulation of T-cell responses. Here we describe the role of costimulation, both positive and negative, in T-cell activation, and discuss recent work demonstrating that blockade of the inhibitory signals mediated by CTLA-4 can be successfully used to enhance anti-tumor responses in mouse and man.

CD28-MEDIATED COSTIMULATION IS REQUIRED FOR INITIATION OF T-CELL RESPONSES

Recognition of antigen by the T-cell antigen receptor (TCR) is by itself not sufficient for full activation of a naïve T cell; additional costimulatory signals are required in order to obtain cytokine production, proliferation, and differentiation to effector function.[1] The major source of these costimulatory signals is provided by engagement of T-cell surface molecule CD28 by members of the classical B7 family (B7.1 and B7.2) on antigen precipitating cells. A large volume of work has established that these CD28/B7 interactions are required for cytokine production and proliferation and in their absence, T cells are not only non-activated, but may be rendered unresponsive. An especially important feature of these costimulatory circuits is that B7 molecules are expressed only on cells with potent antigen presenting activity. These cells include dendritic cells, activated macrophages, and a few other cell types in the hematopoeitic lineage. An encounter by a naïve T cell with its specific antigen on these "professional" antigen-presenting cells (APC) in the lymphoid tissues allows the initiation of T-cell responses. B7 molecules and thus costimulatory activity is not found on other cells in the body. This strict compartmentalization of B7 to "professional" APC in the lymphoid tissues may provide a fail-safe mechanism for the maintenance of T-cell tolerance to peripheral tissue specific antigens.[1] Thus, if a T cell expressing an antigen receptor capable of detecting peptides derived from tyrosinase encounters that peptide on a melanocyte, the T cell will not be activated because melanocytes do not express B7 and cannot provide necessary costimulatory signals.

An important implication of this concept is that tumor cells, even though they might express T-cell epitopes that would be potential targets for T-cell attack, would be invisible to the immune system because of their lack of capacity for costimulation. We and others demonstrated that this is indeed true by showing that many transplantable murine tumor cells which would otherwise grow progressively and kill the host were rejected if the tumor cells were engineered to express B7.[2,3] Rejection was T-cell mediated and resulted in long lasting immunity to rechallenge. The notion was that in the normal situation tumor cells in the emerging cancer would be invisible to the immune system until they outgrow their food supply and began to die or otherwise elicited inflammatory reactions. As a result of the inflammation, professional antigen presenting cells would pick up tumor debris via phagocytic mechanisms, process the acquired tumor antigens, and present tumor-derived peptides on their own major histocompatibility complex (MHC) in the context of the necessary costimulatory signals, thus allowing the initiation of T-cell responses. This process is referred to as cross-priming.[4] The hope was that expression of B7 on the tumor cells would bypass the requirement for cross-priming, thus jumpstarting the anti-tumor responses. Unfortunately, while the B7 approach proved to be very effective in the induction of prophylactic responses to immunogenic mouse tumors, it did not prove to be very effective against poorly immunogenic tumors, or against previously established tumors.[5]

The basic premise that anti-tumor responses are "cross primed" by bone marrow derived host APC rather than the tumor cells themselves has become well established, largely due to a series of elegant experiments that also established that MHC restriction of the response is determined by the host APC and not the tumor cells.[6,7] It has also been shown that functional expression of B7 in the host (or in some cases on the tumors) is critical for anti-tumor response.[8] Thus many current tumor vaccine strategies are ultimately based on costimulation in that the goal is direct or indirect delivery of tumor antigens to professional APC in order to exploit the costimulatory activity and other properties of these cells that make them especially potent in the induction of immune responses.

CTLA-4 Mediates Inhibitory Costimulation

Recent studies have demonstrated a further complexity of costimulation that may provide insight into reasons that many vaccine strategies have been found to have disappointing potency. This insight comes from the realization that there is an inhibitory component to costimulation that is mediated by CTLA-4 (for reviews, see References 9 and 10). CTLA-4 is homologous to CD28, and like CD28, binds B7.1 and B7.2.[11,12] The first notion that CTLA-4 was a negative regulator of T-cell activation came from work showing that soluble antibodies which blocked CTLA-4/B7 interactions enhanced T-cell responses in vitro and in vivo, and that co-cross linking of CTLA-4 together with the TCR and CD28 inhibited T-cell responses.[13–16] Although an inhibitory role for CTLA-4 was initially controversial, the fact that gene targeted CTLA-4 deficient mice suffered massive lymphoproliferation characterized by large numbers of activated T cells resulting in early death supported a critical role for CTLA-4 in the down regulation of T-cell responses.[17–19] The view of CTLA-4 as a negative regulator of T-cell responses has been supported by a large number of subsequent reports (for reviews, see References 9, 10, and 20).

Although the exact mechanism of signaling by CTLA-4 remains to be established, there is a dynamic integration between the T-cell antigen receptor strength in CD28 and CTLA-4 that determines whether, and the extent to which, T cells respond to antigen receptor stimulation.[13] CTLA-4 attenuates proliferation of T cells by inhibiting production of IL-2, an essential growth factor, and also by limiting the induction of cyclin dependent kinases (cdk4 and cdk6) and cyclin D3, factors critical for entry of T cells into the cell cycle.[21,22] The overall effect is to restrict the number of divisions that an activated T cell goes through after activation.

Despite the structural homology of CD28 and CTLA-4, there are certain key differences between them that are relevant to an understanding of their complex interplay in regulating T-cell responses. The first is that CTLA-4 has a much higher affinity for ligand binding than does CD28, as much as 2000-fold higher by some estimates.[23,24] That CD28 can provide positive costimulatory signals given its extreme disadvantage in B7 binding is a result of two additional differences between the molecules. The first is that while CD28 is constitutively present, CTLA-4 expression is induced after TCR signaling.[25,26] The second is cellular localization. CD28 is on the cell surface, while CTLA-4 is primarily found in intracellular stores even after maximal induction and is translocated to the surface only after TCR engagement.[25,27] This temporal and spatial compartmentalization of the costimulatory and inhibitory receptors ensures that T-cell activation can proceed uninhibited for a time, and is then attenuated when CTLA-4 comes into play.

We have recently found that there is an even more subtle level of regulation of CTLA-4 by the TCR. Although even weak TCR signals can result in initiation of synapse formation, recruitment of CD28, and polarization of CTLA-4 toward the site of TCR signaling, the amount of CTLA-4 that is recruited into the synapse is directly proportional to the TCR signal strength.[28] Since only the CTLA-4 in the synapse is likely to be functionally relevant, the implication is that responses initiated by strong stimuli will be more inhibited that those elicited by weaker stimuli. This novel feedback control mechanism suggests a previously unrecognized role for CTLA-4 in regulation of T-cell responses. CTLA-4 might play a fundamental role in maintaining the diversity of early responses to antigens. By preferentially restricting the expansion of strongly responsive clones, CTLA-4 would diminish their competitive advantage over more weakly responsive clones. This would have the effect of keeping the repertoire broad during early stages of the response and allow for a more diverse population of clones of varying specificity and avidity to be involved in clonal selection and affinity maturation. This would serve to prevent a single (or a small number) of high avidity clones from dominating early stages of a response, a situation which favor antigenic selection of a pathogen leading to its escape from the response.[10,28]

CTLA-4 also seems to play an important role in the regulation of T-cell responses to self-antigens. It has been shown that blockade of CTLA-4 with antibodies exacerbates autoimmune encephalomyelitis (EAE); a mouse model of multiple sclerosis which is characterized by T-cell mediated demyelination to which some strains are susceptible.[29–31] Similarly, it has been shown that CTLA-4 blockade can accelerate onset of diabetes in a transgenic mouse system.[32] These results are perhaps not surprising, given the evidence that CTLA-4 attenuates responses and that its blockade by antibody can enhance responses in other systems. However, recent results suggest that CTLA-4 may play a more profound role in regulation of T-cell responses to self-antigens. We have found that CTLA-4 blockade allows induction of EAE in BALB/c mice, a strain normally considered to be inherently resistant to the disease.[33] Under normal conditions BALB/c mice make a small but measurable response to a myelin-derived peptide but do not show clinical signs of disease. However, immunization under conditions of CTLA-4 blockade results in a response of much greater magnitude that is accompanied by both histological and clinical signs of disease.[33] Our interpretation is that chronic stimulation of autoreactive T cells by constant exposure to high avidity self-antigens results in the induction and maintenance of high levels of CTLA-4, thus limiting expansion of the cells and preventing pathogenesis. This could provide a mechanism by which CTLA-4 contributes to the maintenance of peripheral T-cell tolerance to tissue specific self antigens.[10,33]

Blockade of CTLA-4-mediated Attenuation Enhances T-cell Responses to Transplantable and Primary Tumors in Mice

Our studies suggest that blockade of CTLA-4 during immunization will have the effect of preferentially favoring the expansion of those T-cell clones with higher avidity antigen receptors by "removing the brakes" that normally attenuate their proliferative capacity. This has led us to explore the possibility of enhancing anti-tumor T-cell responses by interfering with the inhibitory effects of CTLA-4. Our initial experiments showed that administration of anti-CTLA-4 antibodies was sufficient to obtain rejection of two murine transplantable tumor lines, a colorectal carcinoma and a fibrosarcoma.[34] We found that rejection could be obtained even when treatment was delayed until weeks after tumor implantation and there were sizeable tumor masses (Ref. 34 and unpublished observations). Rejection was accompanied by long lasting immunity to rechallenge. Similar results have been reported in other transplantable murine tumor systems, including renal carcinoma, lymphoma, and prostatic adenocarcinoma.[35–39] Despite these successes, we found that some tumors, such as the B16 melanoma, were not rejected upon treatment with anti-CTLA-4 alone.[40] The important factor seems to be the inherent immunogenicity of the tumor: strongly immunogenic tumors are susceptible to rejection upon CTLA-4 blockade, while poorly immunogenic tumor are resistant.[36]

Although the fact that CTLA-4 blockade as a "single agent" resulted in the rejection of immunogenic tumors established the potential of this approach for immunotherapy, we were interested in determining whether there were ways of making it more effective against poorly immunogenic tumors which are arguably more relevant to human cancer. To this end we have explored a variety of combinatorial therapies. A combination that we have examined extensively is CTLA-4 blockade together with genetically engineered tumor cell vaccines. Our most successful work has employed a vaccine consisting of irradiated tumor cells that have been transduced to express granulocyte monocyte colony stimulating factor (GM-CSF), a cytokine that is a chemoattractant for and induces potent antigen presentation capacity in dendritic cells and macrophages. In a screen in which cytokine gene containing retroviruses were tested for their ability to confer immunogenicity to irradiated B16 melanoma cells, GM-CSF has been reported to prove the most effective by far.[41] However, the effectiveness of the GM-B16 vaccine was limited to prophylaxis; there was little effect on even newly established tumors. We found that while neither CTLA-4 antibodies or a GM-CSF tumor cell vaccine given alone had any significant effect on the growth on a poorly immunogenic mammary carcinoma or on B16, there was a profound synergy when the treatments were combined that resulted in complete tumor rejection.[40,42] In the case of B16, 100% rejection was obtained up to four days after implantation, and significant effects were observed as late as twelve days. These results clearly demonstrate the therapeutic potential of CTLA-4 blockade in combination with GM-CSF in obtaining rejection of transplanted tumors. We have also demonstrated that this combination therapy can delay and reduce the severity of primary tumors in the TRAMP transgenic model of prostate cancer.[43]

An interesting and important aspect of the successful therapy in both the melanoma and prostate models is that tumor rejection is regularly accompanied by tissue-specific autoimmunity.[40,43] This was most apparent in melanoma, where the majority of mice rejecting tumor developed a progressive depigmentation characterized by a lack of normal melanocytes and the presence of inflammatory cells in affected areas of the skin.[40] This syndrome is reminiscent of the vitiligo observed in melanoma patients that have undergone spontaneous remission or that have shown clinical responses to immunotherapy.[44,45] This suggests that tumor rejection induced by the combination therapy was at least in part directed against normal melanocyte antigens. Several normal melanocyte targets (tyrosinase, TRP-1, TRP2, gp100, melanA/MART-1) have been identified as targets of T cells derived from melanoma patients (for review see.[46] T cells from mice that had rejected B16 following CTLA-4 combination therapy were surprisingly restricted in their specificity. We were only able to detect reactivity to a single K^b binding peptide representing residues 180–188 of TRP-2.[47] We have found that immunization of mice with the GM-CSF-B16 cells in combination with CTLA-4 blockade can increase the level of T cells that bind $TRP\text{-}2_{180-188}/K^b$ tetramers from virtually undetectable to levels to over 1% of the total CD8+ T cells in the blood.[47] This is consistent with the notion that CTLA-4 blockade allows the breaking of peripheral T-cell tolerance and the induction of a response of sufficient strength to reject tumors.

Characterization of the cellular mechanisms involved in tumor rejection provided very interesting insights into the mechanisms involved and revealed other potential applications of CTLA-4 in immunotherapy. Earlier work had shown that prophylactic responses induced by the GM-CSF tumor cell vaccine used as a single agent required CD4 T cells, the Th2 cytokines IL-4 and IL-5, and iNOS; CD8 T cells were dispensable.[48] This result was surprising since the tumor cells expressed no class II MHC antigens and therefore would not be expected to be targets of CD4 cells. These observations suggested both "cross-priming" and "cross-effector" mechanisms whereby peptides derived from tumor cells are presented by host dendritic cells in the context of class II MHC leading to the generation of Th-2 CD4 T cells. IL-4 and IL-5 produced by these cells then recruit eosinophils and neutrophils that may be the effector cells that actually result in tumor cell death. In contrast, we found that the combination therapy with CTLA-4 had a totally different mechanism.[47] CD4 cells were completely dispensable, and the only cells required were CD8 cells and natural killer (NK) 1.1+ cells (Whether the latter are bona fide NK cells or are NK-T cells remains to be established). In fact, we found that the effectiveness of the combination therapy was considerably enhanced in the absence of CD4 T cells.[49] This enhancement is most likely due to the removal of CD25+CD4 Treg cells, which seem to play a role in regulation of anti-self responses that is independent of CTLA-4.[49] In any event, these results demonstrate that CTLA-4 blockade can allow the induction of an effective CD8 T-cell response even in the absence of CD4 T-cell help. This has obvious implications to its use in therapeutic settings, such as immunization of AIDS patients, where CD4 T cells are deficient.

RATIONALE FOR CLINICAL APPLICATION OF CTLA-4 BLOCKADE IN TUMOR IMMUNTHERAPY

Our proposal to apply CTLA-4 blockade to the treatment of human cancer is ultimately based on our understanding of the central role that it plays in regulation of T-cell responses, and on our data demonstrating that administration of antibodies to CTLA-4 can greatly enhance T-cell responses in vivo. A scheme for this idea is shown in figure 1. Since tumor cells do not express the B7 costimulatory ligands, the T-cell responses must be initiated by cross-priming of T cells by tumor cell derived antigens expressed on professional APCs (dentritic cells, macrophages) in the context of costimulatory signals. Once initiated, however, CTLA-4 is brought to bear by the mechanisms described above and will attenuate the response by limiting expansion of the relevant cells, with the T cells having the highest avidity antigen receptors and thus the most desirable to have in the antitumor response being attenuated the most. This may diminish the strength of the response and limit the effectiveness of the response obtained to any vaccination strategy. Administration of anti-CTLA-4 antibodies at the appropriate time will block the inhibitory effects of CTLA-4, thus temporarily removing the constraints on T cell expansion and allowing unattenuated expansion of high avidity clones, hopefully with the generation of an effective antitumor response.

There are many ways to obtain priming of T cells in order to initiate a response to amplify via CTLA-4 blockade. In the case of strongly immunogenic and fast growing tumors, as is the case for many of the murine transplantable systems, tumor cell death and inflammation by the mechanisms described above may be sufficient for effective cross-priming to occur. However, in many settings this "spontaneous" cross-priming may not be sufficient and intentional immunization may be required. As described above, we have had considerable success with vaccines engineered to express the immunomodulatory cytokine GM-CSF. It

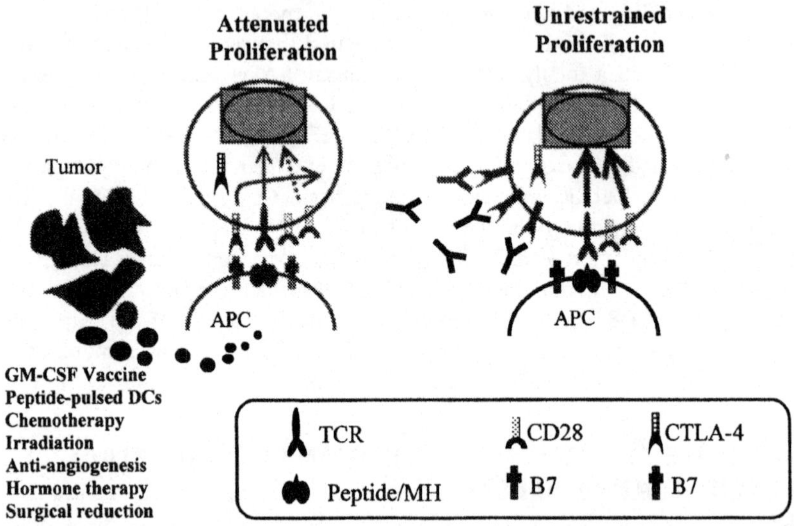

FIGURE 2.1 Model for enhancement of T cell responses to tumors by CTLA-4 blockade. T cells are cross-primed by tumor-derived peptides presented on "professional" antigen presenting cells, which can be increased by several strategies. Normally the responses would be subject to attenuation by CTLA-4 (left). Blockade of CTLA-4 by antibody removes the attenuation, allowing unrestrained expansion of T cells (right).

should also be possible to use cytotoxic chemotherapeutic agents at levels that are non-immunogenic and perhaps sub curative on their own to obtain sufficient tumor cell death to obtain priming. Indeed, others and we have shown synergy between CTLA-4 blockade and low dose treatment with the chemotherapeutic drugs melphalen and cis-platin.[36,50] It should be possible to similarly exploit CTLA-4 blockade to enhance the response of T cells primed as a result of tumor cell death produced by therapeutic radiation treatment. CTLA-4 blockade might also be used in combination with blockers of angiogenesis to exploit tumor cell death and inflammation that occurs as a result of removal of the blood supply. CTLA-4 may also be useful in conjunction with conventional non-cytotoxic therapies. We have shown, for example, that administration of CTLA-4 antibodies following surgical reduction of transplantable prostate tumors in mice can greatly reduce the local reoccurrence and lymph node metastasis.[51] It may also be possible to use CTLA-4 blockade in combination with hormone therapy since it has been shown that androgen withdrawal is accompanied by T cell infiltration and activation in the prostates of patients with prostate cancer,[52] Finally, CTLA-4 blockade may increase the effectiveness of vaccination with known tumor antigens whether by administration of peptides alone, in the context of patient-derived dendritic cells, or other specific immunization strategies.

Safety of CTLA-4 Blockade

An obvious concern in the clinical application of CTLA-4 blockade is the issue of toxicity. The fact that mice in which CTLA-4 expression has been eliminated by gene targeting suffer from a fatal lymphoproliferative disorder raises concerns about the possibility of polyclonal T-cell activation and/or autoimmune reactions following CTLA-4 blockade. However, our extensive experience using antibodies to block CTLA-4 in a number of settings in mice suggested that the treatment would be safe. First, there is no evidence that administration of anti-CTLA-4 antibodies results in polyclonal T-cell activation. In mice treated with anti-CTLA-4 during immunization with antigens or superantigens (e.g. *Staphylcoccus* enterotoxin B), the only observed effect is an increase in number of the responding antigen specific T-cell population. Other T cells show no signs of activation as assessed by display of appropriate markers. Second, we have not observed the appearance of anti-nuclear or dsDNA antibodies, glomerulonephritis, or other signs of autoimmunity (unpublished observations). Thus, the effects of CTLA-4 blockade are limited to T cells that are responding to priming only during the time while the antibody is present.

Another concern is the issue of tissue-specific autoimmunity. In the mouse models we have observed autoimmune destruction of melanocytes and prostatic inflammation after combination immunotherapy in the melanoma and prostate models, respectively. We did not observe depigmentation in the absence of CTLA-4 blockade. It is possible, if not likely, that these side effects are a direct consequence of the mechanism action and may prove to be unavoidable. Until this issue is resolved by additional preclinical work in the mouse models, it will probably be wise to restrict CTLA-4 blockade to the treatment of cancers of cell types that are non-essential and dispensable.

Phase I Clinical Trials of CTLA-4 Blockade in Human Cancer

Medarex, Inc. has generated a panel of antibodies to human CTLA-4. One of these, MDX-010, a fully human anti-human CTLA-4, has recently been tested in phase I trials in hormone refractory prostate cancer and in malignant melanoma.[53,54] Patients were treated by infusion of a single dose of antibody. In all cases, treatments were completed with only mild adverse events. There was no evidence of an increase in the number of activated peripheral T cells, and no evidence of clinical autoimmunity. The most noticeable adverse events were mild, reversible rash or pruritis. In the melanoma patients' biopsies of the rash were consistent with lymphocytic infiltration with targeting to melanocytes. In both trials there were patients who exhibited clinical responses. In the case of prostate cancer, 2 of 6 patients who had not been subjected to prior chemotherapy experienced >50% decrease in PSA lasting from 3–5 months. Several patients in the melanoma trial showed mixed responses, and biopsies showed extensive tumor necrosis with inflammatory infiltrates into the viable tumors. The results of these trials clearly demonstrate that CTLA-4 treatment is well tolerated and there is clear evidence of both immunologic and anti-tumor activity.

Prospectus

Accumulated data in both mouse model systems and in the phase I clinical trials provide optimism that CTLA-4 blockade will be useful in tumor immunotherapy. The ability to combine CTLA-4 blockade with other treatments, both immune-based and conventional, offer the hope that this treatment will be a new and powerful way of mobilizing the immune system to attack cancer. Development of new treatment regimens is underway, and we look forward to rapid progress.

ACKNOWLEDGEMENTS

The author wishes to offer his appreciation for invaluable contributions in terms of both efforts in the laboratory and intellectual contributions to the work described in this paper to former and current members of the Allison lab as well as collaborators, including: Cynthia Chambers, Jackson Egen, Marcella Fassò, Arthur A. Hurwitz, Alan Korman, Michael S. Kuhns, Matthew F. Krummel, Eugene Kwon, Dana R. Leach, Timothy J. Sullivan, Andrea van Elsas, Rebecca Waitz, and Jennifer Ziskin.

The work described here was supported in part by grants from the NCI (CA40041 and CA57986) and CaP CURE. James P. Allison is an Investigator of the Howard Hughes Medical Institute. He is a consultant for Medarex, Inc.

REFERENCES

1. Mueller DL, Jenkins MK, Schwartz RH. Clonal expansion versus functional clonal inactivation: A costimulatory signalling pathway determines the outcome of T cell antigen receptor occupancy. Ann Rev Immunol 1989;7:445–480.
2. Townsend S, Allison JP. Tumor rejection after direct costimulation of CD8+ T cells by B7–transfected melanoma cells. Science 1993;259:368–370.
3. Chen L, Ashe S, Brady WA et al. Costimulation of antitumor immunity by the B7 counterreceptor for the T lymphocyte molecules CD28 and CTLA-4. Cell 1992;71:1093–1102.
4. Bevan MJ. Cross-priming for a secondary cytotoxic response to minor H antigens with H-2 congenic cells which do not cross-react in the cytotoxic assay. J Exp Med 1976;143:1283–1288.
5. Allison JP, Hurwitz AA, Leach DR. Manipulation of costmulatory signals to enhance antitumor T-cell responses. Curr Opin Immunol 1995;7:682–686.
6. Huang AY, Golumbek P, Ahmadzadeh M et al. Role of bone marrow-derived cells in presenting MHC class I-restricted tumor antigens. Science 1994;264:961–965.
7. Huang AYC, Bruce AT, Pardoll DM, Levitsky HI. Does B7–1 expression confer antigen-presenting cell capacity to tumors? J Exp Med 1996;183:769–776.
8. Gajewski TF, Fallarino F, Uyttenhove C, Boon T. Tumor rejection requires a CTLA4 ligand provided by the host or expressed on the tumor: superiority of B7–1 over B7–2 for active tumor immunization. J Immunol 1996;156:2909–2917.

9. Thompson CB, Allison JP. The emerging role of CTLA-4 as an immune attenuator. Immunity 1997;7:445–450.

10. Chambers CA, Kuhns MS, Egen JG, Allison JP. CTLA-4–mediated inhibition in regulation of T cell responses: mechanisms and manipulation in tumor immunotherapy. Ann Rev Immunol 2001; 19:565–594.

11. Harper K, Balzano C, Rouvier E et al. CTLA-4 and CD28 activated lymphocyte molecules are closely related in both mouse and human as to sequence, message expression, gene structure, and chromosomal location. J Immunol 1991;147:1037–1044.

12. Linsley PS, Brady W, Urnes M et al. CTLA-4 is a second receptor for the B cell activation antigen B7. J Exp Med 1991;174:561–569.

13. Krummel MF, Allison JP. CD28 and CTLA-4 have opposing effects on the response of T cells to stimulation. J Exp Med 1995;182:459–465.

14. Krummel MF, Sullivan TJ, Allison JP. Superantigen responses and costimulation: CD28 and CTLA-4 have opposing effects on T cell expansion *in vitro* and *in vivo*. Intl Immunity 1996;8:519–523.

15. Walunas TL, Lenschow DJ, Bakker CY et al. CTLA-4 can function as a negative regulator of T cell activation. Immunity 1994;1:405–413.

16. Kearney ER, Walunas TL, Karr RW et al. Antigen-dependent clonal expansion of a trace population of antigen-specific CD4+ T cells *in vivo* is dependent on CD28 costimulation and inhibited by CTLA-4. J Immunol 1995;155:1033–1036.

17. Tivol EA, Borriello F, Schweitzer AN et al. Loss of CTLA-4 leads to massive lymphoproliferation and fatal multiorgan tissue destruction, revealing a critical negative regulatory role of CTLA-4. Immunity 1995;3:541–547.

18. Waterhouse P, Penninger JM, Timms E et al. Lymphoproliferative disorders with early lethality in mice deficient in CTLA-4. Science 1995;270:985–988.

19. Chambers CA, Sullivan TJ, Allison JP. Lymphoproliferation in CTLA-4–deficient mice is mediated by costimulation-dependent activation of CD4+ T cells. Immunity 1997;7:885–895.

20. Alegre ML, Frauwirth KA, Thompson CB. T-cell regulation by CD28 and CTLA-4. Nat Rev Immunol 2001;1:220–228.

21. Krummel MF, Allison JP. CTLA-4 engagement inhibits IL-2 accumulation and cell cycle progression upon activation of resting T cells. J Exp Med 1996;183:2533–2540.

22. Brunner MC, Chambers CA, Chan F et al. CTLA-4 mediated inhibition of early events of T cell proliferation. J Immunol 1999;162:5813–5820.

23. Greene JL, Leytze GM, Emswiler J et al. Covalent dimerization of CD28/CTLA-4 and oligomerization of CD80/86 regulate T cell costimulatory interactions. J Biol Chem 1996;271:26762–26771.

24. van der Merwe PA, Bodian DL, Daenke S et al. CD80 (B7–1) binds both CD28 and CTLA-4 with a low affinity and very fast kinetics. J Exp Med 1997;185:393–403.

25. Gross JA, St.John T, Allison JP. The murine homolog of the T lymphocyte antigen CD28: Molecular cloning and cell surface expression. J Immunol 1990;144:3201–3210.

26. Lindsten T, Lee KP, Harris ES et al. Characterization of CTLA-4 structure and expression on human T cells. J Immunol 1993;151:3489–3499.

27. Linsley PS, Bradshaw J, Greene J et al. Intracellular trafficking of CTLA-4 and focal localization towards sites of TCR engagement. Immunity 1996;4:535–543.

28. Egen JG, Allison JP. Cytotoxic T lymphocyte associated antigen-4 (CTLA-4) accumulation in the immunological synapse is regulated by TCR signal strength. Immunity 2001;16:23–35.

29. Hurwitz AA, Sullivan TJ, Krummel MF et al. Specific blockade of CTLA-4/B7 interactions results in exacerbated clinical and histologic disease in an actively-induced model of experimental allergic encephalomyelitis. J Neuroimmunol 1997;73:57–62.

30. Karandikar NJ, Vanderlugt CL, Walunas TL et al. CTLA-4: A negative regulator of autoimmune disease. J Exp Med 1996;184:783–788.

31. Perrin PJ, Maldonado JH, Davis TA et al. CTLA-4 blockade enhances clinical disease and cytokine production during experimental allergic encephalomyelitis. J Immunol 1996;157:1333–1336.

32. Lühder FP, Höglund P, Allison JP et al. Cytotoxic T lymphocyte-associated antigen 4 (CTLA-4) regulates the unfolding of autoimmune diabetes. J Exp Med 1998;187:427–432.

33. Hurwitz AA, Sullivan TJ, Sobel RA, Allison JP. Cytotoxic T lymphocyte antigen-4 (CTLA-4) limits the expansion of encephalitogenic T cells in experimental autoimmune encephalomyelitis (EAE)-resistant BALB/c mice. Proc Natl Acad Sci USA 2002;99:3013–3017.

34. Leach D, Krummel M, Allison JP. Enhancement of antitumor immunity by CTLA-4 blockade. Science 1996;271:1734–1736.

35. Yang Y, Zou J, Mu J et al. Enhanced induction of antitumor T-cell responses by cytotoxic T lymphocyte associated molecule-4 blockade: The effect is manifested only at the restricted tumor-bearing stages. Cancer Res 1997;57:4036–4041.

36. Hurwitz AA, van Elsas A, Leach D et al. Manipulation of T cell activation to generate antitumor CTLs. In: Sitovsky MV, Henkart PA, eds., *Cytotoxic Cells: Basic Mechanisms and Medical Applications.* Lippincott Williams & Wilkins, Philadelphia, 1999;385–393.

37. Shrikant P, Khoruts A, Mescher MF. CTLA-4 blockade reverses CD8+ T cell tolerance to tumor by a CD4+ T cell and IL-2 dependent mechanism. Immunity 1999;11:483–493.

38. Sotomayor EM, Borrello IM, Tubb E et al. *In vivo* blockade of CTLA-4 enhances the priming of responsive T-cells but fails to prevent the induction of tumor antigen-specific tolerance. Proc Natl Acad Sci USA 1999;96:11476–11481.

39. Kwon ED, Hurwitz AA, Foster BA et al. Manipulation of T cell costimulatory and inhibitory signals for immunotherapy of prostate cancer. Proc Natl Acad Sci USA 1997;94:8099–8103.

40. van Elsas A, Hurwitz AA, Allison JP. Combination immunotherapy of B16 melanoma using anti-CTLA-4 and GM-CSF producing vaccines induces rejection of subcutaneous and metastatic tumors accompanied by autoimmune depigmentation. J Exp Med 1999;190:355–366.

41. Dranoff G, Jaffee E, Lazenby A et al. Vaccination with irradiated tumor cells engineered to secrete GM-CSF stimulates potent, specific, and long lasting anti-tumor immunity. Proc Natl Acad Sci USA 1993;90:3539–3543.

42. Hurwitz AA, Yu TF, Leach DR, Allison JP. CTLA-4 blockade synergizes with tumor-derived GM-CSF for treatment of an experimental mammary carcinoma. Proc Natl Acad Sci USA 1998;95: 10067–10071.

43. Hurwitz AA, Foster BA, Kwon ED et al. Combination immunotherapy of primary prostate cancer in a transgenic model using CTLA-4 blockade. Cancer Res 2000;60:2444–2448.

44. Rosenberg SA, White DE. Vitiligo in patients with melanoma: normal tissue antigens can be targets for cancer immunotherapy. J Immunotherapy 1996;19:81–84.

45. Rosenberg SA. Cancer vaccines based on the identification of genes encoding cancer regression antigens. Immunol Today 1997;18:175–182.

46. Rosenberg SA. new era for cancer immunotherapy based on the genes that encode cancer antigens. Immunity 1999;10:281–287.

47. van Elsas A, Sutmuller RPM, Hurwitz AA et al. Elucidating the autoimmune and anti-tumor effector mechanisms of a treatment based on cytotoxic T lymphocyte antigen-4 (CTLA-4) blockade in combination with a B16 melanoma vaccine: Comparison of prophylaxis and therapy. J Exp Med 2001;194:427–438.

48. Hung K, Hayashi R, Lafond-Walker A et al. The central role of CD4+ T cells in the antitumor immune response. J Exp Med 1998;188:2357–2368.

49. Sutmuller RPM, van Duivenvoorde L, van Elsas A et al. Synergism of CTLA-4 blockade and depletion of CD25+ regulatory T cells in anti-tumor therapy reveals alternative pathways for suppression of auto-reactive CTL responses. J Exp Med 2001;194:823–832.

50. Mokyr MB, Kalinichenko T, Gorelik L, Bluestone JA. Realization of the therapeutic potential of CTLA-4 blockade in low-dose chemotherapy-treated tumor-bearing mice. Cancer Res 1998;58: 5301–5304.

51. Kwon ED, Foster BA, Hurwitz AA et al. Elimination of residual metastatic prostate cancer following surgery and adjunctive CTLA-4 blockade immunotherapy. Proc Natl Acad Sci USA 1999;96: 15074–15079.

52. Mercader M, Ellis TM, Moser MT et al. T cell infiltration of the prostate induced by androgen withdrawal in patients with prostate cancer. Proc Natl Acad Sci USA 2001;98:14565–14570.

53. Small E, Tchekmedyian ND, Korman A et al. MDZ-010 (Human anti-CTLA4): A phase I trial in hormone refractory prostate carcinoma (CaP) [abstract]. Proc Am Soc Clin Oncol 2002 (in press).

54. Tchekmedyian NS, Hodi S, Glaspy J et al. MDX-010 (Human anti-CTLA4): A phase I trial in malignant melanoma [abstract]. Proc Am Soc Clin Oncol 2002 (in press).

Chapter 3

New Approaches to Gene Therapy for Cancer

Max W. Sung

Shu-Hsia Chen

Savio L.C. Woo

February 2001 was a major landmark in gene research when the results of sequence analyses of the entire human genome were published by two groups, the U.S. Human Genome Project and Celera Genomics, Inc.[1,2] These publications pose a formidable challenge to the scientific community to apply successfully the knowledge of human gene sequences to the treatment, diagnosis, and prevention of disease. Human gene sequences, however, have already been used for the treatment of disease since the discovery of type II restriction enzymes and DNA ligase in the early 1970s. These enzymes enabled the isolation of specific genetic sequences from human DNA; these sequences, when inserted into bacterial plasmid DNA, enabled the propagation and expression of these recombinant plasmids in bacteria, resulting in large-scale production of recombinant human proteins.[3] In 1982, the U.S. Food and Drug Administration approved the commercial production of recombinant human insulin using this technology for the treatment of diabetes mellitus, thereby revolutionizing the management of the millions of diabetic patients who had previously depended on insulin isolated from cows and pigs. Since then, numerous recombinant human proteins produced by this ex vivo technology have been applied to the treatment of cancer, such as interferon-α for melanoma and hairy-cell leukemia; interleukin-2 for kidney cancer; granulocyte colony-stimulating factor for chemotherapy-induced neutropenia; and erythropoietin for cancer-related anemia.

Although ex vivo production of recombinant human proteins uses human genetic sequences for therapeutic purposes, the term *gene therapy* has a more restricted usage and refers to the transfer of genetic sequences into human cells with the intent of treating specific diseases. As in large-scale ex vivo recombinant protein production, specific gene sequences can be isolated and inserted into plasmids or other expression vectors for transfer, not into bacterial cells but into human cells. The resulting human cells, which have been transduced with the expression vector carrying the inserted gene sequence, can initiate the transcription and translation of the transferred genes to the protein product specified by the transgene. When introduced into the human body, these cells take residence and can produce the transgene protein product in vivo.

The advantages of in vivo production of therapeutic proteins as characterized by gene therapy as compared to ex vivo recombinant protein production are being discovered every year. Although many secreted proteins exert their biological effects by binding to membrane receptors, resulting in signal transduction to the nucleus, other proteins require an intracellular or transmembrane localization for their effects. The most successful effort in clinical gene therapy to date is for the treatment of X-linked severe combined immunodeficiency, in which an inherited mutation in the gamma-c cytokine receptor gene results in the production of a dysfunctional receptor protein affecting the binding of many cytokines and produces a total blockade in B- and T-cell development. Restoration of the functional receptor protein by transfer of the normal gamma-c receptor gene into autologous bone marrow stem cells has been shown to be effective in restoring immune function in these patients.[4]

CANCER GENE THERAPY

Can restorative gene therapy, which has been successfully used for the treatment of recessive inherited genetic diseases, be applied to the treatment of cancer? Mutant recessive genes have been identified in cancer cells, the most common of which is the *p53* tumor suppressor gene, which initiates apoptotic cell death and regulates growth.[5] Clinical trials of *p53* gene transfer in tumors with homozygous mutant *p53* genes mediated by replication-defective adenovirus vectors delivered by intratumoral injection have produced tumor necrosis, delayed time to disease progression, but few tumor responses in terms of shrinkage in tumor size.[6,7] Many genetic mutations in cancer involve activation of mutant dominant oncogenes, such as the activated c-Ki-*ras* gene. For these mutations, gene transfer approaches that can antagonize the action of these dominant oncogenes, such as by cleaving *ras* oncogene mRNA using ribozymes or inactivating mRNA by complementary oligonucleotide sequences forming stable mRNA-DNA complexes, have been shown to be effective in preclinical studies.[8] The majority of cancers, however, have multiple genetic defects that were acquired during the process of malignant transformation from normal cells.[9] Gene transfer approaches that target single genetic defects may, therefore, be limited in efficacy against most cancers.

In exploring alternative gene transfer modalities for cancer, the fact that the majority of cancers are either metastatic or are at high risk for metastases to multiple distant organs must be taken into account. Although primary tumors are often amenable to surgical resection or other local ablative methods with the potential for long-term survival, the effective treatment of metastatic disease has been more elusive, and complete remissions are rarely attained except for some less common cancers, such as leukemias, lymphomas, and testis cancer.

One of the earliest investigations in gene transfer for the treatment of cancer was the use of suicide gene transfer to tumor cells to confer susceptibility selectively to a prodrug. For instance, the nucleoside analog ganciclovir is nontoxic unless it has been phosphorylated to ganciclovir triphosphate, which becomes incorporated into elongating DNA strands, interferes with DNA replication, and mediates cell death. Mammalian cells lack the enzyme to initiate the phosphorylation of ganciclovir and are, therefore, not susceptible to its action. The herpes simplex virus (HSV), conversely, produces a thymidine kinase (HSV-tk) that phosphorylates ganciclovir, and virus-infected cells are killed on exposure to ganciclovir. Preclinical studies have shown that transduction of the *HSV-tk* gene to tumor cells induces cell kill with ganciclovir; moreover, only a fraction of cells in a tumor had to be transduced for the entire tumor to necrose after ganciclovir exposure ("bystander" effect).[10,11] Clinical trials of HSV-tk gene transfer by intratumoral injection has been reported for a variety of cancers, including glioblastoma, mesothelioma, prostate cancer, and hepatic metastases from colorectal cancer.[12–15] Although gene transduction and tumor necrosis were demonstrated after intratumoral gene transfer, there was no effect on untreated tumors in the same patient, indicating local rather than systemic anti-tumor activity.

SYSTEMIC STRATEGIES FOR CANCER GENE THERAPY

Alternative gene therapy strategies targeted to cancers with metastatic multiorgan involvement have recently been tested and offer the potential for successful clinical applications. For purposes of discussion, these strategies can be grouped into four broad categories:

1. In vivo gene transfer and expression with replication defective virus vectors in tumor cells at multiple metastatic sites
2. In vivo gene transfer and expression with oncolytic virus mutants to tumor cells at multiple metastatic sites
3. In vivo or ex vivo gene transfer and transgene expression at a single organ site, with production of transgene products with anti-tumor activity delivered to multiple metastatic sites by the systemic circulation

4. In vivo or ex vivo gene transfer and transgene expression at a single organ site, resulting in immunomodulatory effects leading to the induction of effective systemic anti-tumor activity at multiple metastatic sites.

Recent progress of gene therapy strategies in all these categories is discussed but, in view of space limitations, emphasis is placed on the fourth category: immunomodulatory gene therapy.

Tumor- and Tissue-Specific Virus Vectors

In view of the success of in vivo gene transfer by intratumoral delivery of replication-defective adenovirus vectors in producing local anti-tumor effects, a logical next step would be to see whether systemic delivery of these vectors could transduce tumor cells in multiple organ sites and induce tumor necrosis. Several hurdles, however, remain to be overcome before such an approach is clinically feasible. The endothelium is an effective barrier that prevents access of vectors in the systemic circulation to tissue and tumor cells for in vivo transduction.[16] The hepatic sinusoidal system is an exception wherein the endothelium is perforated and permits systemically delivered vectors to come into contact with hepatocytes. In animal studies, however, this phenomenon also accounted for the hepatic toxicities seen with systemically delivered adenovirus vectors. In human studies, intrahepatic arterial infusion of a replication-defective adenovirus vector expressing the ornithine transcarbamoylase gene resulted in multisystem failure and death due to a systemic inflammation syndrome produced by the induction of proinflammatory cytokine production by the vector infusion.[17,18] The use of tumor- or tissue-specific promoters to regulate and limit transgene expression to the respective tumor tissue may enhance the safety of these vectors but has also been limited by low transgene expression.[19,20]

Oncolytic Viruses

In contrast to replication-defective adenovirus vectors, replication-competent viruses have been shown to be effective in infecting tissues in multiple organs via the systemic circulation. Oncolytic viruses are replication-competent virus mutants that have acquired tropism for specific tumor cells, which are selectively infected and killed by the replicating virus. Several oncolytic viruses have been evaluated in preclinical studies and in clinical trials in patients with metastatic cancers.

CI1042 (ONYX-015) is a replication-competent mutant adenovirus that preferentially replicates in tumor cells with the mutant *p53* tumor suppressor gene.[21] The E1B adenovirus protein binds to the normal p53 protein and inhibits p53-mediated cell cycle arrest and apoptosis. CI1042 has a mutation in the E1B region, resulting in the absent production of the E1B protein and inability to bind and interfere with p53-mediated cell cycle arrest and apoptotic cell death.

However, in tumor cells with mutant p53, CI1042 replication is able to proceed and results in subsequent cell lysis by the replicating virus. Phase I trials of CI1042 administered by a number or routes, including intratumoral, intravenous, intracavitary, and intraarterial, have been reported; no dose-limiting toxicities were reported, and viral replication and central tumor necrosis have been noted, although no responses by World Health Organization criteria could be documented.[22,23]

Reovirus is a relatively nonpathogenic double-stranded RNA virus that produces subclinical or mild upper respiratory or gastrointestinal tract infections in humans.[24] In vitro studies have shown that transformation of reovirus-resistant NIH 3T3 cells with the activated *ras* mutant oncogene resulted in acquired sensitivity to the virus. This is possibly due to the inhibition of double-stranded RNA-activated protein kinase by activated *ras,* thereby permitting viral protein synthesis.[25] Intratumoral injection of reovirus in established human U87 glioblastoma cells in SCID or nude mice resulted in significant tumor regression.[26] Clinical trials of reovirus are currently in development.

Cytolytic strains of the Newcastle disease virus (NDV), an avian single-stranded RNA paramyxovirus, have been shown to replicate selectively in and rapidly kill human tumor cells in vitro while sparing normal cells.[27] The mechanism for selectivity is under investigation at this time and may be due to the down-regulation of the interferon pathway in cancer cells, rendering them more susceptible to infection by lytic viruses. Intratumoral injection of NDV strain 73-T produced sustained complete remission of human neuroblastoma and fibrosarcoma xenografts in nude mice.[28] Similar results were seen with xenografts of human epithelial cancers, such as colon, lung, breast, prostate, and epidermoid carcinomas. Systemic delivery by a single intraperitoneal injection of NHV 73-T produced complete regression of IMR-32 neuroblastoma xenografts in 9 of 12 mice without recurrence during the 3- to 9-month follow-up period.[29] Recurrences responded to repeated intraperitoneal (IP) injections of NDV 73-T with complete regression in three of six treated mice. The efficacy of NDV 73-T delivered systemically renders it a candidate for clinical development in patients with metastatic cancers. It should be noted that NDV has been shown to activate interferon and tumor necrosis factor production in the host, and phase II trials of vaccines prepared from NDV-infected melanoma cell lines have shown abatement in disease recurrence 3 years after surgical resection in patients with stage II malignant melanoma (from 95% in historical controls to 12% in the treated patients).[30]

IN VIVO PRODUCTION OF ANTIANGIOGENESIS INHIBITORS

The large-scale production of recombinant human proteins that started in the 1980s has revolutionized the treatment of many human diseases, including diabetes mellitus, growth hormone deficiency, and the hemophilias. Intravenous administration of recombinant human factor IX, for instance, was successful in maintaining adequate serum levels of factor IX and controlling bleeding occurrences in patients with hemophilia IX. Treatment, however, required frequent administrations of the recombinant protein. Recent studies have shown that intramuscular or intraportal injection of an adeno-associated virus vector expressing the factor IX gene was effective in producing sustained elevations of serum factor IX with normalization of coagulation parameters in the blood.[31,32]

Tumor growth has been shown to be associated with and dependent on the recruitment of new blood vessels or angiogenesis that serves to supply oxygen and nutrients to the tumor. Tumor angiogenesis is mediated by angiogenic factors, such as basic fibroblast and vascular endothelial growth factors secreted by the tumor cells.[33,34] Angiogenesis has subsequently been found to be tightly regulated by a balance of activating and inhibiting factors.[35] Endostatin, a 20-kDa C-terminal fragment of collagen XVIII, has been found to be one of the most potent inhibitors of angiogenesis to date and has been shown to inhibit tumor growth in a dose-dependent manner in animal models.[36] The recombinant human endostatin protein has been produced on a large scale for use in clinical trials. However, recombinant endostatin is unstable in the systemic circulation and requires frequent administration in patients.[37]

Recently, a number of investigators have constructed adenovirus vectors expressing the recombinant human endostatin cDNA and have shown that elevated serum levels of endostatin can be produced by a single injection of the adenovirus vector in the systemic circulation.[38–41] Moreover, the elevated levels of endostatin were maintained in the blood for up to 2 weeks after a single injection and resulted in tumor growth inhibition and prevention of disseminated metastases in animal models.[38]

Another approach to angiogenesis inhibitor currently under investigation is the use of ribozymes to target mRNA of angiogenesis-promoting genes. Ribozymes are RNA enzymes that can selectively antagonize specific genes by cleaving mRNA encoded by the gene. Hammerhead ribozymes, derived from plant satellite virus RNA, can selectively degrade mRNA from activated mutant *ras* oncogene in a large variety of cancers and from the *Bcr-Abl* fusion gene associated with chronic myelogenous leukemia.[42,43] Ribozymes can be stabilized by blocking the 3′ end and the 2′ positions of pyrimidines without sacrificing their activity. Stabilized ribozymes have half-lives measured in hours and, because of their low toxicity profile, can be administered by intravenous injection.[44] A ribozyme that targets the Flt-1 receptor for vascular endothelial growth factor and has been shown to block angiogenesis in a corneal model is currently being tested in clinical trials.[45,46]

IMMUNOMODULATORY GENE THERAPY

The Role of Anti-Tumor Immunity

Can gene transfer targeted to only a single tumor site yield anti-tumor effects that are systemic and directed against other tumors in multiple sites and organs in the same host? The transfer of immunomodulatory genes to enhance the induction of effective anti-tumor immune responses that are systemic and long-lasting may offer the potential for the treatment of metastatic cancer. Our preclinical studies in a murine model of established liver and lung metastases from colon cancer have indicated that such an approach targeting a single tumor site can be effective in inducing regression at distant metastatic sites and promoting long-term survival in 80%–100% of treated animals.[47] These studies have provided the basis for clinical testing of this approach in clinical trials.

The existence of humoral and cell-mediated immune responses against autologous tumor cells has been well documented in patients with cancer. For instance, sera and peripheral blood mononuclear cells obtained from patients with colon and other cancers have been shown to inhibit the growth of autologous tumor cells in culture.[48,49] Tumor-infiltrating lymphocytes that have been isolated from colon cancers demonstrate a limited repertoire and react with autologous tumor cells.[50–53] The current concepts in tumor immunology suggest that specific anti-tumor immune responses are elicited against antigens associated with tumor cells and recognized as foreign in the context of class I and class II major histocompatibility complexes (MHC). These antigens may represent differentiation antigens, such as carcinoembryonic antigen, such oncofetal antigens as alpha-fetoprotein, protein products of mutant oncogenes, and such normal antigens as MUC-1, which have become antigenic with the loss of polarization in the cell.[54] Anti-tumor immune responses may result in immune cell-mediated destruction of tumors, in T-cell immune suppression, or in a state of immune tolerance wherein tumor-associated antigens are not recognized as "foreign" and escape immune-mediated destruction.[55]

For effective immune stimulation, two signals must be elicited. The first signal involves the binding of short peptides from tumor-associated antigens on antigen-presenting cells (macrophages, dendritic cells, B cells) in association with the MHC-I and MHC-II complexes to the T-cell receptor on CD8+ and CD4+ T cells, respectively. Ligation of the T-cell receptor leads to signal transduction, to secretion of cytokines that stimulate the proliferation, and to activation of CD4+ and CD8+ T cells in draining lymph nodes.[56] A second signal is elicited when costimulatory molecules, such as B7 in antigen-presenting cells, bind to the receptors on CD4+ or CD8+ T cells in association with peptide-MHC complexes or when high concentrations of secreted cytokines have accumulated in the tumor microenvironment to support the proliferation and activation of T cells.[57] Alternatively, tumor cells can express short peptides derived from tumor-associated antigens in association with MHC-I complex, the binding of which to CD8+ T cells contributes to a first signal for immune stimulation.[58] The induction of an effective immune response, however, requires both first and second signals. Immune stimulation after a first signal without support from a second signal may lead to a state of immune tolerance and escape from immune-mediated destruction.

Barriers to immune-mediated tumor destruction therefore include (1) absence of or suboptimal expression of tumor-associated antigens; (2) spontaneous loss of MHC-I complex expression from tumor cells; (3) suboptimal expression of costimulatory molecules; and (4) inadequate secretion of cytokines to support a second signal for immune stimulation. These barriers could be surmounted by gene transfer strategies that can selectively remedy specific deficiencies responsible for ineffective anti-tumor immune stimulation by enhancing the expression of specific immunomodulatory genes.

Cytokine-Enhanced Tumor Vaccines Prepared Ex Vivo

In patients with metastatic cancers, autologous whole-tumor cell vaccines have been tested for many years with generally disappointing results and weak induction of anti-tumor immunity. The advances in gene transfer technology opened new avenues in the preparation of tumor vaccines and offered possibilities for circumventing some of the mechanisms responsible for the poor efficacy of these vaccines. Dranoff et al[59] reported on their preclinical studies using the MFG retroviral vector to transfer cytokine genes into dividing murine tumor cell lines in culture, which were then irradiated to arrest growth and used to vaccinate syngeneic mice. Cytokines screened in these studies included the interleukins (IL-2, IL-4, IL-5, IL-6), tumor necrosis factor-α, γ-interferon, and granulocyte macrophage colony stimulating factor (GM-CSF). Results from these studies indicated that vaccines prepared from B16 melanoma cells expressing cytokines were superior to those prepared from nontransduced B16 cells in rejecting subsequent challenge of live B16 cells implanted at a distant site. Of the cytokines tested, GM-CSF rejected tumor cell challenge in 10 of 10 animals, whereas IL-4 and IL-6 were successful in only 2 of 5 and 2 of 4 animals, respectively. In comparison, only 1 of 19 animals vaccinated with nontransduced irradiated cells rejected subsequent tumor challenge. The mechanisms by which the immunogenicity of the autologous tumor cell vaccine was enhanced may be related to enhancement of antigen-presenting cell function and activation of granulocytes and monocyte/macrophages. Lymphocyte subset depletion studies indicated that the anti-tumor immunity was dependent on CD4+ and CD8+ T cells but not on natural killer cells. Clinical trials of irradiated autologous tumor cell vaccine in melanoma and prostate cancer have been reported. Specific anti-tumor immune responses were demonstrated in these trials but did not result in sustained clinical remissions in treated patients.[60,61]

Cytokine-Enhanced Antitumor Immunization In Vivo

In clinical trials, vaccines prepared from autologous tumor cells that had been with the GM-CSF gene have been demonstrated to elicit both local and systemic anti-tumor immune responses but did not induce significant tumor regression. The preparation of the vaccine was difficult, as the MFG-based retroviral vector requires dividing cells for transduction. Tumor cells, therefore, had to be isolated from surgical specimens and cultured to achieve logarithmic growth.[62] Retroviral vectors also tended to have relatively low transduction efficiencies and transgene expression, thereby requiring a considerable number of dividing cells to achieve a vaccine preparation. The cells then had to be irradiated to arrest growth while remaining able to secrete the cytokine. Alternatively, adenovirus vectors may be used to transduce tumor cells with the cytokine genes. Adenovirus vectors have high transduction efficiencies with high transgene expression and can transduce both dividing and nondividing cells.[63] In fact, adenovirus vectors can be injected directly into a tumor and are able to transduce these cells in situ. These properties permit the transduction of tumor cells in vivo and thereby preserve the antigenic heterogeneity of tumor cells to elicit immune responses. Adenovirus-transduced cells are usually eliminated by the host immune system in 1–2 weeks, but sustained cytokine secretion was probably not required, as cytokine support of immune stimulation after antigen recognition did not require sustained delivery of the cytokine. We and other investigators have evaluated this approach for inducing anti-tumor immune responses in animal models. Because of the limitations of space, we discuss our more recent work as a paradigm for developing in situ immunization as a potentially effective treatment of metastatic cancer at multiple sites.

We have constructed replication-defective adenovirus vectors that were E1- and E3-deleted and replication-defective.[64] The cDNAs for cytokine genes were prepared and inserted into the E1 region under the control of the Rous sarcoma virus promoter. The vectors were shown to have high transduction efficiency and transgene expression of biologically active cytokines. For our orthotopic murine tumor model, we established metastatic tumors in the livers of Balb/c mice with direct intrahepatic implantation of syngeneic MCA26 colon carcinoma cells at a single site.[65] MCA26 cells were suitable for the testing of immunomodulatory gene therapy because the cells are inherently poorly immunogenic. When the liver tumor size reached 4 × 5 mm, the cells were injected with varying doses of adenovirus vectors expressing cytokine genes, using a 27-gauge needle under direct visual guidance during laparotomy Control animals received either phosphate-buffered saline (PBS) solution or an empty adenovirus vector Adv.DL312. The animals were then followed up for long-term survival or were euthanized to assess for tumor regression, immune responses, and organ toxicities.

The cytokine genes that have been evaluated included IL-2, IL-12, and GM-CSF. We found that the IL-2 vector required concurrent transduction with a vector expressing the HSV-tk gene followed by systemic ganciclovir for optimal tumor regression and anti-tumor immune responses.[66,67] For the IL-2 vector, the combination with GM-CSF and HSV-tk was most effective, with tumor regression, long-term survival, and sustained remissions in up to 20% of treated animals and specific anti-tumor immunity mediated by CD8+ T cells.[67] For the IL-12 vector, we found that a single intratumoral injection induced tumor regression and long-term survival in 20% of treated animals.[47]

Interleukin-12 Gene Therapy

IL-12 is a cytokine secreted by activated antigen-presenting cells (dendritic cells, monocytes, B-cells) that have been successfully produced in large quantities by recombinant DNA technology.[68] Systemic administration of the recombinant IL-12 cytokine has been shown to inhibit tumor growth in mice bearing established tumors.[69] The anti-tumor activity of IL-12 lies in its ability to enhance the cytolytic activity of cytotoxic T lymphocytes, natural killer (NK) cells, and lymphokine activated killer cells; to induce interferon-γ (IFN-γ) production by NK and activated T-cells; and to inhibit tumor angiogenesis by inducing IP-10 and IFN-γ secretion by activated monocytes.[70] Tumor growth inhibition was dose-dependent, and responding animals were found to be immune to subsequent challenge with parental tumor cells.[71] In these animals, the major immune effectors were CD8+ T cells and IFN-γ on the basis of studies in nude mice (T cell–deficient); beige mice (NK cell–deficient); NK cell–depleted mice (by anti-asialoGM1); CD4+ and CD8+ depleted mice, and IFN-γ receptor–deleted knockout mice.

Results of recombinant IL-12 in clinical trials in patients with cancer were less encouraging. After phase I trials that determined the maximal tolerated dose (MTD) of intravenously administered IL-12 to be 500 ng/kg, a phase II trial at the MTD was halted when two patients died from severe systemic toxicities with markedly elevated serum IFN-γ levels.[72,73] No significant tumor responses were seen. Because production of IL-12 by activated antigen-presenting cells provides a strong signal for immune stimulation, we hypothesize that increasing IL-12 production in the tumor microenvironment may enhance the induction of anti-tumor immune responses effective in marshaling the proliferation and activation of specific cytolytic T cells.[74]

These preclinical studies showed significant tumor regression on necropsy evaluation 2 weeks after virus injection.[65] Moreover, 20% of treated animals were long-term survivors without evidence of tumor on necropsy evaluation. Immunopathological examination of the livers 2 days after virus injection showed an early influx of mononuclear cells in the liver. These infiltrating mononuclear cells isolated from these livers and, when assayed for NK cell and cytotoxic T-lymphocyte activities using a chromium release assay on Cr-51-labeled YAC-1 (NK cell–sensitive) and parental MCA26 cells, showed increases in cytotoxicity against YAC-1 and MCA26 cells as compared with results in animals injected with Adv-DL312. NK cell blocking reduced the cytotoxicity of these mononuclear cells, indicating that the immune responses after vector injection were mediated by NK cells. In vivo depletion studies of the major lymphocyte subsets showed that animals surviving long term were substantially reduced with NK cell depletion (anti-asialoGM1) but not with CD4+ (GK1.5) or CD8+ (2.43) T-cell depletion.[75]

To assess whether the anti-tumor immune responses induced by intratumoral vector injection were systemic and long-lasting, we challenged the long-term surviving animals with parental MCA26 or syngeneic JC breast carcinoma cells by subcutaneous implantation at a distant site.[75] Fewer than 10% of animals challenged with MCA26, as compared to 75% of animals challenged with JC, developed tumors. Lymphocyte subset depletion studies showed that both NK and CD8+ T cells were required for protection against tumor rechallenge.

One possible mechanism for the induction of these anti-tumor immune responses after intratumoral vector injection is the high tissue levels of IL-12 produced in the tumor microenvironment as a result of transgene expression of transduced tumor cells. In fact, lysis and resuspension of injected tumors showed IL-12 levels of 25,000 pg/mL. These levels were considerably higher than peak serum levels of IL-12 achieved at the MTD in clinical trials of rhIL-12 (11,135 pg/mL). The kinetic profile of serum cytokines that were assessed daily up to 14 days after intratumoral vector injection showed peak serum IL-12 levels of 644 pg/mL. Induction of IFN-γ production was seen, although serum levels were low (314 pg/mL) as compared to the peak levels (6,000 pg/mL) at the MTD in the rhIL-12 trials. Proinflammatory cytokines IL-6 and tumor necrosis factor-γ were not elevated beyond baseline on kinetic profiling in this murine model, while sustained elevations of serum IL-6 have been reported in a patient who developed fatal multisystem inflammation following hepatic arterial infusion of an adenovirus vector expressing the ornithine transcarbamoylase gene.[17,18]

Other possible mechanisms include the upregulation of MHC class I expression on tumor cells after transduction with the IL-12 gene. MHC-I immunostains were performed on MCA6 liver metastasis before and after intratumoral vector injection showed increase in MHC-1 expression after vector injection, which could enhance the first signal in anti-tumor immune stimulation.

Combination IL-12 Gene Transfer with T-Cell Costimulation

Preclinical studies with a murine model of established hepatic metastases have demonstrated that 20% of animals treated with intratumoral adenovirus-mediated IL-12 gene transfer became long-term survivors with complete pathologic remissions. These studies also indicated that stimulated NK cells were the primary immune effectors after vector injection. We hypothesize that addition of T-cell immune stimulation may enhance the efficacy of IL-12 gene transfer, as NK cell immunity is generally short-lived and T cells are the major effectors for long-term systemic anti-tumor immunity.

4-1BB is a costimulatory molecule expressed in activated CD4+ and CD8+ cells.[76] Ligation of 4-1BB results in a strong second signal for the expansion of TcR-ligated T lymphocytes.[77] The ligation of 4-1BB is accomplished by 4-1BB ligand, a membrane-bound receptor present on antigen-presenting cells. Previous studies have also shown that 4-1BB can be ligated with similar immunomodulatory effects with a monoclonal agonist antibody raised against 4-1BB.[78]

Using our murine tumor model of established hepatic metastasis, we tested 4-1BB ligation with an agonist antibody against 4-1BB (anti-4-1BB), alone and in combination with intratumoral IL-12 gene transfer.[47] Anti-4-1BB at a dose of 50 μg per mouse was injected intraperitoneally at varying doses 1 and 3 days after IL-12 vector injection. In comparison, animals were treated with anti-4-1BB in combination with intratumoral injection of an empty adenovirus vector (Adv-DL312) or intratumoral IL-12 gene transfer in combination with control immunoglobulin or with intratumoral Adv-DL312 in combination with control immunoglobulin. These studies showed that up to 100% of animals treated with combination IL-12 gene transfer and anti-4-1BB achieved long-term survival beyond 120 days after one course of treatment (Fig. 3.1). Reducing the dose of the IL-12 vector from 3.6×10^8 to 0.4×10^8 pfu per mouse resulted in only a mild decrease in long-term survivors to 80% of treated animals. Control animals that received control immunoglobulin and Adv-DL312 died within 30 days with

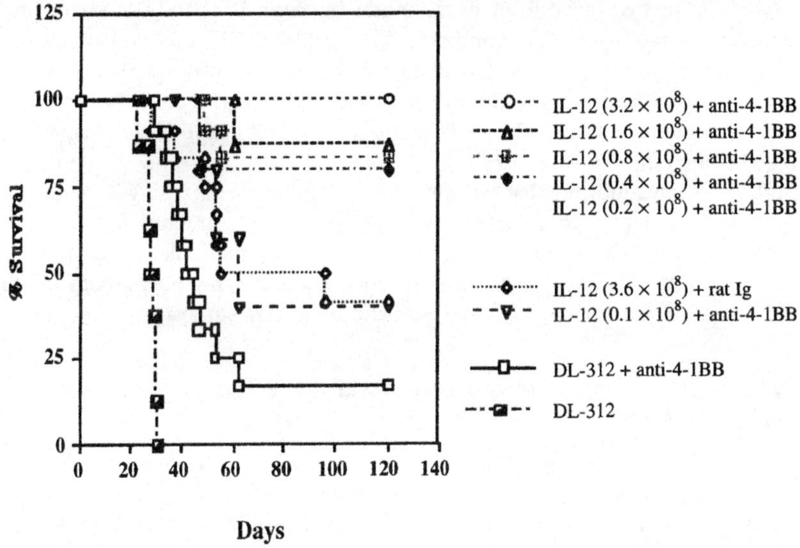

FIGURE 3.1 Survival of tumor-bearing animals after Adv.mIL-12 and anti-4-1BB treatment. Animals were implanted intrahepatically with 7×10^4 MCA26 tumor cells. Seven days later, the animals bearing tumors of size 5×5 mm² were divided into five groups, and those in each group (n = 7–8) were injected intratumorally with various doses of Adv.RSV-mIL-12 (3.2×10^8 to 0.1×10^8 pfu) or with a control vector, Adv.DL312 (3.2×10^8 pfu) in combination with anti-m4-1BB or control Ig. The antibodies were injected intraperitoneally at days 8 and 10 at a dose of 50 μg per mouse. The survival difference between the animals treated with combination Adv.mIL-12 (at 0.2×10^8 pfu or higher) + anti-m4-1BB and the animals treated with either anti-4-1BB or Adv.mIL-12 alone was statistically significant (log rank survival analysis, $P < 0.0001$).

widespread metastatic disease, and only 15% of animals treated with anti-4-1BB in combination with Adv-DL312 survived long term.

The systemic and long-term nature of the anti-tumor immunity induced by the combination treatment was tested in studies of tumor rechallenge at a distant site. Animals surviving long term after the combination treatment were injected subcutaneously in the flank with parental MCA26 cells at tumorigenic doses (7×10^4). Untreated mice were used as controls. The animals were observed for tumor formation over a 4-week period. Of the long-term surviving animals after combination treatment, only one of seven (14%) formed subcutaneous tumor, compared to eight of eight (100%) of controls.

To test whether the combination intratumoral IL-12 gene transfer and anti-4-1BB can be effective against multiple metastases at a distant site, we modified our murine tumor-bearing model to include established multiple macroscopic metastatic nodules in the lung (0.5–0.8 mm) produced by injection of MCA26 cells in the tail vein in addition to the 4 × 5 mm established metastatic MCA26 tumor in the liver produced by intrahepatic implantation. In these studies, the animals were treated with an intratumoral injection of the IL-12 vector and intravenous administration of anti-4-1BB. Control animals received Adv-DL312 and control immunoglobulin, and all died within 32 days with widespread metastatic disease. In contrast, 100% of the animals treated with combination IL-12 gene transfer and anti-4-1BB were long-term survivors beyond 120 days ($P < 0.0011$, log rank test; Fig. 3.2).

These results indicate that targeting a metastatic tumor at a single site for IL-12 gene transfer in combination with systemic administration of an agonist antibody anti-4-1BB ligating the T-cell costimulatory molecule 4-1BB induced anti-tumor immunity that was systemic and effective in producing both tumor regression in metastases at a distant site and long-term survival.

Clinical Translation of Intratumoral IL-12 Gene Transfer and 4-1BB Ligation

To test whether combination intratumoral IL-12 gene transfer and 4-1BB ligation can be safely tolerated and effective in patients with hepatic metastases, we are conducting a phase I trial of escalating doses of an adenovirus vector expressing human IL-12 (Adv.RSV-hIL-12) delivered by intratumoral injection in patients with liver metastases from colorectal or breast cancer. This will be followed with a second phase I trial of escalating doses of anti-4-1BB in combination with a fixed dose of Adv.RSV-hIL-12 determined from the MTD of the vector from the previous trial. Assessment for the induction of specific T-cell-mediated anti-tumor immune responses will be performed by ELISPOT against autologous tumor targets of peripheral blood mononuclear cells obtained before and serially after the study treatment.[79–81] To deliver Adv.RSV-hIL-12 by intratumoral injection, we will use percutaneous placement of three needles with their tips in a metastatic

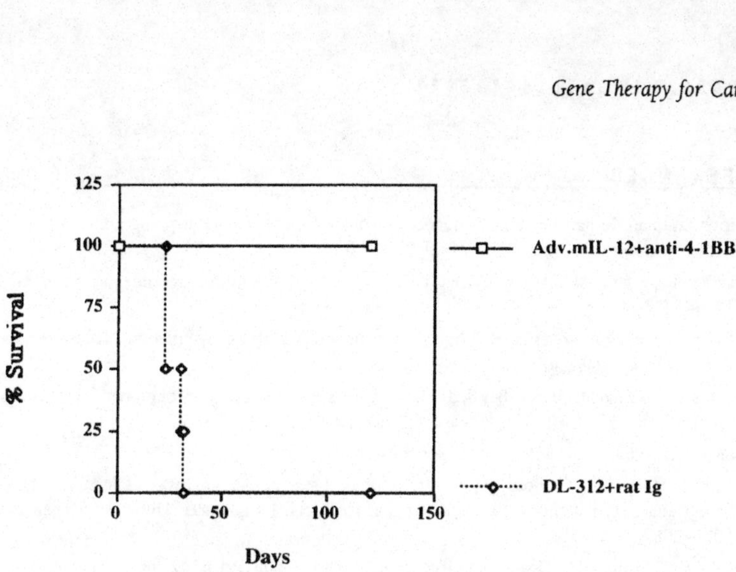

FIGURE 3.2 Effect of Adv.mIL-12 plus anti-4-1BB treatment on macroscopic lung metastases of colon carcinoma. An animal model with both liver tumor and pre-established multiple macroscopic tumor nodules in the lung was subjected to a test of the systemic antitumor effect. Control animals receiving no treatment developed multiple lesions in the lung, and all died within 32 days. However, 100% of the animals receiving the combination treatment (0.4 $\times$ 10^8 pfu Adv.mIL-12 + anti 4-1BB) (n = 6) survived well after 70 days. The results indicate distant protection against pre-existing macroscopic lung metastases by the combination treatment.

tumor in the liver under concurrent ultrasonographic monitoring. We have tested this procedure in a previous phase I trial of intratumoral injection of the adenovirus-mediated HSV-tk gene in 16 patients with hepatic metastases from colorectal cancer and have shown that the procedure was feasible and safely tolerated and did not result in serious hepatic or systemic toxicities.[15] The use of three needles permitted the injection of small aliquots of the vector at multiple sites within the tumor, thereby increasing exposure of tumor cells for virus transduction while minimizing risks of hepatic laceration from needle manipulation.

FUTURE DIRECTIONS

Gene transfer technology offers the potential for effective treatment of metastatic cancer. Moreover, targeting only a single metastatic tumor can minimize the risks of gene transfer without sacrificing the systemic immunomodulatory effects of the treatment. The challenge ahead lies in determining how immunomodulatory gene transfer can be optimized to ensure adequate delivery and expression of the immunomodulatory transgene and in developing other gene transfer strategies for the effective treatment of metastatic cancer in multiple organs.

REFERENCES

1. International Human Genome Sequencing Consortium. Initial sequencing and analysis of the human genome. Nature 2001;409:860–921.
2. Venter JC, Adams MD, Myers EW et al. The sequence of the human genome. Science 2001;291: 1304–1351.
3. Cohen S, Chang A, Boyer H, Helling R. Construction of biologically functional bacterial plasmids in vitro. Proc Natl Acad Sci USA 1973;70:3240–3244.
4. Cavazzana-Calvo M, Hacein-Bey S, de Saint Basile G et al. Gene therapy of human severe combined immunodeficiency (SCID)-X1 disease. Science 2000;288:669–672.
5. Levine AJ. P53, the cellular gatekeeper for growth and division. Cell 1997;88:323.
6. Schuler M, Rochlitz C, Horowitz JA et al. A phase I study of adenovirus-mediated wild-type p53 gene transfer in patients with advanced non-small cell lung cancer. Hum Gene Ther 1998;9: 2075–2082.
7. Swisher SG, Roth JA, Nemunaitis J et al. Adenovirus-mediated p53 gene transfer in advanced non-small-cell lung cancer. J Natl Cancer Inst 1999;91:763–771.
8. Lewin AS, Hauswirth WW. Ribozyme gene therapy: applications for molecular medicine. Trends Mol Med 2001;7:221–228.
8. Gewirtz AM. Oligonucleotide therapeutics: a step forward. J Clin Oncol 2000;18:1812–23.
9. Fujiwara T, Stolker JM, Watanabe T et al. Accumulated clonal genetic alterations in familial and sporadic colorectal carcinomas with widespread instability in microsatellite sequences. Am J Pathol 1998;153:1063–1078.
10. Moolten FL. Tumor chemosensitivity conferred by inserted herpes thymidine kinase genes: paradigm for a prospective cancer control strategy. Cancer Res 1986;46:5276–5281.
11. Freeman SM, Abboud CN, Whartenby KA et al. The bystander effect: tumor regression when a fraction of the tumor mass is genetically modified. Cancer Res 1993;53:5274–5283.
12. Trask TW, Trask RP, Aguilar-Cordova E et al. Phase I study of adenoviral delivery of the HSV-tk gene and ganciclovir administration in patients with recurrent malignant brain tumors. Mol Ther 2000;1:195–203.
13. Sterman DH, Treat J, Litzky LA et al. Adenovirus-mediated herpes simplex virus thymidine kinase/ ganciclovir gene therapy in patients with localized malignancy: results of a phase I clinical trial in malignant mesothelioma. Hum Gene Ther 1998;9:1083–1092.
14. Herman JR, Adler HL, Aguilar-Cordova E et al. In situ gene therapy for adenocarcinoma of the prostate: a phase I clinical trial. Hum Gene Ther 1999;10:1239–1249.
15. Sung MW, Yeh HC, Thung SN et al. Intratumoral adenovirus-mediated suicide gene therapy for hepatic metastases from colorectal adenocarcinoma: results of a phase I clinical trial. Mol Ther 2001;4:182–191.
16. Jain RK. Delivery of novel therapeutic agents in tumors: physiological barriers and strategies. J Natl Cancer Inst 1989;81:570–576.
17. Hollon T. Researchers and regulators reflect on first gene therapy death. Nat Med 2000;6:6.
18. Marshall E. Gene therapy on trial. Science 2000;288:951–957.
19. Humphreys MJ, Ghaneh P, Greenhalf W et al. Hepatic intra-arterial delivery of a retroviral vector expressing the cytosine deaminase gene, controlled by the CEA promoter and intraperitoneal treatment with 5-fluorocytosine suppresses growth of colorectal liver metastases. Gene Ther 2001; 8:1241–1247.
20. Yu D, Chen D, Chiu C et al. Prostate-specific targeting using PSA promoter-based lentiviral vectors. Cancer Gene Ther 2001;8:628–635.

21. Bischoff JR, Kirn DH, Williams A et al. An adenovirus mutant that replicates selectively in p53-deficient human tumor cells. Science 1996;274:373–376.

22. Nemunaitis J, Khuri F, Ganly I et al. Phase II trial of intratumoral administration of ONYX-015, a replication-selective adenovirus, in patients with refractory head and neck cancer. J Clin Oncol 2001;19:289–298.

23. Nemunaitis J, Cunningham C, Buchanan A et al. Intravenous infusion of a replication-selective adenovirus (ONYX-015) in cancer patients: safety, feasibility and biological activity. Gene Ther 2001;8:746–759.

24. Tyler KL, Fields BN. In: NN Fields, DM Knipe, PM Howley, eds. Fields Virology. Philadelphia: Lippincott-Raven, 1996:1597–1623.

25. Coffey MC, Strong JE, Forsyth PA, Lee PW. Reovirus therapy of tumors with activated Ras pathway. Science 1998;282:1244–1246.

26. Wilcox ME, Yang WQ, Senger D et al. Reovirus as an oncolytic agent against experimental human malignant gliomas. J Natl Cancer Inst 2001;12:903–912.

27. Reichard KW, Lorence RM, Cascino CJ et al. Newcastle disease virus selectively kills human tumor cells. J Surg Res 1992;52:448–453.

28. Lorence RM, Katubig BB, Reichard KW et al. Complete regression of human fibrosarcoma xenografts after local Newcastle disease virus therapy. Cancer Res 1994;54:6017–6021.

29. Phuangsab A, Lorence RM, Reichard KW et al. Newcastle disease virus therapy of human tumor xenografts: antitumor effects of local or systemic administration. Cancer Lett 2001;172:27–36.

30. Cassel WA, Nmurray DR, Phillips HS. A phase II study on the postsurgical management of stage II malignant melanoma with a Newcastle disease virus oncolysate. Cancer 1983;52:856–860.

31. High KA. Gene transfer as an approach to treating hemophilia. Circ Res 2001;88:137–144.

32. Wang L Nichols TC, Read MS et al. Sustained expression of therapeutic level of factor IX in hemophilia B dogs by AAV-mediated gene therapy in liver. Mol Ther 2000;1:154–158.

33. Hanahan D, Folkman J. Patterns and emerging mechanisms of the angiogenic switch during tumorigenesis. Cell 1996;86:353–364.

34. Folkman J, D'Amore PA. Blood vessel formation: What is its molecular basis? Cell 1996;87: 1153–1155.

35. Folkman J. Seminars in Medicine of the Beth Israel Hospital, Boston. Clinical applications of research on angiogenesis. N Engl J Med 1995;333:1757–1763.

36. O'Reilly MS, Boehm T, Shing Y et al. Endostatin: an endogenous inhibitor of angiogenesis and tumor growth. Cell 1997;88:277–285.

37. Boehm T, Pirie-Shepherd S, Trinh LB et al. Disruption of the KEX1 gene in *Pichia pastoris* allows expression of full-length murine and human endostatin. Yeast 1999;15:563–572.

38. Sauter BV, Martinet O, Zhang WEJ et al. Adenovirus-mediated gene transfer of endostatin in vivo results in high level of transgene expression and inhibition of tumor growth and metastases. Proc Natl Acad Sci USA 2000;97:4802–4907.

39. Wen XY, Vai Y, Steward AK. Adenovirus-mediated human endostatin gene delivery demonstrates strain-specific antitumor activity and acute dose-dependent toxicity in mice. Hum Gene Ther 2001;12:347–358.

40. Chen CT, Lin J, Li Q et al. Angiogenic gene therapy for cancer via systemic administration of adenoviral vectors expressing secretable endostatin. Hum Gene Ther 2000;11:1983–1996.

41. Feldman AL, Restifo NP, Alexander HR et al. Antiangiogenic gene therapy of cancer utilizing a recombinant adenovirus to elevate systemic endostatin levels in mice. Cancer Res 2000;60: 1503–1506.

42. Kijima H, Scanlon KJ. Ribozyme as an approach for growth suppression of human pancreatic cancer. Mol Biotechnol 2000;14:59–72.

43. Kuwabara T, Hamada M, Warashina M, Taira K. Allosterically controlled single-chained maxizymes with extremely high and specific activity. Biomacromolecules 2001;2:788–799.

44. Lee PA et al. Pharmacokinetics and tissue distribution of a ribozyme directed against hepatitis C virus RNA following subcutaneous or intravenous administration in mice. Hepatology 2000;32: 640–646.

45. Kuwahara T et al. A novel allosterically trans-activated ribozyme, the maxizyme, with exceptional specificity in vitro and in vivo. Mol Cell 1998;2:617–627.

46. Sandberg JA et al. Acute toxicology and pharmacokinetic assessment of a ribozyme (ANGIOZYME) targeting vascular endothelial growth factor mRNA in the cynomolgus monkey. Antisense Nucleic Acid Drug Dev 2000;10:153–162.

47. Chen SH, Pham-Nguyen KB, Martinet O et al. Rejection of disseminated metastases of colon carcinoma by synergism of IL-12 gene therapy and 4-1Bb costimulation. Mol Ther 2000;2:39–46.

48. Hellstrom I, Hellstrom KE, Shepard TN. Cell-mediated immunity against antigens common to human colonic carcinomas and fetal gut epithelium. Int J Cancer 1970;6:346.

49. Hellstrom T, Hellstrom KE, Sjögren H, Warner GA. Demonstration of cell-mediated immunity to human neoplasms of various histologic types. Int J Cancer 1971;7:1–16.

50. Yoo YK, Heo DS, Hata K et al. Tumor-infiltrating lymphocytes from human colon carcinomas. Gastroenterology 1990;98:259–268.

51. Werkmeister JA, Pihl E, Nind APP et al. Immunoreactivity by intrinsic lymphoid cells in colorectal carcinoma. Br J Cancer 1979;40:839–847.

52. Ostenstad B, Sioud M, Schlichting E, Harboe M. Limited heterogeneity in the T-cell receptor V-gene usage in lymphocytes infiltrating human colorectal tumours. Br J Cancer 1994;69:1078–1082.

53. Homm SS, Rosenberg SA, Topalian SL. Specific immune recognition of autologous tumor by lymphocytes infiltrating colon carcinomas: analysis by cytokine secretion. Cancer Immunol Immunother 1993;36:1–8.

54. Houghton AN. Cancer antigens: immune recognition of self and altered self. J Exp Med 1994; 180:1–4.

55. Matzinger P. Tolerance, danger, and the extended family. Annu Rev Immunol 1994;12:991–1045.

56. Bretscher P, Cohn M. A theory of self-nonself discrimination. Science 1970;169:1042–1049.

57. Pardoll D. Immunology: T cells and tumours. Nature 2001;411:1010–1012.

58. Carbone FR, Kurts C, Bennet SRM et al. Cross-presentation: a general mechanism for CTL immunity and tolerance. Immunol Today 1998;19:368–373.

59. Dranoff G, Jaffee E, Lazenby A et al. Vaccination with irradiated tumor cells engineered to secrete murine granulocyte-macrophage colon-stimulating factor stimulates potent, specific and long-lasting anti-tumor immunity. Proc Natl Acad Sci USA 1993;90:3539–3543.

60. Simons JW, Mikhak B, Chang JF et al. Induction of immunity to prostate cancer antigens: results of a clinical trial of vaccination with irradiated autologous prostate tumor cells engineered to secrete granulocyte-macrophage colon-stimulating factor using ex vivo gene transfer. Cancer Res 1999;59:5160–5168.

61. Ellem KA, O'Rourke MG, Johnson GR et al. A case report: immune responses and clinical course of the first human use of granulocyte/macrophage-colony-stimulating-factor-transduced autologous melanoma cells for immunotherapy. Cancer Immunol Immunother 1997;44:10–20.

62. Jaffee EM, Dranoff G, Cohen LK et al High efficiency gene transfer into primary human tumor explants without cell selection. Cancer Res 1993;53[suppl 10]:2221–2226.

63. Jolly D. Viral vector systems for gene therapy. Cancer Gene Ther 1994;1:51–64.

64. Qiao J, Chen SH, Pham-Nguyen KB, Woo SLC. Construction and characterization of a recombinant adenoviral vector expressing human interleukin-12. Cancer Gene Ther 1999;6:373–379.

65. Caruso M, Pham-Nguyen K, Kwon L et al. Adenovirus-mediated interleukin-12 gene therapy for metastatic colon carcinoma. Proc Natl Acad Sci USA 1996;93:11302–11306.

66. Chen SH, Chen XH, Wang Y et al. Combination gene therapy for liver metastasis of colon carcinoma in vivo. Proc Natl Acad Sci USA 1995;28:2577–2581.

67. Chen SH, Kosai K, Xu B et al. Combination suicide and cytokine gene therapy for hepatic metastases of colon carcinoma: sustained antitumor immunity prolongs animal survival. Cancer Res 1996;56:3758–3762.

68. Brunda MJ. Interleukin-12. J Leukoc Biol 1994;55:280–288.

69. Brunda MJ, Luistro L, Warrier RR et al. Antitumor and antimetastatic activity of interleukin-12 against murine tumors. J Exp Med 1993;178:1223–1230.

70. Gately MK, Desai BB, Wolitzky AG et al. Regulation of human lymphocyte proliferation by a heterodimeric cytokine, IL-12 (cytotoxic lymphocyte maturation factor). J Immunol 1991;147: 874–882.

71. Brunda MJ, Luistro L, Rumennik L et al. Interleukin-12: murine models of a potent antitumor agent. Ann NY Acad Sci 1996;765:266–274.

72. Atkins MA, Robertson MJ, DeCoste et al. Phase I evaluation of intravenous recombinant human interleukin-12 in patients with advanced malignancies. Clin Cancer Res 1997;3:409–417.

73. Leonard JP, Sherman ML, Fisher et al. Effects of single-dose interleukin-12 exposure on interleukin-12 associated toxicity and interferon-γ production. Blood 1997;90:2541–2548.

74. Colombo MP, Vaglinai M, Spreafico F et al. Amount of interleukin 12 available at the tumor site is critical for tumor regression. Cancer Res 1996;56:2531–2534.

75. Pham-Nguyen KB, Yang W, Saxena R et al. The role of NK and T cells in IL-12 induced antitumor response against hepatic colon carcinoma. Int J Cancer 1999;81:813–819.

76. Alderson MR, Smith CA, Trough TW et al. Molecular and biological characterization of human 4-1BB and its ligand. Eur J Immunol 1994;24:2219–2227.

77. Hurtaldo J, Kim SH, Pollock KE et al. Potential role of 4-1BB in T-cell activation. Comparison with the costimulatory molecule D28. J Immunol 1995;155:3360–3367.

78. Melero I, Shuford WW, Newby et al. Monoclonal antibodies against the 4-1BB T-cell activation molecule eradicate established tumors. Nat Med 1995;3:682–685.

79. Scheibogen C, Lee KH, Stevanovic et al. Analysis of the T cell response to tumor and viral peptide antigens by an IFN-gamma-ELISPOT assay. Int J Cancer 1997;71:932–936.

80. Schmittel A, Keilhotz U, Scheibenbogen C. Evaluation of the interferon-gamma ELISPOT-assay for quantification of peptide specific T lymphocytes from peripheral blood. J Immunol Methods 1997;210:167–174.

81. Zier K, Johnson K, Maddux JM et al. IFN-γ secretion following stimulation with total tumor peptides from autologous human tumors. J Immunol Methods 2000;241:61–68.

Chapter 4

Regional Cancer Gene Therapy: Principles and Progress in Replication-Competent Tumor-Selective Viruses

Sunil J. Advani

Ralph R. Weichselbaum

Gene therapy for somatic diseases and cancer has grown extensively in the last two decades. Each treatment paradigm operates under different requirements. Whereas successful somatic gene therapy requires survival of the transfected cell with long-term gene expression to correct a genetic defect, cancer gene therapy requires the destruction of tumor cells without long-term gene expression. Cancer gene therapy can be subdivided into two categories: delivery of exogenous genes and oncolysis (virus-mediated tumor cell lysis). The focus of this chapter is the recent progress of replication-competent viruses for cancer therapy. Especially exciting is the recent translation of basic science research in cancer biology and virology to create "tumor-specific" viruses currently under clinical investigation.

One of the most effective means to deliver foreign genes to cells is through the use of viral vectors. Viruses have evolved highly efficient methods to infect human cells, express their gene products, and produce progeny viruses. For gene therapy, viruses have been attenuated to remain effective delivery agents but not to cause disease. Viruses under current investigation for gene therapy are either replication-deficient or replication-competent. Replication-defective viruses can deliver a foreign gene to a cell but do not produce progeny viruses. However, replication-defective viruses also exemplify an important problem in cancer gene therapy: the inability to infect a large proportion of tumor cells. To overcome the problem of viral distribution, replication-competent viruses have been studied in the last decade as potential therapeutic agents for cancer. Replication-competent cancer therapy for the destruction of tumor cells has also been termed *viral oncolysis* or *virotherapy*.

The concept of viral lysis to treat tumors dates back more than a century.[1] A consequence of the replicative cycle of viruses is cell lysis and subsequent spread to and lysis of adjacent tumor cells. In theory, infection of a single cancer cell within a tumor sets up a self-sustaining chain reaction resulting in infection and cell death throughout the tumor. Important to the success of this treatment paradigm is the ability to create a virus that preferentially infects and lyses tumor cells. In the 1950s, wild-type viruses were selected for oncolysis by serial passage in tumor cells such that selective pressure would result in the evolution of tumor-specific viruses; however, this approach failed to generate tumor-selective viruses. In the last 20 years, the viral life cycle of many viruses has been dissected at the molecular biological level such that the genomes of viruses have been sequenced and an understanding of the functions of viral proteins has been obtained. Additionally, the process of malignant transformation has also begun to be unraveled. Thus, the last decade has seen a reemergence of the concept of viral oncolysis. It is now possible to genetically engineer specific genetic alternations into viral genomes to render them tumor-selective.

Two issues are of critical importance in oncolytic viral therapy: safety and efficacy. A proper balance must be achieved to create a clinically effective virus that remains safe. Large viral deletions result in safe viruses; however, such viruses also tend to have decreased efficacy as compared to less attenuated viruses. Safety considerations include an understanding of the disease caused by the wild-type virus and that the mutant, oncolytic virus causes no (or mild) disease. Antiviral drugs should be available to treat adverse outcomes of viral infection. Oncolytic viruses should also be genetically stable and nonintegrating into the host genome.

One important question in oncolytic therapy is how to genetically engineer viruses that infect, replicate in, and destroy tumor cells specifically (Fig. 4.1). In theory, this problem can be resolved at different phases of the virus life cycle, beginning with retargeting the virus to attach to tumor cell–specific receptors (see Fig. 4.1A). This method is more appropriate for creating viruses for systemic delivery to target metastases and is not addressed here. When the virus enters the cell, its lytic program can be controlled by the intracellular environment such that it replicates within rapidly dividing cells (i.e., tumor cells) or tumor cells that harbor certain mutations (see Figs. 4.1, B and C). Further specificity can be

FIGURE 4.1 (A) Tumor targeted viral binding-entry. (B) Deletion virus to target proliferating cells. (C) Attenuated virus to target tumor cell–specific mutations. (D) Transcriptionally targeted viral gene replication.

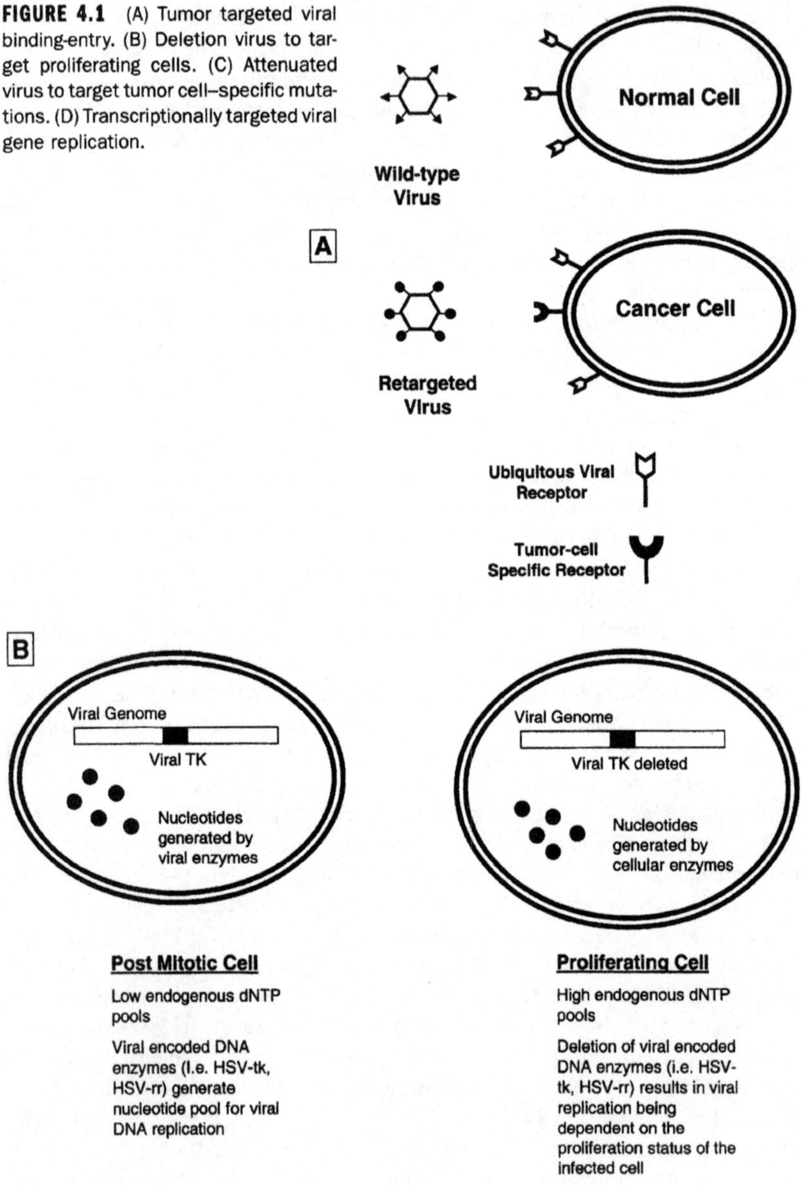

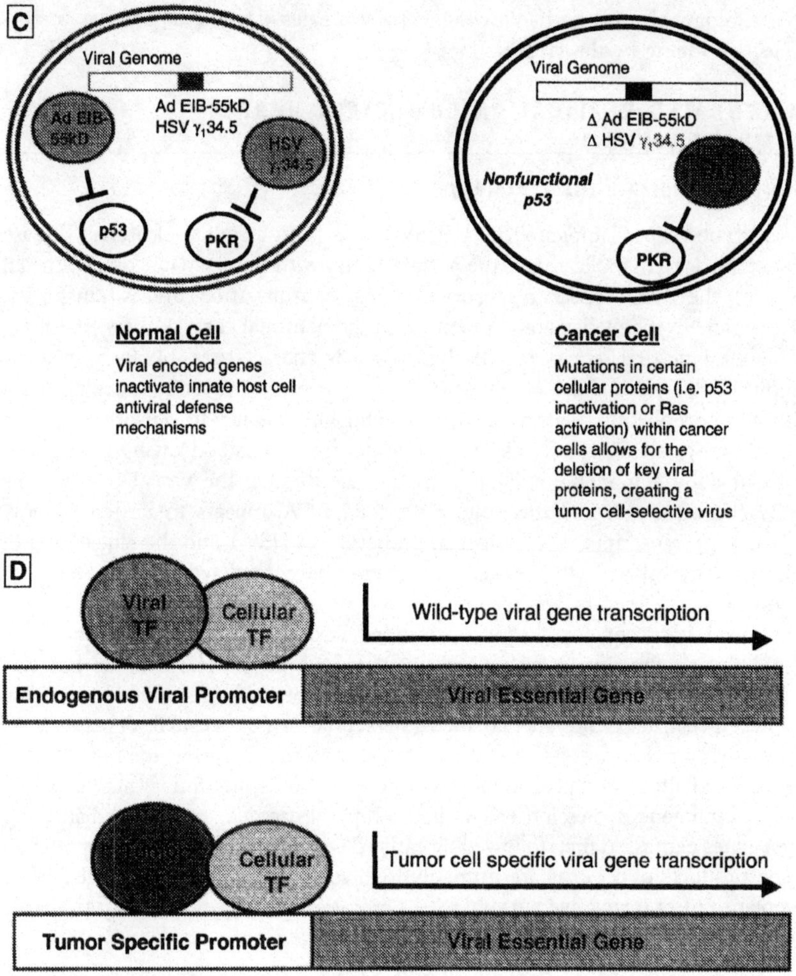

FIGURE 4.1 Continued

attained for specific histologic types of tumors by replacing essential viral gene promoters with tumor type–specific enhancer-promoter elements to control the transcription of viral essential genes (i.e., transcriptional targeting; see Fig. 4.1D). These issues, although complex, have begun to be resolved with the molecular understanding of both cancer and viruses. Replication-competent, attenuated herpesvirus and adenovirus and reovirus are being employed as such anti-tumor agents and have entered the clinical arena. This chapter discusses the development of each of these viruses as oncolytic agents, beginning with a brief summary of the biology of each and following with strategies devised to achieve tumor-selective killing by the viruses.

ATTENUATED REPLICATION-COMPETENT HERPES SIMPLEX VIRUS-1

Herpes Simplex Virus-1 Biology

Wild-type herpes simplex virus-1 (HSV-1) has been a source of human disease for centuries. On replicating at the portal of entry with cell lysis (mucosal epithelial tissue), the virus spreads to sensory neurons (neuroinvasion) and is transported retrograde to the nucleus of the neuron. In the neuronal ganglia, the virus enters either a lytic or latent state. The lytic cycle is characterized by entry into the replication cycle and release of viral progeny. The most drastic outcome results in fatal encephalitis (neurovirulence). Establishing latency in sensory ganglia is a hallmark of HSV-1, yet this process is poorly understood owing to the lack of cell culture models for latency. In the latent state, the viral DNA remains extrachromosomal, and the only transcribed RNA appears to be the latency-associated transcripts. The biological properties of HSV-1 and the elucidation of the function of key viral regulatory proteins have rendered HSV-1 a focus of study for gene therapy applications.

HSV-1 is an enveloped, double-stranded DNA virus with a viral genome of 152 kb encoding more than 84 distinct polypeptides.[2] The genome has two unique stretches—unique long (U_L) and unique short (U_S)—separated by terminal inverted repeats. Genes are classified as essential or nonessential, depending on their requirement for viral replication in cell culture. However, the nonessential genes in all likelihood play an important role in viral replication within its natural host. Viral gene expression occurs in a temporal cascade, with immediate early (α) genes expressed first, followed by early (β), and then late (γ) gene expression. The products of α genes are primarily involved in transcriptional regulation. β gene products are involved in viral DNA replication, and γ gene products primarily encode structural proteins.

Cancer gene therapy with HSV-1 employs attenuated, genetically engineered, replication-competent viruses. Replication-competent viruses have deletions in nonessential genes that attenuate the virus such that replication is dependent on a favorable environment within tumor cells as compared to normal cells.

Targeting Proliferating Cells

Wild-type HSV-1 is able to infect proliferating and quiescent cells efficiently. One method to create tumor-selective, replication-competent HSV-1 is to engineer viral mutations that can be complemented by proteins expressed by proliferating cells. Many viral genes encode proteins that have functional cellular homologs and therefore could be complemented by the tumor cell in trans. The development of attenuated HSV-1 as an antiglioma agent provides a case study for this type of approach. Gliomas grow in an environment surrounded by quiescent neurons. To generate HSV-1 selectivity for gliomas, differences within the intracellular milieu of dividing glioma cells as compared to quiescent neurons has been exploited. HSV-1 encodes multiple genes involved in viral DNA replication and nucleotide production, including viral thymidine kinase (HSV-tk, U_L23) and the large subunit of ribonucleotide reductase (RR), U_L39.[2] Such genes are necessary for wild-type virus to replicate efficiently in cells where deoxynucleotide pools are low (i.e., quiescent neurons). However, proliferating tumor cells contain large pools of deoxynucleotides that the virus can scavenge to replicate its DNA. Deletion of viral genes involved in DNA synthesis has provided a rationale basis to create genetically engineered HSV-1 as an anticancer agent.

On the basis of this reasoning, the HSV-1 viral mutant *dl*sptk containing a deletion in the gene encoding thymidine kinase was shown to have efficacy against experimental gliomas.[3] The striking drawback of deleting viral thymidine kinase is the inability to treat patients with acyclovir if viral replication becomes detrimental. To retain HSV–thymidine kinase but still target proliferating cells, the HSV-1 viral mutant hrR3 containing the *Escherichia coli* lacZ gene inserted within the gene encoding the large subunit of RR was created and used for experimental glioma animal models.[4] The lacZ insertion inactivates expression of the large subunit of RR. This virus has the advantages of being 10-fold more sensitive to ganciclovir along with expression of the lacZ gene to detect the mutant virus within histologic sections. In a similar approach, an HSV-1 deleted of the U_L2 gene encoding uracil DNA glycosylase was shown to have efficacy against tumor xenografts and to have ganciclovir hypersensitivity.[5] These initial studies have spawned much interest in the use of replication-conditional HSV-1 as antiglioma agents and more broadly as anti-tumor agents for a variety of tumors. The pitfall of this approach is that certain normal tissues have high mitotic indices, and such attenuated viruses may not discriminate between rapidly proliferating normal and cancer cells.

Creating a Nonneurovirulent Replication-Competent HSV-1

As replication-competent HSV-1 was beginning to be exploited for cancer therapy, an HSV-1 gene involved in neurovirulence—γ134.5—was uncovered. Deletion of both copies of the γ134.5 gene (virus R3616), present in the repeat regions, reduced HSV-1 neurovirulence by more than five orders of magnitude on direct intracranial inoculation in mice.[6] At least one function has been delineated for the $\gamma_1 34.5$ gene product (ICP34.5). An innate host cell defense mechanism to viral infections is activation of double-stranded RNA-dependent protein kinase (PKR), which phosphorylates the alpha subunit of translation initiation factor 1 (eIF-2α; Fig. 4.2). Phosphorylated eIF-2α blocks the translation of mRNA. HSV-1 has evolved a mechanism to deal with PKR activation. ICP34.5 binds to cellular protein phosphatase-1, dephosphorylates eIF-2α, and prevents host protein syn-

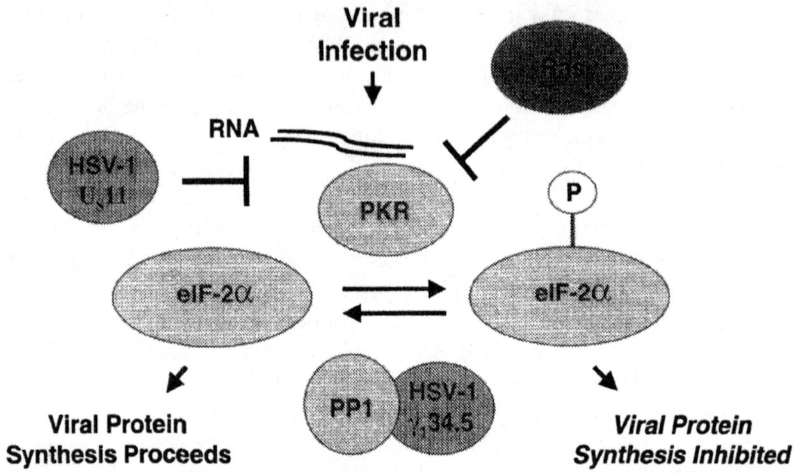

FIGURE 4.2 Cellular RNA-dependent protein kinase antiviral defense mechanism blocks viral protein synthesis. Herpes simples virus–1–encoded $\gamma_1 34.5$ and U_S11 or tumor cell–activated *ras* reverse RNA-dependent protein kinase inhibition and allow viral protein synthesis to proceed.

thesis shutoff.[7,8] Because R3616 is severely attenuated for neurovirulence, R3616 fulfills the safety issue of oncolytic viruses. R3616 is effective in glioma cell killing and glioma xenograft regression in experimental tumor models.[9,10] Although infection with R3616 should result in cessation of viral protein synthesis due to PKR activation, R3616 is able to replicate in certain tumor cells. A resolution to this paradox may involve the Ras signaling pathway in tumor cells as compared to normal cells.[11] The Ras signaling pathway is commonly activated in tumors (see *Oncolytic Reovirus: Targeting Cells with Active ras*, p. 74). R3616 infection of cells with activated Ras results in the synthesis of viral proteins and production of progeny viruses.

Certain cautions should be noted in the use of $\gamma_1 34.5$-deleted HSV-1 for cancer therapy. Viruses deleted for $\gamma_1 34.5$ replicate poorly and are not genetically stable on serial passage in cell culture. In this virus, second-site mutations that have been isolated overcome protein synthesis shutoff characteristic of $\gamma_1 34.5$ viral mutants.[12] One compensatory second-site mutation in HSV-1 lacking $\gamma_1 34.5$ was mapped to the U_S11-12 region.[13] The U_S11 gene is normally expressed as a late gene with γ_2 kinetics, and the U_S11 protein is known to bind RNA, whereas the U_S12 gene (ICP47) is expressed with immediate early (α) kinetics.[2] Viral mutants that link the U_S11 gene with the U_S12 promoter express U_S11 with immediate early kinetics rather than with γ_2 kinetics. U_S11 expressed with α kinetics can compensate for the deletions in $\gamma_1 34.5$, in that eIF-2α is not phosphorylated and protein translation does not cease.[14,15]

Two phenotypes are associated with $\gamma_1 34.5$-deleted HSV-1: eIF-2α phosphorylation and decreased neurovirulence. If these phenotypes are the result of distinct functions of $\gamma_1 34.5$, it may be possible to prevent eIF-2α phosphorylation by expressing $U_S 11$ with α kinetics in a $\gamma_1 34.5$-null virus and yet still retain decreased neurovirulence. This mutant virus would be expected to replicate more efficiently (as protein translation is not blocked) and result in enhanced tumor regression. Recent data support this hypothesis. Viruses with deletions in $\gamma_1 34.5$ but expressing $U_S 11$ with α kinetics replicated close to wild-type levels in tumor cell lines that fail to support appreciable growth of $\gamma_1 34.5$-null virus.[16,17] These genetically engineered viruses are still as nonneurovirulent in mice as the $\gamma_1 34.5$-null parental virus and may serve as more effective oncolytic agents.

Transcriptionally Targeting HSV-1 Replication

Differences in gene expression exist between organs and between tumor and normal cells of the same organ. Identifying specific cellular proteins that are transcriptionally up-regulated in certain cell types allows for the creation of engineered viruses containing cellular promoter-enhancer elements upstream of essential viral genes, thereby restricting expression of the viral essential gene to tumors that express the necessary transcription factors. Infection of cells not expressing the necessary transcription factors would block expression of the viral essential gene, resulting in an abortive infection. Important is the identification of cellular genes that are up-regulated at the transcriptional level in tumor cells but not in surrounding normal tissue. The transcriptional targeting approach has been demonstrated with HSV-1. The α4 gene is essential in cell culture and is expressed with immediate early kinetics.[2] Infected cell protein number 4 (ICP4), the product of the α4 gene, is a major viral regulatory protein and transactivator. The HSV-1 viral mutant d120 contains deletions in both copies of ICP4 but results in apoptosis on infection of cells (i.e., nonproductive infection).[18,19] The first transcriptionally targeted HSV-1, virus G92A, was created by placing the α4 gene under the transcriptional control of the albumin enhancer-promoter elements to restrict viral replication to albumin-expressing cells.[20] Although wild-type HSV-1 replicated efficiently in cells irrespective of albumin expression, virus G92A replicated more efficiently in albumin-expressing cell lines as compared to non-albumin-expressing cell lines. However, G92A replicated more slowly than did wild-type HSV-1, which is the result of delayed accumulation of ICP4 in G92A-infected cells as compared to wild-type infected cells. This result is expected because viral immediate-early promoters have evolved to become transcriptionally active rapidly on infection of cells. The therapeutic potential of G92A was shown in its ability selectively to inhibit tumor xenograft growth of albumin-expressing cells (i.e., hepatomas), compared to non-albumin-expressing tumor xenografts.[21] The problem with the albumin promoter-enhancer element is that it is transcriptionally expressed in the normal adult liver, indicating that normal liver cells may support the replication of G92A by expression of ICP4 off the albumin enhancer-promoter elements and may lyse normal liver cells. To target specific tumors, the human calponin promoter was placed upstream of the $\alpha 4$ gene.[22] Calponin mRNA and protein are aberrantly expressed in human soft tissue and bone tumors, and these tumor histologies could support the replication of such a virus, resulting in tumor type–specific oncolysis.

By using the aforementioned technique, tumor type–specific HSV-1 viruses could be tailored for individual tumor histologies. DNA microarray technology will further aid in identifying novel genes transcribed specifically within tumor cells. This approach has also been employed to create transcription-targeted adenoviruses (see *Attenuated Replication-Competent Adenovirus: Transcriptionally Targeted Adenovirus*, p. 70). However, such a strategy requires multiple viruses to be created, driven by different tumor-specific promoters. Also, tumors consist of a heterogeneous population of cells, and specific promoter elements may not be active in all cancer cells within a tumor. Finally, leaky enhancer-promoter elements may allow replication in nontargeted cells, and cellular promoter-enhancer elements in the context of the viral genome may not behave as they do in the human genome.

Replication-Competent HSV-1 in Clinical Trials

After intensive preclinical studies of the efficacy and safety of replication-competent HSV-1 as an anti-tumor agent, these viruses have entered clinical trials. At least three clinical trials are underway using replication-competent genetically engineered HSV-1 as anti-tumor agents. These attenuated HSV-1 viruses are 1716, G207, and NV1020.

1716 and G207 Glioblastoma multiforme (GBM) is the most aggressive form of primary brain tumor. Certain characteristics of this tumor render it an ideal candidate for novel therapy. The median survival from diagnosis is 1 year. Treatment failure is local in that 90% of patients have tumor recurrence within 2 cm of the initial lesion, and metastases are rare. Given the rapid mortality and local therapy failure, direct intratumoral inoculation with genetically engineered HSV-1 has been tested in patients with recurrent glioma. As mentioned, R3616 deleted in both copies of $\gamma_1 34.5$ is significantly neuroattenuated and mediates tumor xenograft regression.[6,9,10] The genetically engineered HSV-1 1716 is also deleted of both copies of $\gamma_1 34.5$.[23,24] A phase I clinical trial has been completed in Glasgow assessing the safety of 1716 on intratumoral inoculation in nine patients with recurrent GBM.[25] Dose escalation from 10^3 to 10^5 plaque-forming units (pfu) was delivered by stereotactic intratumoral injection. No evidence of encephalitis, HSV-1 reactivation, or adverse clinical outcomes was seen in this clinical trial. Tissue samples after viral inoculation were available from three of the patients who underwent subsequent tumor resection, with the earliest time being 3.5 weeks after inoculation. However, immunohistochemistry or polymerase chain reaction analyses of the tissues did not reveal the presence of 1716.

The malignant glioma phase I clinical trial in the United States used the genetically engineered HSV-1 G207.[26] G207 is deleted for $\gamma_1$34.5 and has a lacZ insertion in the U_L39 gene that inactivates the large subunit of RR (ICP6). The $\gamma_1$34.5 deletion renders the virus nonneurovirulent (identical to 1716), and inactivation of ICP6 targets the virus to replicate in proliferating cells. For safety reasons, it may be beneficial to create attenuated viruses with several different genes mutated to reduce the probability of second-site mutations or recombination that can restore functions of deleted genes. G207 has been extensively studied as having oncolytic activity against a variety of tumor histologies, and its safety was characterized in *Aotus nancymae* primates by intracerebral inoculation at doses up to 10^9 pfu.[26–29] Twenty-one patients with malignant glioma were enrolled in a dose-escalating study with G207, 10^6 pfu to 3×10^9 pfu.[30] As with the Glasgow trial, no patient developed HSV encephalitis or adverse toxicity directly ascribed to G207 after intratumoral inoculation of G207, even at the highest dose. Tissue samples available from two patients were positive for HSV-1 and lacZ by polymerase chain reaction, indicating the presence of G207.

Both these clinical trials established the safety of stereotactic intracranial inoculation of attenuated, replication-competent HSV-1 for malignant glioma. This is an important accomplishment because of the safety concerns associated with replication-competent HSV-1. Both trials used a $\gamma_1$34.5-null virus, with the difference in the viruses being whether ICP6—a large subunit of RR—was functional (1716) or inactivated (G207). Each viral mutant has advantages and disadvantages that have to be considered in terms of anti-tumor efficacy and patient safety. Although deletion of $\gamma_1$34.5 creates a highly attenuated virus in terms of neurovirulence, it was later recognized that such viruses can evolve second-site mutations to overcome the protein synthesis shutoff phenotype. As the molecular basis for attenuated neurovirulence of $\gamma_1$34.5-deleted HSV-1 is unresolved, certain safety features should be engineered into the virus. Deletion of ICP6 in G207 creates a multimutated HSV-1 with the benefit of being hypersensitive to ganciclovir.

HSV-1 deleted in $\gamma_1$34.5 does not replicate very efficiently in experimental tumor models as compared to wild-type HSV-1. Inactivation of ICP6 further impedes viral replication. As tumor volume is the net effect of tumor cell division and death, effective clinical responses require a virus the replication of which outstrips tumor growth. Deletion of ICP6 creates a replication-conditional virus that preferentially replicates in proliferating cells. G207 may effectively replicate in the fraction of cancer cells within a tumor that are actively dividing. However, a significant proportion of cells within a tumor may not divide at such a rate to complement the virus in trans with nucleotide precursors, leading to abortive infection. The multimutated genotype of G207 is one reason 1716 was dose-escalated to 1×10^5 pfu as compared to 3×10^9 pfu for G207. It appears that toxicity-limiting doses of 1716 or G207 were not attained in either clinical trial, implying that higher viral inocula could be tolerated. Although higher titers of 1716 may be given in follow-up trials, it is unlikely that clinical-grade viral stocks will allow for delivery of more that 3×10^9 pfu in future clinical trials with G207. Owing to the location of these tumors, it is also difficult to assess whether viral replication occurred within the tumor. It is hoped that demonstration of tumor-specific viral replication and clinical efficacy will be resolved in future clinical trials.

NV1020 NV1020 is also known as R7020. Genetically engineered HSV-1 R7020 is an intertypic virus, initially constructed for immunization against both HSV-1 and HSV-2.[31] It contains deletions of the internal inverted repeat as well as the U_L24 promoter, U_L55, and U_L56. In place of this deletion were inserted genes encoding HSV-2 glycoproteins G, J, D, and I. R7020 has been studied for genetic stability and safety in rodents and primates.[31,32] Due to the fact that viral vaccines are created with an overriding regard for patient safety, this virus appears to satisfy the safety criteria for a potential oncolytic agent. Although this virus retains one copy of the $\gamma_1 34.5$ gene, it is attenuated for neuroinvasiveness and has been studied as an oncolytic virus for non–central nervous system tumors. R7020 grew to higher titers in tumor xenografts than did R3616.[33] In experimental tumor models, intratumoral and intrahepatic artery inoculation of R7020 (NV1020) results in tumor regression for head and neck squamous cell carcinoma, prostate adenocarcinoma, pancreatic carcinoma, and metastatic hepatic cancer.[34–36] A key feature of R7020 is its attenuation for neuroinvasion. Whereas wild-type HSV-1 injection of flank grown tumors resulted in tumor regression but also mouse death, R7020 injection resulted in tumor regression without mouse death.[34] NV1020 is multimutated and nonneuroinvasive and replicates more robustly than does R3616 or G207, therefore providing a second genetically engineered HSV-1 anti-tumor agent for tumors located outside the central nervous system. NV1020 has entered phase I clinical trials for liver metastases from colon adenocarcinoma (*www.clinicaltrials.gov*).

Multimodality Therapy with HSV-1

Complete tumor regression with attenuated replication-competent viruses is rarely seen in experimental tumor xenograft models when intratumoral viral inoculation is given after the establishment of relatively large tumor xenografts. Combining other treatment modalities offers a way to increase the therapeutic efficacy of oncolytic viruses. Therapeutic genes can be inserted into the viral genome, or conventional cancer therapies (i.e., chemotherapy or radiotherapy) can be combined with viral therapy. The interplay of different therapies in addition to attacking cancer cells by differing methods of cell kill may translate into clinically meaningful tumor responses. However, such approaches may seem counterintuitive in that additional cytotoxic agents may interfere with viral replication, thereby limiting the efficacy of replication-competent viruses. In combining treatment modalities, it is critical to determine the impact of the additional therapy on the ability of the virus to replicate within the tumor.

Foreign Gene Insertion Within HSV-1

Immune Modulation Cancer immunotherapy remains under active clinical investigation. Identification of tumor-associated antigens has not translated into significantly beneficial clinical therapies. To overcome dose-limiting toxicities associated with systemic administration of immunomodulatory cytokines, viral vectors are employed. Replication-competent viruses encoding cytokines offer potential advantages in that viral replication, local overexpression of cytokines, and tumor cell debris after viral lysis may combine to result in a potent antitumor immune response. Interleukin-4 has been inserted into $\gamma_1$34.5-deleted HSV-1.[37] Infection of cells with an interleukin-4-encoding virus resulted in a 1,300-fold increase in interleukin-4 production. Intracranial inoculation of this virus in a syngeneic murine glioma model resulted in increased accumulation of macrophages, CD8+, and CD4+ T cells along with enhanced mouse survival. Interleukin-12 has also been inserted into $\gamma_1$34.5-deleted HSV-1 virus, virus M002.[38] In a murine syngeneic model for neuroblastoma, intratumoral inoculation of M002 prolonged survival with abundant immune cell infiltration as compared to the parental $\gamma_1$34.5-deleted HSV-1.

Many viruses encode proteins that allow the virus to evade the immune system. ICP47, the product of the U_S12 gene, is known to block major histocompatibility complex class I expression of antigenic peptides.[39] ICP47 binds to the transporter associated with antigen processing and inhibits loading of major histocompatibility complex class I molecules with antigen. In strategies employing replication-competent HSV-1 with immunomodulatory cytokines, deletion of the U_S12 gene may prove advantageous. An additional benefit of a virus deleted for U_S12 gene is decreased neurovirulence.[40] U_S12 has been deleted from two viruses in clinical trials, G207 and NV1020.[17,41] As mentioned, deletion of the U_S12 gene and placement of the U_S12 α kinetic promoter in juxtaposition with the U_S11 gene precludes phosphorylation of eIF-2α associated with $\gamma_1$34.5-deleted virus (G207). An additional advantage of U_S12 deletion is that major histocompatibility complex class I surface expression is not blocked in infected cells.[17] A parallel approach has also been undertaken with NV1020. The viruses NV1034 and NV1042 do not produce ICP47, owing to the insertion of the *E. coli* lacZ gene within the U_S12 gene, and encode either granulocyte macrophage colony stimulating factor or interleukin-12, respectively.[41] In studies using a syngeneic murine squamous cell carcinoma model, preestablished tumors injected with NV1042 had enhanced regression as compared to the parental virus that does not encode interleukin-12.

Prodrug-Converting Enzymes The prodrug-converting enzyme treatment paradigm involves viral delivery of a gene encoding a prodrug-converting enzyme to tumor cells, followed by systemic administration of a relatively nontoxic prodrug that is converted to toxic metabolites in cells expressing the prodrug-converting enzyme. This approach has also been termed *suicide gene therapy.* Certain prodrugs are converted to soluble toxic metabolites that can diffuse out of the cell that encodes the prodrug-converting enzyme and be taken up by uninfected surrounding cells (bystander effect). The bystander effect greatly enhances the therapeutic potential of this strategy.

HSV-1 thymidine kinase (HSV-1 tk) has often been used as a prodrug-converting enzyme with the prodrugs acyclovir and ganciclovir. HSV-1 tk delivered to tumor cells by multiple transfection methods effectively destroys tumor cells. All current replication-competent HSV-1 viruses being studied encode HSV-1 tk; however, acyclovir or ganciclovir administration to HSV-1-infected cells inhibits viral replication. Two additional prodrug-converting enzymes—cytochrome P-450 2B1 and cytosine deaminase—have been inserted in replication-competent HSV-1 to improve tumor cell kill while not impairing the ability of the virus to replicate.[42,43]

Cytochrome P-450 2B1 converts the prodrugs cyclophosphamide and ifosfamide to the toxic metabolites phosphoramide mustard (a DNA alkylator) and acrolein (a protein alkylator). The replication-competent HSV-1 rRp450 was constructed by insertion of the rat cytochrome P450 2B1 gene into the U_L39 gene locus, resulting in loss of expression of the viral large subunit of RR (ICP6).[42] Cytosine deaminase (CD) is not expressed in mammalian cells and deaminates cytosine to uracil. CD can, therefore, convert nontoxic 5-fluorcytosine (5-FC) to 5-fluorouracil (5-FU). 5-FU is metabolized to deoxynucleotide monophosphate and poisons thymidylate synthetase. 5-FU triphosphate, produced from phosphorylation of 5-FU, also is incorporated into RNA and disrupts mRNA and rRNA function. Though 5-FU is an effective cytotoxic agent, the therapeutic index of this drug could be enhanced by confining 5-FU production to the tumor bed through the CD/5-FC combination. 5-FU is also freely diffusible such that surrounding non-CD-transduced cells can be exposed to 5-FU. The replication-competent HSV-1 HSV1yCD was created by insertion of the yeast CD gene into the U_L39 gene, thereby inactivating ICP6.[43] By virtue of the inactivation of ICP6 in rRp450 and HSV1yCD, both viruses replicate preferentially in tumor cells as compared to normal cells.[4] Treatment with either of these prodrug-converting enzymes containing viruses enhanced tumor cell cytotoxicity and tumor xenograft regression on administration of the prodrug.[42–44] Importantly, the toxic metabolites of cyclophosphamide or 5-FC did not impair the ability of the virus to replicate, whereas treatment with ganciclovir drastically reduced viral replication.[43,44]

Replication-Competent HSV-1 in Combination with Conventional Cancer Therapies

The application of replication-competent genetically engineered HSV-1 in combination with either radiotherapy or chemotherapy may provide a simple means of enhancing the anti-tumor efficacy of oncolytic viruses. Given that radiotherapy is routinely employed for GBM and in more than 50% of all cancer patients and given its ability to be specifically targeted to the tumor bed, it may prove to be a useful adjuvant to intratumoral HSV-1 inoculation. The combination of ionizing radiation with either R3616 or R7020 has been shown to result in enhanced tumor regression and survival in experimental tumor models for gliomas, squamous cell epithelial carcinomas, and prostate adenocarcinoma.[33,34,45] Studies indicate that ionizing radiation enhanced viral replication and distribution within experimental glioma xenografts.[33,45]

Chemotherapeutic agents have also been combined with replication-competent HSV-1. The chemotherapeutic agent cisplatin was used in combination with G207 for human squamous cell carcinomas.[46] Cisplatin did not adversely affect viral growth and, in certain tumor cell xenografts, cisplatin combined with G207 resulted in supra-additive effects on xenograft regression. Mitomycin C in combination with 1716 for non-small-cell lung cancer xenografts had additive effects.[47] Fluorodeoxyuridine has been shown to enhance replication and cytotoxicity of G207 in colorectal adenocarcinoma cell lines.[48] Fluorodeoxyuridine appears to aid G207 replication by targeting the activity of cellular RR. G207 is deleted for $\gamma_1 34.5$ and lacks functional ICP6 (a large subunit of RR). A potential benefit of fluorodeoxyuridine for G207 replication is inactivation of cellular thymidylate synthetase, causing depletion of dTTP and an imbalance of intracellular deoxynucleotide pools and up-regulation of cellular RR activity. Enhanced cellular RR activity may complement inactive viral RR of G207. Though mode of action of enhanced tumor cell eradication in combination with replication-competent HSV-1 is speculative, radiotherapy and chemotherapy could increase the therapeutic ratio of oncolytic HSV-1 and translate into clinically significant tumor regression.

ATTENUATED REPLICATION-COMPETENT ADENOVIRUS

Adenovirus Biology

Wild-type adenoviruses tend to infect epithelial cells and are usually associated with mild human disease, such as respiratory infection. Approximately 50 serotypes of adenovirus have been identified and are classified into six groups, A to F. Adenoviruses gained attention in the cancer field for the ability of adenovirus serotype 12 (group A) to induce tumors in rodents. For gene therapy, group C adenoviruses have been the most extensively studied (serotypes 1, 2, 5, and 6), and these are not oncogenic in rodent models.

Adenoviruses are nonenveloped, double-stranded DNA viruses with a genome of approximately 36 kb. The linear genome is flanked on the ends by inverted terminal repeats of 100–150 bases, which facilitate circulation of the genome during viral replication. As with HSV-1, adenoviral gene transcription occurs in a temporal cascade. Early (E) gene expression occurs in the absence of viral DNA replication, and transcription of late (L) genes commences with the onset of viral DNA replication. The regions of the genome that transcribe early genes are designated E1A, E1B, E2A, E2B, E3, E4, and L1. In general, early gene products encode for regulatory proteins to facilitate viral replication, and late gene products encode for structural proteins of the virion. Of particular interest in the development of replication-selective adenoviruses for cancer gene therapy are the proteins encoded by the E1A and E1B regions of the viral genome. Polypeptides of the E1A and E1B region are the first to be made and affect the cell cycle and cellular apoptotic pathways to create a conducive environment for viral replication.

After replication, the viral genome is packaged in an icosahedron capsid (20 surfaces with 12 vertices). Fiber projections extend from each vertex and end in a knob. The cellular receptor identified for adenoviruses is the coxsackie-adenovirus receptor. Recent modifications within the fiber-knob of adenovirus have resulted in the ability to retarget the virus, which may hold potential for creating a virus that can be systemically injected and seek out tumor cell–specific receptors. As with HSV-1, elucidation of the functions of adenoviral proteins has resulted in the creation of genetically engineered adenoviruses to replicate selectively within certain tumor cell environments.

Targeting Tumor Cells with Mutations in the p53 Pathway

One function of the adenoviral E1B-55K protein is inactivating cellular p53. This function is thought to be important in adenoviral infection, as transfection of the E1A gene into cells can result in p53-dependent apoptosis. Because p53 is commonly mutated in tumor cells, the E1B-55K protein may not be necessary for adenoviral infection of such tumor cells. A virus deleted in the E1B-55K protein would be predicted to replicate efficiently in tumor cells with an inactive p53 pathway; however, this mutant virus could not replicate in cells harboring a functional p53 pathway.

The adenovirus mutant dl1520 (Onyx-015) was constructed on this basis. Initial studies showed a correlation between cellular p53 status and dl1520 viral replication.[49] Tumor cells with nonfunctional p53 supported dl1520 replication and underwent tumor xenograft regression on intratumoral dl1520 injection; in contrast, tumor cells and xenografts with functional p53 were relatively resistant to dl1520 infection. Conflicting studies by other groups have failed to confirm the correlation between p53 status and the ability of dl1520 to replicate.[50–52] The role of p53 in adenovirus infection is further confounded by recent results suggesting that wild-type adenovirus can replicate efficiently even in the presence of an active, nondegradable form of p53.[53]

A further understanding of the relationship between E1B-55K-deleted adenovirus and the p53 pathway of tumor cells has implicated $p14^{ARF}$. The $p14^{ARF}$ protein is a member of the INK4 proteins and is a negative regulator of MDM2. MDM2 binds p53 and mediates its degradation. Loss of $p14^{ARF}$ in tumor cells results in the unopposed action of MDM2, rendering p53 functionally inactive. In tumor cells that do not have functional p14^{ARF}, MDM2 could complement for E1B-55K deletion. Therefore, dl1520 should be able to replicate in tumor cells with functional p53 if the tumor cells have nonfunctional p14^{ARF}. Studies appear to support this hypothesis. In colon carcinoma and mesothelioma, dl1520 was shown to replicate cell lines that have loss of p14^{ARF}.[54,55] These series of studies on the E1B-55K-deleted adenovirus for cancer therapy highlight an important lesson. Our current understanding of viral-host cell interactions is incomplete. Further basic science knowledge of how viral and cellular proteins interact with each other is needed. The other issue centers on the multifunctionality of viral proteins. Deletion of the entire E1B-55K, although intended to target the p53 pathway, may also have unexpected consequences. For example, the E1B-55K also modulates the transport of mRNA during viral infection.[56] Point mutations within viral proteins may result in the ability to knock out specific functions while sparing other functions of the protein.

Targeting the G_1-S Checkpoint

The adenoviral E1A protein has at least two functions: S-phase induction and transactivation of the remaining viral early genes. E1A is able to induce S phase in cells by binding to the retinoblastoma (Rb) family of proteins and releasing the inhibition on E2F proteins.[57] Amino acids 121–127 of the E1A protein are required for binding to Rb. The ability of adenovirus E1A to bind and inactivate Rb allows the virus to replicate in both quiescent and cycling cells by overcoming the G_1-S checkpoint. Deletion of the E1A amino acids responsible for Rb binding prevents S-phase induction in quiescent cells and blocks viral replication. Therefore, such a mutant virus preferentially replicates in proliferating cells, and it may replicate more efficiently in tumor cells, routinely containing mutations in the G_1-S checkpoint. Two groups have independently created such E1A mutant viruses.[58,59]

The Delta24 adenovirus has a 24-bp deletion in the region of E1A responsible for Rb binding. Importantly, the E1A protein produced by Delta24 did not associate with Rb, and intratumoral injections into glioma xenografts experienced significant tumor regression.[58] The other E1A adenoviral mutant is dl922-947.[59] Infection of nonproliferating normal cells by dl922-947 failed to induce S phase and had delayed and reduced viral protein expression as compared to wild-type adenovirus. However, in a variety of tumor cells, dl922-947 grew as efficiently as did wild-type adenovirus and was effective in tumor xenografts on intratumoral injection. A significant advantage of the dl922-947 virus is that it is a more potent oncolytic virus than is dl1520 (E1B-55K-deleted). This is an expected result given the nature of the deletions created in each virus. Although dl1520 is deleted of the entire E1B-55K protein (with loss of functions unrelated to p53 inactivation), dl922-947 is deleted in only a small portion of E1A (the Rb-binding region).

The dl922-947 mutant virus produces the remainder of the E1A protein such that the virus can use the protein for its other known (i.e., p300 binding and adenoviral early gene transactivation) and unknown functions.

Enhancing the Lytic Capacity of the Virus

To achieve meaningful tumor responses with oncolytic viruses, viral replication must outstrip tumor cell growth. One method is to create viruses that lyse tumor cell more rapidly. Quicker cell lysis and spread of the virus would also enable it to operate more efficiently before a host immune response is activated to destroy the virus. One strategy to enhance the tumor cell kill efficacy of replication-competent adenoviruses is by manipulating viral genes implicated in cell survival. Viral genes promoting cell death can be overexpressed, whereas genes that are cytoprotective can be deleted. Of course, altered expression of these viral genes should not be detrimental to adenoviral replication. At least two adenoviral gene products fit into this category: E1B-19K and the adenoviral death protein (ADP).

The ADP is a nuclear membrane glycoprotein required for efficient cell lysis and release of viral progeny. ADP normally accumulates late in the infectious life cycle.[60] The adenoviral mutant KD1 expressed higher levels of ADP earlier in infection than did wild-type adenovirus.[61] To achieve tumor cell selectivity, KD1 also has two mutations in the E1 region, precluding binding to Rb and p300 and resulting in targeting the virus to replicate in proliferating tumor cells (see the section Targeting Tumor Cells with Mutations in the p53 Pathway). The key phenotype is the ability to lyse tumor cells and spread more rapidly than wild-type virus to adjacent cells.

The EIB-19K gene product, conversely, is an inhibitor of apoptotic pathways. The adenoviral mutant Ad 337 is deleted of the E1b-19K gene.[62] This virus is reported to kill tumor cells more efficiently. This phenotype may be due to more rapid release of progeny viruses from the infected cell with quicker spread to neighboring tumor cells. In cell culture, deletion of the antiapoptotic gene does not appear detrimental to viral replication. In tumor xenografts, Ad337 mediated enhanced tumor xenograft regression as compared to the parental adenovirus.[63]

Transcriptionally Targeted Adenovirus

The concept of creating viruses having essential genes linked to cellular promoters to restrict viral replication was discussed earlier for HSV-1. Similar strategies have been employed for adenovirus. The E1a and E1b promoter regions of adenovirus have been placed under the control of tumor- and tissue-specific promoters. Again, the cellular promoter-enhancer selected to regulate viral essential gene transcription must be transcriptionally up-regulated in the targeted tumors to which viral replication is to be restricted. In other tissues, failure to transcribe the viral essential gene will lead to nonproductive infection.

One such adenoviruses created was CN706.[64] In this adenovirus mutant, E1A gene expression is driven from the prostate-specific antigen (PSA) promoter-enhancer elements. Cn706 replicated selectively in PSA expressing prostate cancer lines (LNCaP) but not in prostate cancer cells that do not express PSA (DU145). In tumor xenograft models, CN706 mediated LNCaP xenograft regression after intratumoral inoculation. Other tumor-specific promoters linked to the E1a gene include α-fetoprotein for hepatocellular carcinomas; DF3/MUC1 for MUC1-positive breast cancer cells; estrogen response elements for estrogen receptor–positive tumors; and bone matrix protein osteocalcin for prostate cancer and bone stroma.[65–68]

Two other viruses that have been created regulate transcription of both the E1a and E1b genes from tumor-specific promoter elements. CV787 has prostate-specific response elements in front of E1a and E1b, and CV890 has E1a and E1b gene expression under the control of the α-fetoprotein transcriptional response elements.[69,70] Restricting transcription of two viral essential gene open reading frames may provide further tumor cell selectivity. An extension of this strategy combined gene mutations in the E1A protein with transcriptional targeting. The KD1 adenovirus mutant already described has mutations in E1a, preventing binding to Rb or p300, and it also overexpressed the adenoviral death protein. The E1a mutations render KD1 selective for proliferating cells, and tissue cell specificity was achieved by introducing the surfactant protein B promoter to transcribe the E4 region, virus KD1-SPB.[71] The virus is proposed to replicate selectively in alveolar and bronchial cancer cells that can bypass the G_1-S checkpoint (E1a mutation) and have surfactant B promoter transactivation (for E4 transcription).

Replication-Competent Adenovirus in Combination with Conventional Cancer Therapies

The use of replication-restrictive adenovirus in combination with standard cancer therapies has also been investigated. (The concepts of this treatment paradigm were introduced in the section *Attenuated Replication-Competent Herpes Simplex Virus-1.*) All the chemotherapeutic agents (cisplatin, 5-FU, and paclitaxel) have been shown to enhance tumor cell killing in combination with dl1520 (ONYX-015) both in cell culture and in tumor xenograft models.[72,73] Transcriptional targeted adenoviral mutants CV787 (PSA-specific) and CV890 (α-fetoprotein-specific) also have enhanced anti-tumor effects when given in combination with paclitaxel, docetaxel, or doxorubicin.[70,74] Significantly, chemotherapeutic agents did not inhibit viral replication.[74] The other conventional cancer therapy, radiotherapy, also has been demonstrated to augment the anti-tumor efficacy of the adenoviral mutants ONYX-015 (E1B-55K-deleted) and CN706 (E1a driven by PSA promoter).[75,76] As has been reported with HSV-1 and ionizing radiation, ionizing radiation has recently been shown to enhance the viral burst size of CN706.[33,76] The preclinical results obtained with combining replication-competent adenoviruses with chemotherapy have been supported by clinical trial results (see *Replication-Competent Adenoviruses in Clinical Trials*, p. 72), in that dl1520 has minimal anti-tumor efficacy as a single agent but appears more effective in combination with chemotherapy.

To increase the therapeutic index, a variety of exogenous genes have been inserted into replication-competent adenovirus. Such genes include immunomodulatory cytokines or prodrug-converting enzymes. The drawback of adenovirus as compared to HSV-1 is that the adenovirus capacity to carry foreign genes is smaller. Replication-competent adenoviruses encoding foreign genes may also be amenable to combinations with conventional cancer therapies to result in enhanced tumor control. One example of this "trimodal" approach is combining replication-competent adenovirus with prodrug-converting enzymes and radiotherapy.[77] An E1B-attenuated replication-competent adenovirus that was created expresses the prodrug-converting enzymes cytosine deaminase and HSV-thymidine kinase. This approach results in cancer cell kill by the viral oncolysis, conversion of the prodrugs 5-FC and ganciclovir to toxic metabolites. Because cytosine deaminase converts 5-FC to 5-FU (a radiosensitizer), radiotherapy in this treatment paradigm resulted in a further augmentation of tumor cell kill. The results of this trimodal approach are promising in experimental tumor models and warrant consideration in future clinical trials. Along similar lines, tumor necrosis factor-α has been placed under the promoter of the radiation-inducible promoter Egr-1.[78] In this strategy, cytotoxic gene expression encoded by the virus is controlled by ionizing radiation, providing a means to restrict gene expression to the irradiated tumor bed.

Replication-Competent Adenoviruses in Clinical Trials

The E1B-55K-deleted adenovirus (dl1520, ONYX-015) was first reported in 1996 and has rapidly proceeded to clinical trials. There are numerous clinical trials with ONYX-015, and we highlight some of the more interesting lessons learned and focus on more recent results from clinical trials combining ONYX-015 with chemotherapeutic agents. Whereas clinical trials with HSV-1 have focused on gliomas, clinical trials with ONYX-015 initially focused on head and neck cancers. Treatment of head and neck cancers has characteristics that allow for easier analysis of certain parameters important in understanding the successes and failures of clinical trial with oncolytic viruses. Tumor accessibility allows for repeated intratumoral viral inoculation and for biopsies to determine whether the virus is replicating within the tumor.

A phase I trial to determine the safety and tolerance of ONYX-015 was performed in patients with recurrent head and neck cancer.[79] Twenty-two patients received a single intratumoral injection of 1×10^7 to 1×10^{11} pfu of ONYX-015. Although initial viral inocula were reported as plaque-forming units, more recent studies have switched to particles injected, infectious and noninfectious (1 pfu = 20 particles). This study established the feasibility and safety of ONYX-015. Treatment was well tolerated with grade 1 and grade 2 flulike symptoms, and dose-limiting toxicity did not occur at the highest viral inoculum (10^{11} pfu or 2×10^{12} particles). In 21 of 22 patients, neutralizing antibodies to adenovirus increased, and in situ hybridization of tumor biopsies to adenoviral DNA were positive in 4 of 22 patients. A follow-up phase II study was performed in 37 patients with recurrent head and neck cancer to determine whether ONYX-015 replicated selectively in tumor cells.[80] Patients received either 2×10^{11} particles during week 1 (5 days) in 3-week cycles or 2×10^{11} particles twice daily for 10 days (weeks 1 and 2) with week 3 off. Both protocols were well tolerated, with mild to moderate fevers and pain at the site of intratumoral injection. Important results of this study included demonstrating that of 11 patient tumor biopsies, 7 were positive for ONYX-015, whereas none of 11 biopsies of adjacent normal tissue were positive, demonstrating tumor selectivity of ONYX-015. Although initial tumor regression was observed in 21% of patients, complete responses were rare. A phase I study of intratumoral inoculation of ONYX-015 for pancreatic tumors has also been completed. Although this approach was tolerated at doses up to 2×10^{12} particles, no evidence of viral replication was documented.[81]

These studies established the safety and feasibility of direct intratumoral inoculation of ONYX-015. However significant, sustainable responses were not achieved despite aggressive inoculation schedules. For this reason and on the basis of preclinical data, ONYX-015 was administered in combination with cisplatin and 5-FU to patients with recurrent head and neck cancer.[72,82] An important feature of this study was the ability to have an internal control for each patient. Patients with multiple tumor recurrences were treated with chemotherapy, but only the larger tumor was injected with ONYX-015. In an individual patient, a tumor received 5-FU and cisplatin, and another tumor received 5-FU and cisplatin with intratumoral inoculation of ONYX-015. The time to tumor progression of the virus-inoculated tumor was significantly longer than that of the noninjected tumor (11 patients). Viral replication was also documented in tumor tissue exposed to 5-FU and cisplatin. This result underscores the necessity to initiate multimodality therapy with replication-competent viruses as a method to enhance the therapeutic response in patients. ONYX-015 has also been delivered to patients by other routes (i.e., intraperitoneally, intravenously, and into the hepatic artery). A review of these clinical trials was recently published.[83]

A second adenoviral mutant CV706 (CN706; PSA-driven transcription of E1a) was used in a recently completed phase I clinical trial for recurrent prostate cancer.[84] Twenty patients with recurrent prostate cancer and rising serum PSA were injected intraprostatically with 1×10^{11} to 1×10^{13} viral particles in a single dose. CV706 was deemed safe at all doses tested, with at most reversible grade 3 toxicities. Viral replication was documented, and preliminary results indicated that a fraction of patients treated at the higher doses had a greater than 50% reduction in their PSA levels.

ONCOLYTIC REOVIRUS

Reovirus Biology

Reovirus is an acronym for *r*espiratory *e*nteric *o*rphan virus. As its name implies, it is usually isolated from respiratory or gastrointestinal tracts. The term *orphan* was added because it was not associated with any known disease states in humans and may cause mild upper respiratory infections or enteritis. It is ubiquitous in the human population, with more than 50% of adults having antibodies to reovirus. In a study in which patients were intranasally infected with reovirus, only 9 of 27 patients developed symptoms consisting of mild sneezing and pharyngitis.[85]

Reovirus is a nonenveloped segmented double-stranded virus with 10 segments encoding 4.5 kb. The genome is packaged in an icosahedron capsid, and viral binding to the cell is mediated by sialic acid. The virus is taken into the cell through endosomes and is released into the cytoplasm. Viral replication occurs within the cytoplasm, where the negative strand of the genome is transcribed and used both as mRNA for protein translation and as a template to replicate genomic dsRNA for viral progeny. On completion of the replicative cycle, the cell is lysed, and viral progeny is released. Although sialic acid is ubiquitously expressed, reovirus is not capable of replicating in many cells. The implication is that a certain intracellular environment is necessary for reovirus replication to proceed. Recent insight into the virus-host cell interactions has elucidated a key cellular pathway critical to reovirus replication and provides a rational basis for the use of reovirus as an oncolytic agent.

Targeting Cells with Active Ras

On infection with reovirus, viral mRNA is generated within cells that do not support viral replication (NIH-3T3); however, viral protein synthesis is inhibited.[86] The block of viral protein synthesis in the infected cell is due to the activation of double-stranded PKR. As mentioned, PKR phosphorylates the α-subunit of translation initiation factor 2 (eIF-2α), which inhibits mRNA translation and blocks viral protein synthesis. If PKR is deleted from nonpermissive NIH-3T3 cells, the cells become susceptible to reovirus.

Previous studies have shown that cells that do not support reovirus (type 3) replication can be made susceptible to infection by activation of the cellular ras pathway. Cells resistant to reovirus infection when transfected with the receptor tyrosine kinases, epidermal growth factor receptor, or v-erbB support reovirus replication.[87,88] These receptor tyrosine kinases mediate the activation of the ras pathway. Furthermore, NIH-3T3 cells transfected with ras or sos are permissive to reovirus replication.[86] Transfection of ras, sos, or v-erbB into resistant cells prevented the activation of PKR after reovirus infection and resulted in reovirus replication. These studies indicated that antagonization of the PKR pathway by the ras pathway allows for reovirus replication to occur. What remains unclear is how exactly activation of the ras pathway inhibits PKR activation, although studies indicate that ras induces an inhibitor of PKR.[89] Many tumors have mutations that result in activation of the ras pathway; with either activating mutations of ras or up-regulation of receptor tyrosine kinases, epidermal growth factor receptor, or platelet-derived growth factor receptor.[90] The utility of reovirus as an oncolytic virus has, therefore, been proposed for tumors with active ras (see Fig. 4.2). The efficacy of reovirus as an oncolytic agent for human glioma cells has been demonstrated both in cell culture and in animal models.[91,92] Human glioma tumor xenografts grown either subcutaneously or intracranially in mice demonstrated significant tumor regression after intratumoral injection with reovirus. Clinical phase I trials with reovirus are in progress.

CONCLUSIONS

Although researchers have experimented for more than a century with replicating viruses for cancer therapy, the elucidation of viral-host cell interactions has resulted in the reemergence of this treatment paradigm within the last 10 years. It should be remembered that viruses are obligate parasites that require cells for replication. To infect and overtake cellular machinery, the virus must deal with innate cellular antiviral mechanisms. Understanding the interplay of viral proteins with cellular proteins has provided a rational basis for creation of genetically engineered viruses (HSV-1 and adenovirus) and reovirus as tumor-selective agents. Although these viruses are effective in a variety of experimental tumor models, many issues remain to be addressed in viral oncolytic therapy for local tumor control before it is effective in the clinical setting. Finally, with a further evolution in the development of tumor-selective, replication-competent viruses, it may be eventually possible to develop effective viruses that target metastatic disease.

REFERENCES

1. Russell SJ. Replicating vectors for gene therapy of cancer: risks, limitations, and prospects. Eur J Cancer 1994;30(8):1165–1171.
2. Roizman B, Sears AE. Human herpes viruses and their replication. In: BN Fields, DM Knipe, PM Howley, eds. Fields Virology, 3rd ed. Philadelphia: Lippincott-Raven, 1996:2231–2296.
3. Martuza RL, Malick A, Markert JM et al. Experimental therapy of human glioma by means of a genetically engineered virus mutant. Science 1991;252:854–856.
4. Mineta T, Rabkin SD, Martuza RL. Treatment of malignant gliomas using ganciclovir-hypersensitive, ribonucleotide reductase–deficient herpes simplex viral mutant. Cancer Res 1994;54(15): 3963–3966.

5. Pyles RB, Warnick RE, Chalk CL et al. A novel multiply-mutated HSV-1 strain for the treatment of human brain tumors. Hum Gene Ther 1997;8(5):533–544.

6. Chou J, Kern ER, Whitley RJ, Roizman B. Mapping of herpes simplex virus-1 neurovirulence to γ134.5, a gene nonessential for growth in cell culture. Science 1990;250:1262–1266.

7. Chou J, Gross M, Roizman B. Association of a M(r) 90,000 phosphoprotein with protein kinase PKR in cell exhibiting enhanced phosphorylation of translation initiation factor eIF-2 alpha and premature shutoff of protein synthesis after infection with gamma 134.5-mutants of herpes simplex virus 1. Proc Natl Acad Sci USA 1995;92(23):10516–10520.

8. He B, Gross M, Roizman B. The $\gamma_1$34.5 protein of herpes simplex virus 1 complexes with protein phosphatase 1α to dephosphorylate the α-subunit of the eukaryotic translation initiation factor 2 and preclude the shutoff of protein synthesis by double-stranded RNA-activated protein kinase. Proc Natl Acad Sci USA 1997;94(3):843–848.

9. Chambers R, Gillespie GY, Soroceanu L et al. Comparison of genetically engineered herpes simplex viruses for the treatment of brain tumors in a SCID mouse model of human malignant glioma. Proc Natl Acad Sci USA 1995;92(5):1411–1415.

10. Andreansky S, Soroceanu L, Flotte ER et al. Evaluation of genetically engineered herpes simplex viruses as oncolytic agents for human malignant brain tumors. Cancer Res 1997;57(8):1502–1509.

11. Farassati F, Yang AD, Lee PW. Oncogenes in ras signaling pathway dictate host-cell permissiveness to herpes simplex virus 1. Nat Cell Biol 2001;3(8):745–750.

12. Mohr I, Gluzman Y. A herpesvirus genetic element which affects translation in the absence of the viral GADD34 function. EMBO J 1996;15(17):4759–4766.

13. He B, Chou J, Brandimarti R et al. Suppression of the phenotype of $\gamma_1$34.5 herpes simplex virus 1: failure of activated RNA-dependent protein kinase to shut off protein synthesis is associated with a deletion in the domain of the α47 gene. J Virol 1997;71(8):6049–6054.

14. Cassady KA, Gross M, Roizman B. The second-site mutation in the herpes simplex virus recombinants lacking the gamma 134.5 genes precludes shutoff of protein synthesis by blocking the phosphorylation of eIF-2alpha. J Virol 1998;72(9):7005–7011.

15. Cassady KA, Gross M, Roizman B. The herpes simplex virus US11 protein effectively compensates for the gamma1(34.5) gene if present before activation of protein kinase R by precluding its phosphorylation and that of the alpha subunit of eukaryotic translation initiator factor 2. J Virol 1998;72(11):8620–8626.

16. Mohr I, Sternberg D, Ward S et al. A herpes simplex virus type 1 gamma34.5 second-site suppressor mutant that exhibits enhanced growth in cultured glioblastoma cells is severely attenuated in animals. J Virol 2001;75(11):5189–5196

17. Todo T, Martuza RL, Rabkin SD, Johnson PA. Oncolytic herpes simplex virus vector with enhanced MHC class I presentation and tumor cell killing. Proc Natl Acad Sci USA 2001;98(11):6396–6401.

18. DeLuca NA, McCarthy AM, Schaffer PA. Isolation and characterization of deletion mutants of herpes simplex virus type 1 in the gene encoding immediate-early regulatory protein ICP4. J Virol 1985;56(2):558–570.

19. Leopardi R, Roizman B. The herpes simplex virus major regulatory protein ICP4 blocks apoptosis induced by the virus or by hyperthermia. Proc Natl Acad Sci USA 1996;93(18):9583–9587.

20. Miyatake SI, Iyer A, Martuza RL, Rabkin SD. Transcriptional targeting of herpes simplex virus for cell- specific replication. J Virol 1997;71(7):5124–5132

21. Miyatake SI, Tani S, Feigenbaum F et al. Hepatoma-specific antitumor activity of an albumin enhancer/promoter regulated herpes simplex virus in vivo. Gene Ther 1999;6(4):564–572.

22. Yamamura H, Hashio M, Noguchi M et al. Identification of the transcriptional regulatory sequences of human calponin promoter and their use in targeting a conditionally replicating herpes vector to malignant human soft tissue and bone tumors. Cancer Res 2001;61(10):3969–3977.

23. MacLean AR, ul-Fareed M, Robertson L et al. Herpes simplex virus type 1 deletion variants 1714 and 1716 pinpoint neurovirulence-related sequences in Glasgow strain 17+ between immediate early gene 1 and the 'a' sequence. J Gen Virol 1991;72(3):631–639.

24. Kesari S, Randazzo BP, Valyi-Nagy et al. Therapy of experimental human brain tumors using a neuroattenuated herpes simplex virus mutant. Lab Invest 1995;73(5):636–648.

25. Rampling R, Cruickshank G, Papanastassiou V et al. Toxicity evaluation of replication-competent herpes simplex virus (ICP 34.5 null mutant 1716) in patients with recurrent malignant glioma. Gene Ther 2000;7(10):859–866.

26. Mineta T, Rabkin SD, Yazaki T et al. Attenuated multi-mutated herpes simplex virus-1 for the treatment of malignant gliomas. Nat Med 1995;1(9):938–943.

27. Martuza RL. Conditionally replicating herpes vectors for cancer therapy. J Clin Invest 2000;105(7): 841–846.

28. Hunter WD, Martuza RL, Feigenbaum F et al. Attenuated, replication-competent herpes simplex virus type 1 mutant G207: safety evaluation of intracerebral injection in nonhuman primates. J Virol 1999;73(8):6319–6326.

29. Todo T, Feigenbaum F, Rabkin SD et al. Viral shedding and biodistribution of G207, a multimutated, conditionally replicating herpes simplex virus type 1, after intracerebral inoculation in Aotus. Mol Ther 2000;2(6):588–595.

30. Markert JM, Medlock MD, Rabkin SD et al. Conditionally replicating herpes simplex virus mutant, G207 for the treatment of malignant glioma: results of a phase I trial. Gene Ther 2000;7(10): 867–874.

31. Meignier B, Longnecker R, Roizman B. In vivo behavior of genetically engineered herpes simplex viruses R7017 and R7020: construction and evaluation in rodents. J Infect Dis 1988;158(3): 602–614.

32. Meignier B, Martin B, Whitley RJ, Roizman B. In vivo behavior of genetically engineered herpes simplex viruses R7017 and R7020: II. Studies in immunocompetent and immunosuppressed owl monkeys (*Aotus trivirgatus*). J Infect Dis 1990;162(2):313–21.

33. Advani SJ, Sibley GS, Song PY et al. Enhancement of replication of genetically engineered herpes simplex virus by ionizing radiation: a new paradigm for destruction of therapeutically intractable tumors. Gene Ther 1998;5(2):160–165.

34. Advani SJ, Chung SM, Yan SY et al. Replication-competent, nonneuroinvasive genetically engineered herpes virus is highly effective in the treatment of therapy-resistant experimental tumors. Cancer Res 1999;59(9):2055–2058.

35. Delman KA, Bennett JJ, Zager JS et al. Effects of preexisting immunity on the response to herpes simplex–based oncolytic viral therapy. Hum Gene Ther 2000;11(18):2465–2472.

36. McAuliffe PF, Jarnagin WR, Johnson P et al. Effective treatment of pancreatic tumors with two multimutated herpes simplex oncolytic viruses. J Gastrointest Surg 2000;4(6):580–588.

37. Andreansky S, He B, van Cott J et al. Treatment of intracranial gliomas in immunocompetent mice using herpes simplex viruses that express murine cytokines. Gene Ther 1998;5(1):121–130.

38. Parker JN, Gillespie GY, Love CE et al. Engineered herpes simplex virus expressing IL-12 in the treatment of experimental murine brain tumors. Proc Natl Acad Sci USA 2000;97(5):2208–2213.

39. Hill A, Jugovic P, York I et al. Herpes simplex virus turns off the TAP to evade host immunity. Nature 1995;375:411–415.

40. Goldsmith K, Chen W, Johnson DC, Hendricks RL. Infected cell protein (ICP)47 enhances herpes simplex virus neurovirulence by blocking the CD8+ T cell response. J. Exp Med 1998;187(3): 341–348.

41. Wong RJ, Patel SG, Kim S et al. Cytokine gene transfer enhances herpes oncolytic therapy in murine squamous cell carcinoma. Hum Gene Ther 2001;12(3):256–265.

42. Chase M, Chung RY, Chiocca EA. An oncolytic viral mutant that delivers the CYP2B1 transgene and augments cyclophosphamide chemotherapy. Nat Biotechnol 1998;16(5):444–448.

43. Nakamura H, Mullen JT, Chandrasekhar S et al. Multimodality therapy with a replication-conditional herpes simplex virus 1 mutant that expresses yeast cytosine deaminase for intratumoral conversion of 5-fluorocytosine to 5-fluorouracil. Cancer Res 2001;61(14):5447–5452.

44. Pawlik TM, Nakamura H, Yoon SS et al. Oncolysis of diffuse hepatocellular carcinoma by intravascular administration of a replication-competent, genetically engineered herpesvirus. Cancer Res 2000;60(11):2790–2795.

45. Bradley JD, Kataoka Y, Advani S et al. Ionizing radiation improves survival in mice bearing intracranial high-grade gliomas injected with genetically modified herpes simplex virus. Clin Cancer Res 1999;5(6):1517–1522.

46. Chahlavi A, Todo T, Martuza RL, Rabkin SD. Replication-competent herpes simplex virus vector G207 and cisplatin combination therapy for head and neck squamous cell carcinoma. Neoplasia 1999;1(2):162–169.

47. Toyoizumi T, Mick R, Abbas AE et al. Combined therapy with chemotherapeutic agents and herpes simplex virus type 1 ICP34.5 mutant (HSV-1716) in human non-small cell lung cancer. Hum Gene Ther 1999;10(18):3013–3029.

48. Petrowsky H, Roberts GD, Kooby DA et al. Functional interaction between fluorodeoxyuridine-induced cellular alterations and replication of a ribonucleoside reductase–negative herpes simplex virus. J Virol 2001;75(15):7050–7058.

49. Bischoff JR, Kirn DH, Williams A et al. An adenovirus mutant that replicates selectively in p53-deficient human tumor cells. Science 1996;274:373–376.

50. Rothmann T, Hengstermann A, Whitaker NJ et al. Replication of ONYX-015, a potential anticancer adenovirus, is independent of p53 status in tumor cells. J Virol 1998;72(12):9470–9478.

51. Harada JN, Berk AJ. p53-independent and -dependent requirements for E1B-55K in adenovirus type 5 replication. J Virol 1999;73(7):5333–5344.

52. Vollmer CM, Ribas A, Butterfield LH et al. p53 selective and nonselective replication of an E1B-deleted adenovirus in hepatocellular carcinoma. Cancer Res 1999;59(17):4369–4374.

53. Koch P, Gatfield J, Lober C et al. Efficient replication of adenovirus despite the overexpression of active and nondegradable p53. Cancer Res 2001;61(15):5941–5947.

54. Ries SJ, Brandts CH, Chung AS et al. Loss of p14ARF in tumor cells facilitates replication of the adenovirus mutant dl1520 (ONYX-015). Nat Med 2000;6(10):1128–1133.

55. Yang CT, You L, Uematsu K et al. p14ARF modulates the cytolytic effects of ONYX-015 in mesothelioma cells with wild-type p53. Cancer Res 2001;61(16):5959–5963.

56. Pilder S, Moore M, Logan J, Shenk T. The adenovirus E1B-55K transforming polypeptide modulates transport or cytoplasmic stabilization of viral and host cell mRNAs. Mol Cell Biol 1986;6(2): 470–476.

57. Whyte P, Williamson NM, Harlow E. Cellular targets for transformation by the adenovirus E1A proteins. Cell 1989;56(1):67–75.

58. Fueyo, J, Gomez-Manzano C, Alemany R et al. A mutant oncolytic adenovirus targeting the Rb pathway produces anti-glioma effect in vivo. Oncogene 2000;19(1):2–12.

59. Heise C, Hermiston T, Johnson L et al. An adenovirus E1A mutant that demonstrates potent and selective systemic anti-tumoral efficacy. Nat Med 2000;6(10):1134–1139.

60. Tollefson AE, Ryerse JS, Scaria A et al. The adenovirus death protein (E3-11.6K) is required at very late stages of infection for efficient cell lysis and release of adenovirus from infected cells. J Virol 1996;70(4):2296–2306.

61. Doronin K, Toth K, Kuppuswamy M et al. Tumor-specific, replication-competent adenovirus vectors overexpressing the adenovirus death protein. J Virol 2000;74(13):6147–6155.

62. Sauthoff H, Heitner S, Rom WN, Hay JG. Deletion of the adenoviral E1b-19kD gene enhances tumor cell killing of a replicating adenoviral vector. Hum Gene Ther 2000;11(3):379–388.

63. Harrison D, Sauthoff H, Heitner S et al. Wild-type adenovirus decreases tumor xenograft growth, but despite viral persistence complete tumor responses are rarely achieved-deletion of the viral E1b-19kD gene increases the viral oncolytic effect. Hum Gene Ther 2001;12(10):1323–1332.

64. Rodriguez R, Schuur ER, Lim GY et al. Prostate attenuated replication competent adenovirus (ARCA) CN706: a selective cytotoxic for prostate-specific antigen-positive prostate cancer cells. Cancer Res 1997;57(13):2559–2563.

65. Hallenbeck PL, Chang YN, Hay C et al. A novel tumor-specific replication-restricted adenoviral vector for gene therapy of hepatocellular carcinoma. Hum Gene Ther 1999;10(10):1721–1733.

66. Kurihara T, Brough DE, Kovesdi I, Kufe DW. Selectivity of a replication competent adenovirus for human breast carcinoma cells expressing the MUC1 antigen. J Clin Invest 2000;106(6): 763–771.

67. Hernandez-Alcoceba R, Pihalja M, Wicha MS, Clarke MF. A novel, conditionally replicative adenovirus for the treatment of breast cancer that allows controlled replication of E1a-deleted adenoviral vectors. Hum Gene Ther 2000;11(14):2009–2024.

68. Matsubara S, Wada Y, Gardner TA et al. A conditional replication-competent adenoviral vector, AD-OC-E1a, to cotarget prostate cancer and bone stroma in an experimental model of androgen-independent prostate cancer bone metastasis. Cancer Res 2001;61(16):6012–6019.

69. Yu DC, Chen Y, Seng M et al. The addition of adenovirus type 5 region E3 enables calydon virus 787 to eliminate distant prostate tumor xenografts. Cancer Res 1999;59(17):4200–4203.

70. Li Y, Yu DC, Chen Y et al. A hepatocellular carcinoma-specific adenovirus variant, CV890, eliminates distant human liver tumors in combination with doxorubicin. Cancer Res 2001;61(17): 6428–6436.

71. Doronin K, Kuppuswamy M, Toth K et al. Tissue-specific, tumor-selective, replication-competent adenovirus vector for cancer gene therapy. J Virol 2001;75(7):3314–3324.

72. Heise C, Sampson-Johannes A, Williams A et al. ONYX-015, an E1B gene-attenuated adenovirus, causes tumor-specific cytolysis and antitumoral efficacy that can be augmented by standard chemotherapeutic agents. Nat Med 1997;3(6):639–644.

73. You L, Yang CT, Jablons DM. ONYX-015 works synergistically with chemotherapy in lung cancer cell lines and primary cultures freshly made from lung cancer patients. Cancer Res 2000;60(4): 1009–1013.

74. Yu DC, Chen Y, Dilley et al. Antitumor strategy synergy of CV787, a prostate cancer-specific adenovirus, and paclitaxel and docetaxel. Cancer Res 2001;61(2):517–525

75. Rogulski KR, Freytag SO, Zhang K et al. In vivo antitumor activity of ONYX-015 is influenced by p53 status and is augmented by radiotherapy. Cancer Res 2000;60(5):1193–1196.

76. Chen Y, DeWeese T, Dilley J et al. CV706, a prostate cancer–specific adenovirus variant, in combination with radiotherapy produces synergistic antitumor efficacy without increasing toxicity. Cancer Res 2001;61(14):5453–5460.

77. Rogulski KR, Wing MS, Paielli DL et al. Double suicide gene therapy augments the antitumor activity of a replication-competent lytic adenovirus through enhanced cytotoxicity and radiosensitization. Hum Gene Ther 2000;11(1):67–76.

78. Hallahan DE, Mauceri HJ, Seung LP et al. Spatial and temporal control of gene therapy using ionizing radiation. Nat Med 1995;1(8):786–791.

79. Ganly I, Kirn D, Eckhardt et al. A phase I study of ONYX-015, an E1B attenuated adenovirus, administered intratumorally to patients with recurrent head and neck cancer. Clin Cancer Res 2000;6(3):798–806.

80. Nemunaitis J, Ganly I, Khuri F et al. Selective replication and oncolysis in p53 mutant tumors with ONYX-015, an E1B-55kD gene-deleted adenovirus, in patients with advanced head and neck cancer: a phase II trial. Cancer Res 2000;60(22):6359–6366.

81. Mulvihill S, Warren R, Venook A et al. Safety and feasibility of injection with an E1B-55 kDa gene-deleted, replication selective adenovirus (ONYX-015) into primary carcinomas of the pancreas: a phase I trial. Gene Ther 2001;8(4):308–315.

82. Khuri FR, Nemunaitis J, Ganly I et al. A controlled trial of intratumoral ONYX-015, a selectively-replicating adenovirus, in combination with cisplatin and 5-fluorouracil in patients with recurrent head and neck cancer. Nat Med 2000;6(8):879–885.

83. Kirn D. Clinical research results with dl1520 (ONYX-015), a replication-selective adenovirus for the treatment of cancer: what have we learned? Gene Ther 2001;8(2):89–98.

84. DeWeese TL, van der Poel H, Li S et al. A phase I trial of CV706, a replication-competent PSA selective adenovirus for the treatment of locally recurrent prostate cancer following radiation therapy. Cancer Res 2001;61(20):7464–7472.

85. Rosen L, Evans HE, Spickard A. Reovirus infections in human volunteers. Am J Hygeine 1963; 77:29–37.

86. Strong JE, Coffey MC, Tang D et al. The molecular basis of viral oncolysis: usurpation of ras signaling pathway by reovirus. EMBO J 1998;17(12):3351–3362.

87. Strong JE, Tang D, Lee PW. Evidence that the epidermal growth factor receptor on host cells confers reovirus infection efficiency. Virology 1993;197(1):405–411.

88. Strong JE, Lee PWK. The v-erbB oncogene confers enhanced cellular susceptibility to reovirus infection. J Virol 1996;70(1):612–616.

89. Mundschau LJ, Faller DV. Oncogenic ras induces an inhibitor of double-stranded RNA-dependent eukaryotic initiation factor 2 alpha-kinase activation. J Biol Chem 1992;267(32):23092–23098.

90. Bos J. Ras oncogenes in human cancer: a review. Cancer Res 1989;49(17):4682–4689.

91. Coffey MC, Strong JE, Forsyth PA, Lee PWK. Reovirus therapy of tumors with activated ras pathway. Science 1998;282:1332–1334.

92. Wilcox ME, Yang WQ, Senger D et al. Reovirus as an oncolytic agent against experimental human malignant gliomas. J Natl Cancer Inst 2001;93(12):903–912.

Chapter 5

The Role of the Anti-Apoptotic *Survivin* Gene in Bladder Cancer

Dario C. Altieri

Robert M. Weiss

The ability of tumor cells to evade apoptosis, or programmed cell death,[1] and to exhibit deregulated proliferative capacity comprise two of the genetic abnormalities that are probably common to all human cancers.[2] Positioned at the interface between the control of apoptosis and the regulation of mitosis, survivin is a recently described molecule that is differentially expressed in cancers *versus* normal tissues and is required to maintain cancer cell viability.[3] The dramatic upregulation of the *survivin* gene that has been observed in most, if not all, human cancers suggests that this is a pathway commonly used to promote the survival of tumor cells at various stages of tumorigenesis and to promote their unrestricted proliferation. As detailed later, recent progress has been made in the elucidation of the survivin pathway in bladder cancer. These studies have offered new principles for molecular diagnosis and follow-up protocols and novel therapeutic opportunities for the treatment of bladder cancer patients.

BLADDER CANCER: IMPACT AND UNRESOLVED ISSUES

In the United States, bladder cancer is the fourth most common cancer in men and the eighth most common cancer in women. Each year, 54,400 Americans receive new diagnoses of bladder cancer, and 11,200 people are expected to die from the disease.[4] Usually, bladder cancer is heralded by insidious symptoms, including painless hematuria or irritating voiding symptoms. Bladder cancer can occur at any age, but it is generally a disease of the middle-aged and elderly populations, with a median age at diagnosis of 70 years. Bladder cancer is approximately two times more common in white males than in black males and is 1.5 times more common in white females than in black females. The known risk factors for bladder cancer are cigarette smoking, occupational exposure to dyes, dietary exposure to nitrates, chronic inflammation, use of the chemotherapeutic agent cyclophosphamide, and pelvic irradiation.

Most cancers of the bladder are histopathologically identified as transitional cell carcinomas. These tumors exhibit a broad range of biologic behavior, from the relatively benign, superficial, low-grade papillary lesions to the highly malignant and aggressive anaplastic carcinomas.[5] Seventy to eighty percent of patients are found to have low-grade, nonaggressive tumors confined to the superficial mucosa. Although generally amenable to treatment with local excision and selective intravesical immunotherapy or chemotherapy,[6] these tumors recur in up to 80% of patients, thus posing formidable challenges for the accurate follow-up of treated patients. Ten to fifteen percent of these recurrences exhibit a more aggressive and invasive tumor type carrying a dismal clinical outcome due to metastatic dissemination. The molecular abnormalities underlying bladder cancer have been intensely investigated[7] and involve loss of tumor suppressor genes, including *p53*[8] and the retinoblastoma proteins; aberrant expression of oncogenes involved in the growth factor receptor signaling pathway, such as *ras*[9] and epidermal growth factor receptor[10]; and ablation of cyclin-dependent kinase inhibitors p15 and p16 resulting from abnormal methylation and promoter silencing.[11,12] Some of the genetic defects appear to influence disease progression in a temporal fashion. For instance, loss of *p53* has been associated with more aggressive and evolved forms of bladder cancer,[13] whereas deletion of chromosomes 9p and 9q has been implicated in the earliest molecular abnormalities of normal urothelium during progression to transitional cell carcinoma. Consistent with the idea that dysregulation of apoptosis is a phenotype common to all cancers,[2] a potential role of the cell death–cell viability balance in the diagnosis and treatment of bladder cancer has been investigated. This has important therapeutic implications. Indeed, manipulation of apoptotic pathways recently emerged as a potential modality for sensitizing tumor cells to chemotherapy or radiotherapy treatments.[14] In this context, in situ analysis of apoptosis has been shown to predict clinical outcome of bladder cancer patients treated with radiotherapy,[15] and expression of apoptosis regulators Bcl-2 and Rb may influence clinical outcome and response to therapy via different and nonoverlapping pathways.[16] In addition, increased expression of antiapoptotic bcl-2 family protein Bcl-2,[17] Bcl-X[1] and, more recently, survivin[1] (see later) has been demonstrated in bladder cancer, and the implications of the latter in the diagnosis and treatment of the disease are reviewed in detail in the following sections.

SURVIVIN STRUCTURE AND FUNCTION

Survivin is a 16.5-kD intracellular protein that belongs to the inhibitor of apoptosis (IAP) gene family.[3] IAP molecules are found in the genomes of all metazoans and are characterized by the presence of one to three copies of a ~70 amino acid zinc finger fold, designated baculovirus IAP repeat (BIR).[20] Other structural motifs found in certain IAPs include a caspase-recruitment domain, a RING finger, a ubiquitin-conjugating domain, and a nucleotide-binding P loop motif.[20] Originally described in the baculovirus for their ability to thwart the host suicidal response to viral infection, several IAPs are now acknowledged to block cell death in mammalian cells by functioning as endogenous inhibitors of caspases. Caspases are intracellular cysteine proteases that are processed by limited proteolysis to a catalytically active state[21] and mediate the executioner phase of apoptotic cell death by cleaving various cellular substrates, preserving cytoskeletal integrity, repair processes, and energy production.[22] The structural requirements of IAP-dependent cytoprotection have been elucidated in detail and involve the formation of a physical complex between IAPs and effector caspases, which results in suppression of the enzyme's catalytic activity or proteolytic maturation[20] (or both). Consistent with this ability to counteract the common executioner phase of apoptosis, IAPs have been shown to suppress multiple cell death stimuli initiated via the extrinsic, i.e., death receptor, or intrinsic, mitochondrial, apoptotic pathways.[1]

Survivin is a structurally and functionally unique member of the IAP gene family in that it has a single BIR and an extended carboxyl terminal α-helix,[3,23] a stable dimeric architecture in solution,[24] and a cell cycle–regulated expression that peaks at mitosis.[25] The cell cycle periodicity of survivin expression is transcriptionally controlled,[26,27] and a mechanism of ubiquitin-dependent survivin destruction in interphase cells has been described.[28] On a > 40-fold upregulation in G2/M, survivin localizes to various components of the mitotic apparatus. These include centrosomes (also called *microtubule-organizing centers*), microtubules of the metaphase and anaphase spindle, and the remnants of the mitotic apparatus (i.e., midbodies) at telophase. A fraction of survivin also localizes to the nucleus in close association with kinetochores of metaphase chromosomes.[29] The various subcellular pools of survivin that localize to different mitotic compartments are immunochemically distinct, thus potentially reflecting posttranslational modifications modulating epitope accessibility and intracellular trafficking of the mature protein.[30]

ROLE OF SURVIVIN IN CELL DEATH

Three lines of experimental evidence support a critical role of survivin in the modulation of apoptotic cell death pathways. First, recombinant expression of survivin in cell culture systems has been shown to inhibit apoptosis induced by various stimuli acting through the extrinsic or the intrinsic pathway of apoptosis.[3,27,31–35] Second, the antiapoptotic function of survivin has been demonstrated in vivo using genetically engineered animals. Transgenic expression of survivin in the basal layer of the epidermis did not affect developmental programs of keratinocyte differentiation or proliferation but blocked ultraviolet radiation-induced apoptosis and substituted for the loss of a second p53 allele in promoting apoptosis resistance.[36] A third line of evidence pointing to a critical role of survivin in apoptosis inhibition comes from experiments targeting the integrity-function of the survivin pathway using antisense or a Cys^{84}→Ala dominant negative mutant. Overexpression of these molecular antagonists was sufficient to cause spontaneous apoptosis, increased caspase activity, and inhibition of cell proliferation in cell culture systems in vitro and in various experimental animal models of tumor growth and progression in vivo.[25,37–42] The apoptosis inhibitory function of survivin is evolutionary conserved, and a survivin homolog in *Drosophila*—Deterin—functions to block apoptosis in flies.[43] In addition, survivin and Deterin are functionally interchangeable in inhibiting apoptosis in mammalian or insect cells.[44] The reported ability to associate with caspases[27,31,35] suggests that survivin cytoprotection may fall into the general paradigm of other IAPs with respect to the overall mechanism of apoptosis inhibition. However, alternative possibilities also are plausible. The ability of survivin to inhibit caspase-3 activity in vitro has been openly debated, and conflicting results reported in the literature have been attributed to differences in experimental protocols or differential stability-folding of the recombinant survivin protein.[24,35,45] In addition, survivin lacks a "hook" region upstream of the BIR that acts as a caspase-binding domain in other IAPs,[46] suggesting that a survivin-caspase complex may use different structural requirements as compared to other IAP family members.

ROLE OF SURVIVIN IN CELL DIVISION

In addition to causing spontaneous apoptosis,[25] antisense suppression of survivin in various cancer cell types produced a second phenotype of aberrant mitotic progression characterized by supernumerary centrosomes, formation of multipolar mitotic spindles, failure of cytokinesis, and generation of multinucleated cells.[39,47,48] The phenotype of survivin knockout mice is consistent with a critical role of survivin in controlling mitosis, which is indispensable during development.[49] Beginning at embryonic (E) day 3.5 (E3.5), homozygous deletion of the *survivin* gene resulted in a catastrophic defect of microtubule assembly, with absence of mitotic spindles, formation of multinucleated cells, and 100% embryonic lethality by E4.5.[49] Along the same line, ablation of potential survivin-like molecules in the worm *C. elegans* and in budding and fission yeast also resulted in lethal defects of mitosis and meiosis.[50,51] However, in contrast to the survivin-like molecules in lower organisms, survivin appears positioned to influence multiple aspects of cell division, in agreement with its multiple sites of subcellular localization.[30] Accordingly, targeting of survivin by cytosolic microinjection or lipid-based delivery of antibodies did not affect cytokinesis but caused dysregulation of the mitotic spindle checkpoint with abnormal sister chromatid separation[48] and catastrophic defects in microtubule assembly and function.[30]

EXPRESSION OF SURVIVIN IN CANCER

One of the most significant features of survivin is its differential distribution in cancer *versus* normal tissues.[3] Reminiscent of "oncofetal" antigens, survivin is strongly expressed in embryonic and fetal organs[27,52] but undetectable in most terminally differentiated normal tissues.[3] Adult normal tissues reported to express survivin included thymus,[3] $CD34^+$ bone marrow–derived stem cells in low levels,[53,54] and the basal colonic epithelium.[55] In contrast, survivin was not expressed in basal keratinocytes.[36,56] By contrast, dramatic overexpression of survivin was demonstrated in tumors of lung,[57] breast,[58] colon,[59] stomach,[60] esophagus,[61] pancreas,[62] uterus,[63] and ovaries[64] and in large-cell non-Hodgkin's lymphoma,[65] leukemias,[66,67] neuroblastoma,[34,68] soft tissue sarcomas,[69] melanoma,[38] and non-melanoma [56] skin cancers. In genome-wide searches, survivin was identified as the fourth most common "transcriptome" expressed in cancers of the colon, lung, brain, and breast and in melanoma but was undetectable or was found in very low levels in the normal tissues of the same organs.[70]

Despite its role in mitosis, survivin overexpression in cancer clearly does not simply reflect the presence of a higher number of proliferating cells. In melanoma, survivin expression was indistinguishable in cases with a low (1.9) or high (38.2) mitotic index.[38] In addition, survivin is typically observed in nearly all tumor cells and not just in the mitotic fraction, thus suggesting a potential deregulation of *survivin* gene expression in cancer. Two molecular abnormalities that have been reported may contribute to aberrant survivin expression in cancer. First, amplification of the survivin locus on 17q25 has been described in neuroblastoma by fluorescence in situ hybridization,[34] and gain of chromosome 17q has long been recognized as the most common genetic abnormality of neuroblastoma.[71] In addition, survivin exon 1 sequences are largely silenced by methylation in normal ovaries but become unmethylated—thus transcriptionally active—in most ovarian cancers overexpressing survivin.[72] To account for the broad overexpression of survivin in many cancers, possibly multiple oncogenic pathways may contribute to the reactivation of the *survivin* gene in neoplasia.

When analyzed retrospectively, cancer patients expressing survivin exhibited a shortened survival,[57–59,61,64,65,69,73] an association with unfavorable markers of disease progression,[34,66,68] and an increased resistance to therapy.[61] In some studies, expression of survivin correlated with bcl-2,[65] or reduced apoptotic index, in vivo.[58,59,62] It is unclear whether a correlation exists between survivin expression and p53 status. A potential expression of survivin in bladder cancer and its implications for disease progression has been intensely investigated. In an immunohistochemical study, survivin expression was detected in 78% of all cases of bladder cancer and was more frequently observed in higher-grade tumors as compared with low-grade tumors: survivin-positive grade I tumors, 65% (13 of 20); grade II tumors, 90% (9 of 10); grade III tumors, 100% (6 of 6).[19] Consistent with the expression of survivin in cancer, but not in normal tissues, normal urothelium was consistently negative for survivin expression as assessed by immunohistochemistry.[19] In retrospective analysis for disease recurrence, which is the overwhelming feature of bladder cancer, the average time to first recurrence of grade I tumors was 35.5 ± 16.3 months in survivin-negative cases as opposed to 11.5 ± 6.2 months in survivin-positive cases ($P < 0.001$).[19] In the same tumor series, expression of antiapoptotic bcl-2 (3 of 36) or p53 (9 of 36) did not correlate with disease recurrence, whereas all tumors exhibited low apoptotic index (0.8%–1.0%) by internucleosomal DNA fragmentation.[19]

SURVIVIN AND MOLECULAR DIAGNOSIS OF BLADDER CANCER

The foregoing studies suggested that simple detection of survivin in tumor specimens by immunohistochemistry, in situ hybridization, or reverse transcriptase–polymerase chain reaction may provide a quick, one-step assessment to identify patients at high risk of invasive disease with unfavorable outcome. Recently, additional approaches have emerged to further exploit the survivin pathway for molecular diagnosis of cancer. One of these strategies was to measure an immune response to survivin in cancer patients. The rationale was that if survivin is undetectable in most normal tissues, cancer patients might recognize it as a "non-self" protein and mount an immune response to it. Indeed, circulating antibodies to survivin have been demonstrated in patients with cancers of colon and lung but not in normal volunteers.[74] The possibility that cancer patients may mount an immune response to survivin may have important implications that go beyond cancer diagnostics. Specifically, it was demonstrated recently that T cells mount a vigorous cytolytic response to survivin peptides in vitro and in vivo[75,76] and that human leukocyte antigen class I–restricted cytolytic T cells against survivin peptides exist in patients with breast cancer, leukemia, and melanoma in vivo.[76] These data suggest that survivin may be therapeutically used for cancer vaccination strategies, wherein its selective expression in cancer (but not in normal tissues) is likely to minimize further the risks of undesirable autoimmune effects.

A second approach was to test for the presence of survivin in biological fluids of cancer patients. Although survivin is not a secreted protein, the rationale was that exfoliated tumor cells from the primary site may release survivin in the extracellular milieu. This has been tested in bladder cancer, in which sensitive and specific tumor markers are urgently needed to improve early detection and to facilitate follow-up protocols of treated patients. Apart from categories of patients at occupational risk, the overall prevalence of bladder cancer is too low to make general screening practical or effective, and diagnosis is largely made as a result of manifestations of potentially indicative symptoms. Traditionally, patients presenting with microhematuria, gross hematuria, or irritating voiding symptoms in the absence of infection undergo upper urinary tract radiographic imaging, cystoscopy, and urine cytology to rule out malignancy. In addition, patients who previously have been given a diagnosis of and treated for bladder cancer are monitored for recurrence via cystoscopy and urine cytology as often as every 3 months. The frequency of follow-up depends on the grade and stage of the initial tumor and the patient's history of remission or recurrence. Cystoscopy and cytology are currently considered the gold standard for diagnosis and follow-up. The primary goal of these modalities is to recognize flat, superficial lesions prior to invasion and the 10% of papillary lesions that are destined to invade.

Cystoscopy involves insertion of a cystoscope through the urethra and into the bladder, thus allowing for a full visual inspection of the bladder mucosa. Additionally, laser fibers and cutting or cautery devices can be inserted through the cystoscope to obtain a biopsy or to resect suspicious areas of erythema or mucosal irregularity. A recent study of endoscopic procedures concluded that the sensitivity of traditional white-light cystoscopy ranged from 47.2% to 53%, with a reasonable estimate of 46.7%.[77] Because it is essentially a naked-eye assessment, this examination engenders a great deal of inter- and intrapersonal variability in cystoscopic results, which may account for the modest evaluation of what is generally considered a valuable diagnostic tool. Cystoscopy can be performed in the urologist's office and carries a low risk of complications, but it is invasive, uncomfortable, and costly. Urine cytology carries an estimated sensitivity of only 40%–60%, but a positive cytology is highly predictive of transitional cell carcinoma and may even precede cystoscopic diagnosis. Specificity is considered to be 95%.[78] Urine cytology is extremely effective in the detection of high-grade lesions, rendering it an important screening and surveillance tool. However, its overall sensitivity is variable (range, 0%–100%, depending on the study) largely because cytology is inconsistent in the detection of low-grade lesions. The application of strict criteria during analysis has improved sensitivity up to 85% in some series. However, difficulty remains in interpreting somewhat ambiguous cytology reports characterized by the presence of "atypical urothelial cells," which may originate from low-grade tumors or may be unrelated to neoplasia.

Because of the drawbacks associated with cystoscopy and cytology, there has been considerable effort to develop urine-based markers of bladder cancer that may provide high sensitivity and specificity. The goal has been to integrate urine cytology and molecular markers to improve their diagnostic potential and to relegate cystoscopy to a second line of modality for diagnosis and follow-up of transitional cell carcinoma of the urinary tract.[79,80] In this context, urine determination of nuclear matrix protein-22,[81] telomerase activity,[82] microsatellite analysis,[83] and hyaluronic acid–hyaluronidases[84] have been investigated for their suitability as markers in bladder cancer detection and follow-up. A similar approach recently was applied to the detection of survivin in urine samples of bladder cancer patients. To this effect, an antibody-based detection method has been developed and tested in an initial series of patients and normal controls.[85] In these studies, urine survivin was not detected in normal volunteers or in patients with nonneoplastic genitourinary disease. In contrast, all patients with new or recurrent bladder cancers tested positive for urine survivin, and 32 of 35 patients successfully treated for bladder cancer as assessed by cystoscopy became negative for urine survivin.[85] Intriguingly, one of the three patients with a positive urine test for survivin had a positive cytology, and another subsequently developed a recurrent tumor. Another potential useful aspect of immunologic detection of urine survivin was the implementation of a quantitative "survivin score" in tested individuals.[85] Accordingly, patients with carcinoma in situ, which may portend an unfavorable prognosis, had the highest urine survivin score.[85]

Studies are underway to validate the urine survivin detection system in much larger patient populations and to extend this approach to more mechanistic models of carcinogen-induced bladder cancer in rodents. Combined with histopathologic analysis of tumor samples, these studies will tell whether quantitative measurement of urine survivin may eventually provide an easily implemented, point-of-service test with prognostic implications for disease progression. No formal or quantitative comparison has yet been made between the urine survivin test and the other experimental urine-based markers for bladder cancer.[79] However, some aspects of the urine survivin test, including its simplicity, its sensitivity, and its specificity combined with its low cost, render it a potentially attractive first-line diagnostic test to detect early recurrences in treated patients. As suggested, this is an inherently serious problem for bladder cancer, given the extremely high rate of recurrences (up to 90%) and the uncomfortable and expensive nature of follow-up procedures (i.e., cystoscopy). A second potential application of the urine survivin test could be as a first-line screening of individuals at risk of bladder cancer resulting from chronic environmental exposure to urothelial carcinogens. Currently, this is conducted by urine cytology, with all its limitations and potential concerns with respect to sensitivity as outlined.

SURVIVIN AS A MOLECULAR THERAPEUTIC TARGET IN BLADDER CANCER

In addition to the potential benefits of exploiting the survivin pathway for early diagnosis and outcome prediction in bladder cancer, a therapeutic application for cancer treatment can be envisioned. This stems from a large of body of experimental work, both in cell culture systems and in in vivo animal models of cancer progression, which suggests that the integrity of the survivin pathway is required to maintain cancer cell viability. Consistent with this scheme, molecular antagonists of the survivin pathway, including antisense or dominant negative mutant constructs, exhibited convincing anti-tumor activity in vivo, suppressing tumor formation, inhibiting growth of established tumors, causing apoptosis of cancer cells, and sensitizing tumor cells to chemotherapy-induced cell death. From in vitro mechanistic studies, one of the critical requirements of survivin-dependent cytoprotection was identified as the cell cycle–dependent phosphorylation of survivin on Thr^{34} by the main mitotic kinase $p34^{cdc2}$-cyclin B1.[86] This phosphorylation site is evolutionary conserved in survivin homologs and is ideally positioned in the crystal structure to stabilize potential antiapoptotic protein-protein interactions mediated by the survivin BIR.[24] The rationale of targeting Thr^{34} phosphorylation for therapeutic intervention came from experiments using a phosphorylation-defective survivin Thr^{34}→Ala mutant (survivinT34A), which acts as a dominant-negative antagonist of this pathway and prevents phosphorylation of the endogenous protein. Loss of Thr^{34} phosphorylation resulted in the activation of the mitochondrial apoptotic pathway with activation of the upstream caspase-9 and caspase-dependent apoptosis of cells traversing mitosis.[86] In pre-clinical xenograft models of melanoma in immunodeficient (SCID) mice, expression of survivin(T34A) prevented melanoma tumor formation and suppressed the growth of existing tumors by 60%–70% in a reaction associated with loss of proliferating cells and with tumor cell apoptosis in vivo.[87] To render survivin (T34A) a potentially more flexible therapeutic tool, a replication-deficient adenovirus encoding survivinT34A (pAd-T34A) was recently generated. Administration of pAd-T34A promoted caspase-dependent apoptosis in a variety of cancer lines, exhibited no toxicity for normal primary cells, and inhibited tumor growth in three distinct xenograft breast cancer models in mice.[88]

Gene therapy has recently emerged as a viable treatment in solid tumors by reestablishing apoptosis and checkpoint function. A similar indication may be envisioned for the survivin mutant virus,[88] alone or in combination with chemotherapy. In this context, bladder cancer may provide an amenable target for a gene therapy approach. Already several studies have demonstrated that adenoviral transfer of various cell cycle–apoptosis modulators, including p53,[89] H-Ras dominant negative mutant,[90] interleukin-2,[91] antisense basic fibroblast growth factor,[92] antisense interleukin-8,[93] and antisense telomerase,[94] resulted in sizable anticancer activity in bladder cancer models both in vitro and in vivo. One advantage of bladder cancer gene therapy is the intravesical administration of molecular antagonists, which may improve the efficacy and magnitude of gene delivery and limit undesirable systemic side effects of viral exposure.

FUTURE DIRECTIONS AND CHALLENGES

Although identified only 5 years ago, survivin has generated considerable interest from various viewpoints of biomedical research. The complexity of subcellular localization, the evidence for a dual role in both apoptosis and cell division, and the far-reaching consequences of overexpression in cancer define the existence of a "survivin pathway." Bladder cancer has provided a paradigm for the exploitation of the survivin pathway for early detection and long-term monitoring and has offered some intriguing therapeutic opportunities to interfere locally with the survivin pathway in the transformed urothelium. Clearly, several questions about the basic biology of survivin remain to be answered. From a more translational perspective, the next set of challenges will be to integrate the survivin pathway in the global genetic fingerprinting of cancer patients, including those with bladder cancer, linking individual patterns of gene expression to prediction of clinical outcome and response to therapy. As the survivin pathway continues to gain credentials, the identification of additional critical requisites for apoptosis inhibition or cell division will likely increase and, with that, more options for molecular diagnosis and therapeutic intervention will become available.

ACKNOWLEDGMENTS

This work is dedicated to the memory and spirit of Shannon D. Smith, M.D. This work was supported by NIH Grants CA78810 and CA90917 (D.C.A.) and DK47548 and DK38311 (R.M.W.).

REFERENCES

1. Hengartner MO. The biochemistry of apoptosis. Nature 2000;407:770–776.
2. Hanahan D, Weinberg RA. The hallmarks of cancer. Cell 2000;100:57–70.
3. Ambrosini G, Adida C, Altieri DC. A novel anti-apoptosis gene, survivin, expressed in cancer and lymphoma. Nat Med 1997;3(8):917–921.
4. Ozen H. Bladder cancer. Curr Opin Oncol 1998;10:273–278.
5. Farrow GM. Pathology of carcinoma in situ of the urinary bladder and related lesions. J. Cell Biochem Suppl 1992:39–43.
6. Alexandroff AB, Jackson AM, O'Donnell MA, James K. BCG immunotherapy of bladder cancer: 20 years on. Lancet 1999;353:1689–1694.
7. Brandau S, Bohle A. Bladder cancer: I. Molecular and genetic basis of carcinogenesis. Eur Urol 2001;39(5):491–497.
8. Slaton JW, Benedict WF, Dinney CP. P53 in bladder cancer: mechanism of action, prognostic value, and target for therapy. Urology 2001;57(5):852–859.
9. Przybojewska B, Jagiello A, Jalmuzna P. H-RAS, K-RAS, and N-RAS gene activation in human bladder cancers. Cancer Genet Cytogenet 2000;121(1):73–77.
10. Theodorescu D, Laderoute KR, Gulding KM. Epidermal growth factor receptor-regulated human bladder cancer motility is in part a phosphatidylinositol 3-kinase-mediated process. Cell Growth Differ 1998;9(11):919–928.
11. Cordon-Cardo C. Molecular alterations in bladder cancer. Cancer Surv 1998;32:115–131.
12. Adshead JM, Kessling AM, Ogden CW. Genetic initiation, progression and prognostic markers in transitional cell carcinoma of the bladder: a summary of the structural and transcriptional changes, and the role of developmental genes. Br J Urol 1998;82(4):503–512.
13. Dahse R, Utting M, Werner W et al. Prognostic significance of mutations in the p53 gene in superficial bladder cancer. Oncol Rep 2000;7(5):931–936.
14. Nicholson DW. From bench to clinic with apoptosis-based therapeutic agents. Nature 2000;407: 810–816.

15. Lara PC, Perez S, Rey A, Santana C. Apoptosis in carcinoma of the bladder: relation with radiation treatment results. Int J Radiat Oncol Biol Phys 1999;43:1015–1019.

16. Pollack A, Wu CS, Czerniak B et al. Abnormal bcl-2 and pRb expression are independent correlates of radiation response in muscle-invasive bladder cancer. Clin Cancer Res 1997;3(10):1823–1829.

17. Lipponen PK, Aaltomaa S, Eskelinen M. Expression of the apoptosis suppressing bcl-2 protein in transitional cell bladder tumours. Histopathology 1996;28(2):135–140.

18. Kirsh EJ, Baunoch DA, Stadler WM. Expression of bcl-2 and bcl-X in bladder cancer. J Urol 1998;159(4):1348–1353.

19. Swana HS, Grossman D, Anthony JN et al. Tumor content of the antiapoptosis molecule survivin and recurrence of bladder cancer. N Engl J Med 1999;341(6):452–453.

20. Deveraux QL, Reed JC. IAP family proteins-suppressors of apoptosis. Genes Dev 1999;13(3): 239–252.

21. Thornberry NA, Lazebnik Y. Caspases: enemies within. Science 1998;281:1312–1316.

22. Budihardjo I, Oliver H, Lutter M et al. Biochemical pathways of caspase activation during apoptosis. Annu Rev Cell Dev Biol 1999;15:269–290.

23. Li F, Altieri DC. The cancer antiapoptosis mouse survivin gene: characterization of locus and transcriptional requirements of basal and cell cycle-dependent expression. Cancer Res 1999; 59(13):3143–3151.

24. Verdecia MA, Huang H, Dutil E et al. Structure of the human anti-apoptotic protein survivin reveals a dimeric arrangement. Nat Struct Biol 2000;7(7):602–608.

25. Li F, Ambrosini G, Chu EY et al. Control of apoptosis and mitotic spindle checkpoint by survivin. Nature 1998;396(6711):580–584.

26. Li F, Altieri DC. Transcriptional analysis of human survivin gene expression. Biochem J 1999; 344 Pt 2:305–311.

27. Kobayashi K, Hatano M, Otaki M et al. Expression of a murine homologue of the inhibitor of apoptosis protein is related to cell proliferation. Proc Natl Acad Sci USA 1999;96(4):1457–1462.

28. Zhao J, Tenev T, Martins LM et al. The ubiquitin-proteasome pathway regulates survivin degradation in a cell cycle-dependent manner. J Cell Sci 2000;113(23):4363–4371.

29. Wheatley SP, Carvalho A, Vagnarelli P, Earnshaw WC. INCENP is required for proper targeting of Survivin to the centromeres and the anaphase spindle during mitosis. Curr Biol 2001;11(11): 886–890.

30. Fortugno P, Wall NR, Giodini A et al. Survivin exists in immunochemically distinct subcellular pools and is involved in spindle microtubule function. J Cell Sci 2001;115:575–585.

31. Tamm I, Wang Y, Sausville E et al. IAP-family protein survivin inhibits caspase activity and apoptosis induced by Fas (CD95), Bax, caspases, and anticancer drugs. Cancer Res 1998;58(23): 5315–5320.

32. Mahotka C, Wenzel M, Springer E et al. Survivin-deltaEx3 and survivin-2B: two novel splice variants of the apoptosis inhibitor survivin with different antiapoptotic properties. Cancer Res 1999;59(24):6097–6102.

33. Suzuki A, Ito T, Kawano H et al. Survivin initiates procaspase 3/p21 complex formation as a result of interaction with Cdk4 to resist Fas-mediated cell death. Oncogene 2000;19(10): 1346–1353.

34. Islam A, Kageyama H, Takada N et al. High expression of Survivin, mapped to 17q25, is significantly associated with poor prognostic factors and promotes cell survival in human neuroblastoma. Oncogene 2000;19(5):617–623.

35. Kasof GM, Gomes BC. Livin, a novel inhibitor-of-apoptosis (IAP) family member. J Biol Chem 2001;276:3238–3246.

36. Grossman D, Kim PJ, Blanc-Brude OP et al. Transgenic expression of survivin in keratinocytes counteracts UVB-induced apoptosis and cooperates with loss of p53. J Clin Invest 2001;108: 991–999.

37. Ambrosini G, Adida C, Sirugo G, Altieri DC. Induction of apoptosis and inhibition of cell proliferation by survivin gene targeting. J Biol Chem 1998;273(18):11177–11182.

38. Grossman D, McNiff JM, Li F, Altieri DC. Expression and targeting of the apoptosis inhibitor, survivin, in human melanoma. J Invest Dermatol 1999;113(6):1076–1081.

39. Chen J, Wu W, Tahir SK et al. Down-regulation of survivin by antisense oligonucleotides increases apoptosis, inhibits cytokinesis and anchorage-independent growth. Neoplasia 2000;2(3):235–241.

40. Olie RA, Simoes-Wust AP, Baumann B et al. A novel antisense oligonucleotide targeting survivin expression induces apoptosis and sensitizes lung cancer cells to chemotherapy. Cancer Res 2000; 60(11):2805–2809.

41. Shankar SL, Mani S, O'Guin KN et al. Survivin inhibition induces human neural tumor cell death through caspase-independent and -dependent pathways. J Neurochem 2001;79(2):426–436.

42. Kanwar JR, Shen WP, Kanwar RK et al. Effects of survivin antagonists on growth of established tumors and b7-1 immunogene therapy. J Natl Cancer Inst 2001;93(20):1541–1552.

43. Jones G, Jones D, Zhou L et al. Deterin, a new inhibitor of apoptosis from *Drosophila melanogaster.* J Biol Chem 2000;275(29):22157–22165.

44. Jiang X, Wilford C, Duensing S et al. Participation of Survivin in mitotic and apoptotic activities of normal and tumor-derived cells. J Cell Biochem 2001;83(2):342–354.

45. Shin S, Sung BJ, Cho YS et al. An anti-apoptotic protein human survivin is a direct inhibitor of caspase-3 and -7. Biochemistry 2001;40(4):1117–1123.

46. Huang Y, Park YC, Rich RL et al. Structural basis of caspase inhibition by XIAP: differential roles of the linker versus the BIR domain. Cell 2001;104(5):781–790.

47. Li F, Ackermann EJ, Bennett CF et al. Pleiotropic cell-division defects and apoptosis induced by interference with survivin function. Nat Cell Biol 1999;1(8):461–466.

48. Kallio MJ, Nieminen M, Eriksson JE. Human inhibitor of apoptosis protein (IAP) survivin participates in regulation of chromosome segregation and mitotic exit. FASEB J 2001.

49. Uren AG, Wong L, Pakusch M et al. Survivin and the inner centromere protein INCENP show similar cell-cycle localization and gene knockout phenotype. Curr Biol 2000;10(21):1319–1328.

50. Uren AG, Beilharz T, O'Connell MJ et al. Role for yeast inhibitor of apoptosis (IAP)-like proteins in cell division. Proc Natl Acad Sci USA 1999;96(18):10170–10175.

51. Speliotes EK, Uren A, Vaux D, Horvitz HR. The survivin-like *C. elegans* BIR-1 protein acts with the Aurora-like kinase AIR-2 to affect chromosomes and the spindle midzone. Mol Cell 2000; 6(2):211–223.

52. Adida C, Crotty PL, McGrath J et al. Developmentally regulated expression of the novel cancer anti-apoptosis gene survivin in human and mouse differentiation. Am J Pathol 1998;152(1): 43–49.

53. Carter BZ, Milella M, Altieri DC, Andreeff M. Cytokine-regulated expression of survivin in myeloid leukemia. Blood 2001;97(9):2784–2790.

54. Fukuda S, Pelus LM. Regulation of the inhibitor-of-apoptosis family member survivin in normal cord blood and bone marrow CD34(+) cells by hematopoietic growth factors: implication of survivin expression in normal hematopoiesis. Blood 2001;98(7):2091–2100.

55. Gianani R, Jarboe E, Orlicky D et al. Expression of survivin in normal, hyperplastic, and neoplastic colonic mucosa. Hum Pathol 2001;32(1):119–125.

56. Grossman D, McNiff JM, Li F, Altieri DC. Expression of the apoptosis inhibitor, survivin, in

nonmelanoma skin cancer and gene targeting in a keratinocyte cell line. Lab Invest 1999;79(9): 1121–1126.

57. Monzo M, Rosell R, Felip E et al. A novel anti-apoptosis gene: re-expression of survivin messenger RNA as a prognosis marker in non-small-cell lung cancers. J Clin Oncol 1999;17(7):2100–2104.

58. Tanaka K, Iwamoto S, Gon G et al. Expression of survivin and its relationship to loss of apoptosis in breast carcinomas. Clin Cancer Res 2000;6(1):127–134.

59. Kawasaki H, Altieri DC, Lu CD et al. Inhibition of apoptosis by survivin predicts shorter survival rates in colorectal cancer. Cancer Res 1998;58(22):5071–5074.

60. Lu CD, Altieri DC, Tanigawa N. Expression of a novel antiapoptosis gene, survivin, correlated with tumor cell apoptosis and p53 accumulation in gastric carcinomas. Cancer Res 1998;58(9): 1808–1812.

61. Kato J, Kuwabara Y, Mitani M et al. Expression of survivin in esophageal cancer: correlation with the prognosis and response to chemotherapy. Int J Cancer 2001;95(2):92–95.

62. Satoh K, Kaneko K, Hirota M et al. Expression of survivin is correlated with cancer cell apoptosis and is involved in the development of human pancreatic duct cell tumors. Cancer 2001;92(2): 271–278.

63. Saitoh Y, Yaginuma Y, Ishikawa M. Analysis of Bcl-2, Bax and Survivin genes in uterine cancer. Int J Oncol 1999;15(1):137–141.

64. Yoshida H, Ishiko O, Sumi T et al. Survivin, bcl-2 and matrix metalloproteinase-2 enhance progression of clear cell- and serous-type ovarian carcinomas. Int J Oncol 2001;19(3):537–542.

65. Adida C, Haioun C, Gaulard P et al. Prognostic significance of survivin expression in diffuse large B-cell lymphomas. Blood 2000;96(5):1921–1925.

66. Adida C, Recher C, Raffoux E et al. Expression and prognostic significance of survivin in de novo acute myeloid leukaemia. Br J Haematol 2000;111(1):196–203.

67. Kamihira S, Yamada Y, Hirakata Y et al. Aberrant expression of caspase cascade regulatory genes in adult T-cell leukaemia: survivin is an important determinant for prognosis. Br J Haematol 2001;114(1):63–69.

68. Adida C, Berrebi D, Peuchmaur M et al. Anti-apoptosis gene, survivin, and prognosis of neuroblastoma. Lancet 1998;351(9106):882–883.

69. Kappler M, Kohler T, Kampf C et al. Increased survivin transcript levels: an independent negative predictor of survival in soft tissue sarcoma patients. Int J Cancer 2001;95(6):360–363.

70. Velculescu VE, Madden SL, Zhang L et al. Analysis of human transcriptomes. Nat Genet 1999; 23(4):387–388.

71. Plantaz D, Mohapatra G, Matthay KK et al. Gain of chromosome 17 is the most frequent abnormality detected in neuroblastoma by comparative genomic hybridization. Am J Pathol 1997;150:81–89.

72. Hattori M, Sakamoto H, Satoh K, Yamamoto T. DNA demethylase is expressed in ovarian cancers and the expression correlates with demethylation of CpG sites in the promoter region of c-erbB-2 and survivin genes. Cancer Lett 2001;169(2):155–164.

73. Sarela AI, Scott N, Ramsdale J et al. Immunohistochemical detection of the anti-apoptosis protein, survivin, predicts survival after curative resection of stage II colorectal carcinomas. Ann Surg Oncol 2001;8(4):305–310.

74. Rohayem J, Diestelkoetter P, Weigle B et al. Antibody response to the tumor-associated inhibitor of apoptosis protein survivin in cancer patients. Cancer Res 2000;60(7):1815–1817.

75. Schmitz M, Diestelkoetter P, Weigle B et al. Generation of survivin-specific CD8+ T effector cells by dendritic cells pulsed with protein or selected peptides. Cancer Res 2000;60(17):4845–4849.

76. Andersen MH, Pedersen LO, Becker JC, Straten PT. Identification of a cytotoxic T lymphocyte response to the apoptosis inhibitor protein survivin in cancer patients. Cancer Res 2001;61(3): 869–872.

77. Schneeweiss S, Kriegmair M, Stepp H. Is everything all right if nothing seems wrong? A simple method of assessing the diagnostic value of endoscopic procedures when a gold standard is absent. J Urol 1999;161(4):1116–1119.

78. Brown FM. Urine cytology. It is still the gold standard for screening? Urol Clin North Am 2000; 27(1):25–37.

79. Ramakumar S, Bhuiyan J, Besse JA et al. Comparison of screening methods in the detection of bladder cancer. J Urol 1999;161:388–394.

80. Soloway MS, Briggman V, Carpinito GA et al. Use of a new tumor marker, urinary NMP22, in the detection of occult or rapidly recurring transitional cell carcinoma of the urinary tract following surgical treatment. J Urol 1996;156(2):363–367.

81. Miyanaga N, Akaza H, Tsukamoto T et al. Urinary nuclear matrix protein 22 as a new marker for the screening of urothelial cancer in patients with microscopic hematuria. Int J Urol 1999; 6(4):173–177.

82. Rahat MA, Lahat N, Gazawi H et al. Telomerase activity in patients with transitional cell carcinoma: a preliminary study. Cancer 1999;85:919–924.

83. Steiner G, Schoenberg MP, Linn JF et al. Detection of bladder cancer recurrence by microsatellite analysis of urine. Nat Med 1997;3(6):621–624.

84. Lokeshwar VB, Obek C, Pham HT et al. Urinary hyaluronic acid and hyaluronidase: markers for bladder cancer detection and evaluation of grade. J Urol 2000;163:348–356.

85. Smith SD, Wheeler MA, Plescia J et al. Urine detection of survivin and diagnosis of bladder cancer. JAMA 2001;285(3):324–328.

86. O'Connor DS, Grossman D, Plescia J et al. Regulation of apoptosis at cell division by $p34^{cdc2}$ phosphorylation of survivin. Proc Natl Acad Sci USA 2000;97(24):13103–13107.

87. Grossman D, Kim PJ, Schechner JS, Altieri DC. Inhibition of melanoma tumor growth in vivo by survivin targeting. Proc Natl Acad Sci USA 2001;98(2):635–640.

88. Mesri M, Wall NR, Li J et al. Cancer gene therapy using a survivin mutant adenovirus. J Clin Invest 2001;108:981–990.

89. Pagliaro LC. Gene therapy for bladder cancer. World J Urol 2000;18(2):148–151.

90. Watanabe T, Shinohara N, Sazawa A et al. Adenovirus-mediated gene therapy for bladder cancer in an orthotopic model using a dominant negative H-ras mutant. Int J Cancer 2001;92(5):712–717.

91. Freund CT, Sutton MA, Dang T et al. Adenovirus-mediated combination suicide and cytokine gene therapy for bladder cancer. Anticancer Res 2000;20(3A):1359–1365.

92. Inoue K, Perrotte P, Wood CG et al. Gene therapy of human bladder cancer with adenovirus-mediated antisense basic fibroblast growth factor. Clin Cancer Res 2000;6(11):4422–4431.

93. Inoue K, Wood CG, Slaton JW et al. Adenoviral-mediated gene therapy of human bladder cancer with antisense interleukin-8. Oncol Rep 2001;8(5):955–964.

94. Koga S, Kondo Y, Komata T, Kondo S. Treatment of bladder cancer cells in vitro and in vivo with 2-5A antisense telomerase RNA. Gene Ther 2001;8(8):654–658.

Chapter 6

Imatinib (STI571, Gleevec™) as Therapy to Target the Molecular Pathophysiology of Gastrointestinal Stromal Tumors: A Model for Rational Drug Development

George D. Demetri, MD

Our understanding of the histogenesis, cellular differentiation, and molecular biology of gastrointestinal stromal tumors (GIST), the most common mesenchymal neoplasms of the gastrointestinal tract, has advanced tremendously over the last four years. Key pathologic features of GIST have been described that have been linked to the genetic and molecular features characteristic of the disease. In less than five years, an entirely new understanding of the pathophysiology and molecular basis of GIST has been developed; these insights have fostered the development of effective new therapeutic approaches to the disease. It is critical for clinicians from the fields of oncology, gastroenterology, surgery, pathology, and radiology to understand how quickly this field has evolved and to incorporate this understanding into practice as soon as possible.

BACKGROUND

Insightful pathologists noted the histopathological similarity between a subset of spindle cell tumors of the gastrointestinal tract and the interstitial cells of Cajal as early as 1993.[1] Other pathologists also suspected a relationship of these spindle cell tumors of the GI tract to the myenteric/neural plexus cells and proposed calling these tumors by the rather cumbersome, though logical, name of "GI Pacemaker Cell Tumors."[2] It now appears clear that GISTs are derived from primitive precursor cells in the wall of the gut (and rarely, elsewhere in the body); it is likely that these are the same precursor cells that would ordinarily give rise to the interstitial cells of Cajal. GISTs can occur throughout the digestive system, though they have been noted most commonly in the stomach (60% to 70%), followed by the small intestine (20% to 25%), colon or rectum (5%), and rarely in the esophagus (< 5%).[3] Although the majority of GISTs may *appear* to be benign by conventional criteria of light microscopic histopathology, it is critical to recognize that at least 20%–30% of even the most histopathologically bland-appearing GISTs will ultimately prove malignant in the patient by metastasizing or recurring in an infiltrative, unresectable manner. Pathologists now recognize that even the most histologically "benign" GIST lesions have a risk of recurrence with liver metastases or multifocal unresectable disease; the magnitude of this risk may be correlated with such factors as size of the primary lesion, number of mitoses, etc.[4] In fact, it is unclear whether any specific histopathologic criteria of GIST can reliably predict future biologic behavior.[4,5] Certainly, some GISTs present with histopathologic criteria of a high grade malignancy, such as nuclear atypia, necrosis, etc. The recognition that there probably is no truly "benign" GIST is a new consensus amongst pathogists, and it is probably safer to regard the bland GISTs as possessing uncertain malignant potential, rather than being "benign."

No one would argue that malignant GIST (an entity synonymous with Gastrointestinal Stromal Sarcoma) is associated with significant morbidity and a rapidly fatal course if unresectable. Certainly no cytotoxic chemotherapy or radiotherapy regimen has proven effective in GIST once the disease has gone beyond surgical resectability.[6,7] The median duration of survival for patients with unresectable or metastatic GIST has been reported to be less than 2 years following the diagnosis of metastases.[6,8,9]

This review will summarize recent advances in the pathology, molecular biology, and therapy of GIST, with particular focus on the fast-moving clinical development of imatinib mesylate (previously known as STI571), a selective tyrosine kinase inhibitor that targets the molecular pathogenesis of GIST and that was approved in early 2002 as an effective therapy for patients with advanced unresectable disease.

EVOLUTION OF THE UNDERSTANDING OF GIST PATHOLOGY

Clinical and Pathologic Features

GIST is a disease that can affect patients of any age, although it has been most widely reported in patients in middle age or later. In localized disease, the lesions of GIST tend to be primarily intramural and submucosal, often evading clinical diagnosis until their size impacts GI function, unless they rupture and bleed.[3,7] Similar to other soft tissue sarcomas, GISTs rarely metastasize to locoregional draining lymphatics. The pattern of metastatic spread is characterized by hepatic metastases or multifocal omental tumor implants. Distant extra-abdominal metastases are extremely rare, except in cases of bulky disease, and pulmonary parenchymal metastases are even less common, in contrast to other soft tissue sarcomas such as true leiomyosarcomas, which exhibit high rates of pulmonary metastatic spread.

GISTs are a heterogenous set of diseases that can confuse clinicians by the variety of presentations possible. GIST lesions can be single or multiple (as in the multifocal GISTs that have been reported in Carney's triad); the histology can also be that of a spindle cell neoplasm, an epithelioid cancer, or even a mixed cell type (Fig. 6.1).[7] It has been proposed that at least 30% of GISTs at presentation are clearly malignant, with clear histopathologic features of malignancy or clinical behavior indicative of malignancy (such as intra-abdominal spread or liver metastases at presentation). However, the "benign" appearance of many GISTs at presentation can be highly misleading, and no single histopathologic feature has yet been identified in GIST that can fully predict the course of the disease. One of the most important prognostic factors is definitely the size of the primary lesion, with far better prognosis for lesions < 1 cm in size.[4] More recent data indicate that even these tiny GIST lesions (< 1 cm) have been noted to possess mutations in the *c-kit* gene that are identical to the mutations noted in large, high grade malignant GISTs (J. Fletcher, M. Heinrich, and C. Corless, pers. comm., 2002). This strongly suggests the molecular identity of GISTs regardless of the histopathologic appearance, and it also indicates that mutations of the *c-kit* gene likely represent a very early event in the pathogenesis of GIST. Given this lack of ability to predict with reasonable certainty how any GIST will behave following resection, patients with GIST should be followed closely over the long-term, since even "benign"-appearing tumors can recur and ultimately prove fatal.[4]

Until recently, malignant GIST was often classified as a tumor of smooth muscle derivation, thought to be related to leiomyosarcomas. In the mid-1980s, however,

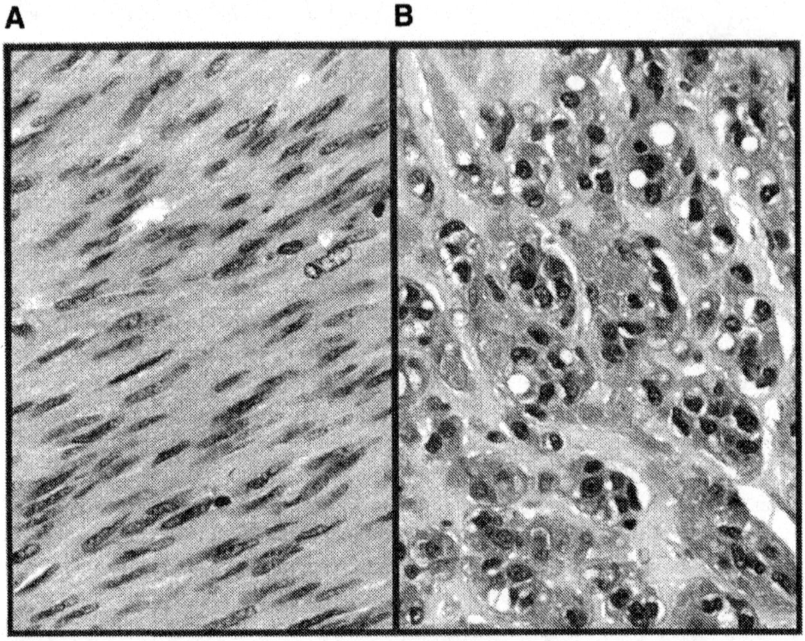

FIGURE 6.1 Variety of histologic appearances of GIST: spindle cell (A) versus epithelioid (B) morphologies. Courtesy of Drs. Brian Rubin and Christopher Fletcher, Department of Pathology, Brigham and Women's Hospital, Harvard Medical School, Boston MA.

electron microscopic studies revealed that GISTs fail to exhibit typical smooth muscle differentiation.[10] GISTs have subsequently been shown to share immunohistochemical and ultrastructural similarities with the interstitial cells of Cajal.[3] The interstitial cells of Cajal—the myenteric complex of "pacemaker cells" responsible for the coordinated peristalsis and movement of the GI tract—has been suggested to be closely related to the histogenesis of GIST, likely by sharing a precursor cell of origin.[1,2,11,12] It is now clear that GIST is a pathogenetically distinct entity and needs to be differentiated from other spindle cell tumors of the GIST tract, such as leiomyosarcomas, true leiomyomas (which occur predominantly in the esophagus, colon, and rectum), or schwannomas (spindle cell tumors that express the S100 antigen and often are benign) (Table 6.1).[3] Some spindle cell tumors of the GI tract, which were previously known by other names, are in fact GISTs. For example, most tumors previously labeled as "leiomyoblastomas" or "gastrointestinal autonomic nerve tumors" (GANT), with modern techniques have in fact been proven to be GISTs. It is only through recent advances in molecular pathology and the more widespread application of diagnostic tools, such as immunohistochemistry for the KIT protein, that it has become possible

TABLE 6.1 Differential diagnoses of GIST (other spindle cell tumors of the abdomen)

Tumor	Differentiating Features
Esophageal leiomyoma	Well-differentiated smooth muscle cells; + for desmin and SMA
Uterine-type leiomyoma	Usually pelvic; + for desmin, SMA and E+, P+ receptors
Leiomyosarcoma	Smooth muscle tumor; + for desmin and SMA; CD117-negative
Inflammatory fibroid polyp	Slender spindle cells, admixed lymphoid cells, and eosinophils
Inflammatory Myofibroblastic Tumor	Children or young adults; expresses ALK
Melanoma	S100+, may mimic the epithelioid GISTs
Mesenteric desmoid	Characteristic pattern of myofibroblasts in collagenous background;
Dedifferentiated liposarcoma	May have lipomatous component or myxoid/ pleomorphic fibrosarcoma-like features;
Schwannoma	Usually small, yellow circumscribed submucosal tumors S100+ spindle cells in S100- fibrous background

Adapted from Ref. 3 with permission.

to distinguish GIST definitively from other spindle cell tumors of the GI tract. The diagnosis of GIST should be made by a pathologist with experience in this area. Specifically, since GIST can exhibit either a spindle cell or epithelioid histology, it is important for pathologists to keep GIST on the list of differential diagnoses of intra-abdominal or pelvic malignancies (Fig. 2). In the proper histologic context, a key diagnostic test for GIST is immunohistochemistry directed at detection of the CD117 antigen, which detects the KIT protein. The CD117 assay, like any immunohistochemical test, should be performed by a laboratory with experience and with proven validated methodology, ideally controlled by standardizing with molecular assays of the KIT protein by immunoblotting. Strong and diffuse expression of the CD117 (KIT) antigen is generally found in the vast majority of GIST tumor cells.[4,7]

KIT Activation and the Molecular Biology of GIST

In 1998, Hirota and colleagues from Osaka, Japan, described an important molecular mechanism that appeared likely to contribute to the pathogenesis of GIST.[13] This was critical to the subsequent development of new therapeutic interventions,

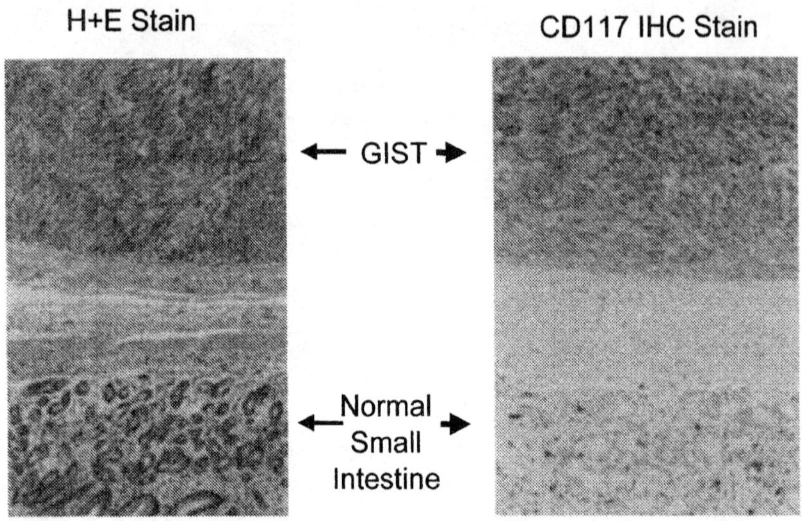

FIGURE 6.2 H+E and anti-CD117 immunohistochemical staining of GIST. The small dark flecks within the small intestine noted by anti-CD117 immunostaining represent normal intestinal mast cells, not metastatic tumor. (Courtesy of Dr. Christopher D.M. Fletcher, Department of Pathology, Brigham and Women's Hospital and Dana-Farber Cancer Institute, Harvard Medical School, Boston, MA).

since it identified KIT tyrosine kinase signal transduction as a potential target by which one might be able to interrupt the proliferation and accumulation of GIST cells.[13] Sequencing of the c-*kit* proto-oncogene revealed mutations in five human GIST specimens. The authors observed that in the presence of these mutations, the corresponding KIT protein was activated even in the absence of the physiologic ligand of KIT (stem cell factor). The logical connection was completed by their mechanistic studies, which showed that transfection and expression of these mutant variants of KIT induced malignant transformation of murine cells and caused uncontrolled tumor growth in nude mice. More recently, the group of Rubin and Fletcher at Harvard reported that 100% of human GIST cells studied exhibited constitutive phosphorylation of the KIT protein, independent of ligand regardless of whether c-*kit* mutations were detected.[14]

Today, GIST is generally defined as a spindle cell or epithelioid mesenchymal tumor of the gastrointestinal tract with constitutive phosphorylation of the KIT protein. The simplest surrogate marker for GIST has been positive immunohistochemical detection of the CD117 antigen (KIT), recognizing that this must be noted in the proper histopathologic context.[4,7] Approximately 70% of GISTs are also positive for expression of CD34, 20% to 30% are positive for smooth muscle actin, 10% for S100 protein, and < 5% for desmin. The specific genetic mutations characterizing GIST have been described as being highly variable between GIST lesions from different individuals. Often these mutations represent small in-frame deletions that maintain an intact reading frame, but point mutations leading to amino acid substitutions are also noted commonly. The experience of Fletcher and Heinrich has shown that an individual GIST generally possesses only a single mutation in the c-*kit* gene, and that the specific mutation will vary greatly between GISTs from different patients (J. Fletcher, M. Heinrich, pers. comm. 2002). The most frequently noted mutations of c-*kit* have clustered within exon 11 (thereby affecting the juxtamembrane domain of the KIT protein); however, mutations in exon 9, exon 13, exon 17, or even other loci have been described.[14-16] The structural biology of these different mutations in the KIT gene is beginning to be elucidated, and there is a great deal of research ongoing to understand how these minor structural changes in KIT protein lead to constitutive activation. Cytogenetic analyses of GISTs often show a normal karyotype. However, it is not uncommon for GISTs to possess losses in 14q and 22q; these chromosomal changes appear unrelated to whether the GISTs have exhibited either benign or malignant clinical courses. Aneuploidy is noted in some GISTs with more obviously malignant histopathologic features, often with several extra copies of chromosomes.[3] Overall, although complex molecular changes can be a feature of certain high-grade malignant GISTs, the majority of molecular and cytogenetic evidence points to GIST as a disease in which a single critical signaling pathway (KIT) goes awry early in the pathogenesis of the neoplasm. The current hypothesis is that activation of KIT is the event that is fundamental to the pathogenesis of GIST. While other distinct molecular aberrations probably develop over time, the crucial dependence upon the uncontrolled KIT signaling is an important characteristic of GIST. This understanding of the molecular pathophysiology of the disease made GIST an ideal candidate in which to test the activity of a selective signal transduction inhibitor.

Understanding Signal Transduction Pathways and Changes in the Management of GIST

The identification of critical molecular biologic aberrancies in GIST and the elucidation of their relationship to signal transduction pathways generated a new focus for targeted therapeutic research. The initial preclinical data were further supported with the report of a Japanese family that manifested an autosomal dominant pattern of GISTs and shared a germline mutation in the locus for c-*kit*, further linking genetic mutations, KIT signal transduction, and pathogenesis of GIST in humans.[17] Based on this substantial understanding of their molecular pathophysiology, sarcomas such as GIST represent highly informative proof-of-concept models for cancer research.

Concurrent with the advances in the molecular understanding of GIST, other advances were being made in leukemia research that would soon come to have direct relevance to GIST. Dr. Brian Druker reasoned that the uncontrolled tyrosine kinase activity of the BCR-ABL chimeric oncoprotein of chronic myelogenous leukemia (CML) was likely pathogenetically critical for the development and maintenance of the leukemia in humans; this conclusion was based on many years of elegant research since the 1960s, ranging from the identification of the Philadelphia chromosome, the later identification of the BCR-ABL chimera as an uncontrolled tyrosine kinase, and the neoplasia induced by BCR-ABL in mouse model systems. Dr. Druker and colleagues screened a panel of small molecules of the 2-phenylaminopyrimidine class and identified a potent inhibitor of Bcr-Abl kinase activity in vitro.[18] In subsequent preclinical studies, this compound called STI571 (shorthand for "Signal Transduction Inhibitor 571," now known by the generic name of imatinib mesylate, or by the trade names of Gleevec™ in the USA and Glivec® in the rest of the world) (Fig. 6.3) was noted to selectively inhibit the Bcr-Abl tyrosine kinase, leading to reduction in leukemic cell proliferation and inhibition of tumor formation associated with Bcr-Abl positive cells.[18-20] By 1999, the first results from the use of this signal transduction inhibitor as anticancer therapy of chronic myelogenous leukemia were reported to an enthusiastic audience at the American Society of Hematology annual meeting by Dr. Druker. The inhibitory activity of imatinib was highly selective and did not broadly affect kinases that functioned in normal cell growth and proliferation. These early clinical trials of imatinib in CML patients found that the drug was impressively safe, causing only mild to moderate nausea, myalgia, edema, and diarrhea, while inducing complete hematologic response in 53 of 54 patients with CML treated at daily oral doses of 300 mg or greater.[21]

Further laboratory evaluation by Dr. Druker in Oregon and colleagues at Novartis Pharmaceutical Corporation in Switzerland demonstrated that imatinib

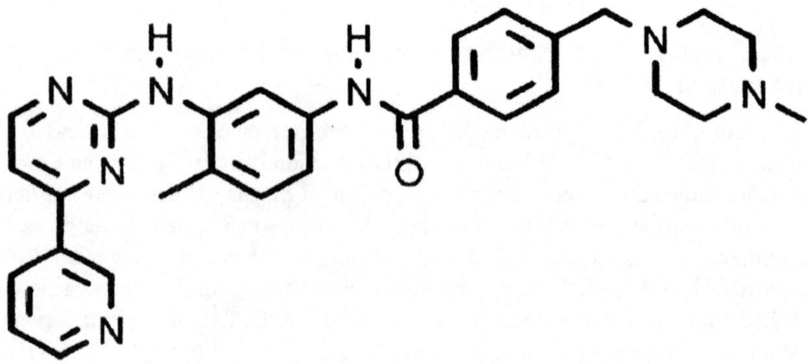

FIGURE 6.3 Chemical structure of STI571, now called imatinib mesylate, trade names Gleevec™ or Glivec®. The chemical is (4-[(4-methyl-1-piperazinyl)methyl]-N-[4-methyl-3-[{4-(3-pyridinyl)-2-pyrimidinyl}amino] phenyl] benzamide methanesulfonate (see Ref. 32).

was selective, but not totally specific, for Bcr-Abl or the Abl class of tyrosine kinases. Imatinib was found also to block the tyrosine kinase activity of two other receptors: KIT and the platelet-derived growth factor receptor (PDGF-R). Importantly, Heinrich and colleagues at the Oregon Cancer Institute reported that the imatinib could inhibit both the wild type (non-mutated) and several different mutated versions of KIT.[22] Heinrich and colleagues studied the in vitro inhibitory effects of imatinib on the human myeloid leukemia cell line, M-07C, expressing KIT.[22] In these preclinical studies, imatinib was found to decrease KIT autophosphorylation and inhibit KIT-dependent cellular proliferation, without inhibiting other signaling pathways (such as the GM-CSF receptor-dependent proliferation that characterizes this cell line). Heinrich also noted that certain human mast cell lines could not be inhibited by imatinib despite the fact that these cells had demonstrable expression of mutated KIT proteins. The KIT mutations in the mast cell leukemia cell lines involved exon 17, which encodes the kinase domain of the enzyme. This was predicted to be the actual binding site of imatinib, and it was likely that the exon 17 mutation led to structural changes that prevented functional binding of the drug to the KIT protein. These data further strengthened the mechanistic link between the tyrosine kinase inhibition of imatinib and the anticancer activity of this agent.

The efficacy of the compound in blocking cellular proliferation in hematologic malignancies, however, did not necessarily predict similar behavior in a solid tumor. Preclinical evidence specific to GIST came from Tuveson et al,[16] who reported that addition of imatinib to cell cultures of human GIST with known activating KIT mutations abolished the constitutive tyrosine phosphorylation of KIT, stopped cellular proliferation, and ultimately induced apoptosis of GIST cells.[16] These results, in conjunction with the prior work identifying KIT as a critical pathogenic factor in GIST and the exploration by Dr. Druker of imatinib in hematologic malignancies, provided a scientific rationale that was more than sufficient to justify the testing of imatinib in the clinical management of patients with advanced GIST.

CLINICAL EXPERIENCE USING IMATINIB IN THE TREATMENT OF GIST

The clinical activity of imatinib in advanced GIST was quickly shown to be exceptional, beginning with the first patient who received this agent for this disease. A 50-year-old Finnish woman presented with progressive, life-threatening, multiply recurrent, widely metastatic, unresectable GIST that had failed all prior attempts at therapy, including multiple surgical resections, combination chemotherapy, and even an attempt at investigational anti-angiogenic therapy. The patient's GIST had been analyzed and was shown to express a deletion in exon 11 of the c-*kit* gene, which is a relatively common mutation leading to activation of the KIT tyrosine kinase activity. Beginning in March 2000, the patient received imatinib orally at the dose of 400 mg daily, continuously for 11 months at the time of the first report.[23] Prior to the start of imatinib therapy, the summed cross-sectional measurement of eight hepatic GIST metastases totaled more than 112 cm^2. Subsequent MRI scans during treatment revealed rapid and sustained tumor regression of 28 liver metastases, including complete elimination of six (Fig. 6.4). Serial needle biopsy specimens of a metastatic lesion within the liver revealed a markedly reduced density of viable tumor cells with myxoid degeneration and scarring, consistent with the anticancer effect shown on the imaging studies. Complete metabolic response in the tumors was apparent on PET scan, as evidenced by rapid decrease in tumor-related accumulation of ^{18}FDG (fluorodeoxyglucose) in all sites of metastatic disease. The patient's performance status also improved from 1 to 0, demonstrating the clinical benefits suggested by these imaging and pathology studies. Toxicity was minimal, comprised only of some mild dyspepsia and minimal increased frequency of bowel movements. The positive response has continued for more than 21 months (H. Joensuu, pers. comm., 2002).

Therefore, all the pieces were in place to foster a rapid clinical development plan to prove the worth of this agent for patients with GIST. The compelling scientific rationale was supported by preclinical tests on GIST cells as well as by this dramatic and sustained response in the first GIST patient. By July 2000, a multicenter, dose-randomized clinical trial was initiated to assess the safety, efficacy, and biologic activity of two different doses of imatinib given orally to adult patients with unresectable and/or metastatic malignant GIST expressing CD117.[24] All patients had previously failed conventional therapy including surgery, chemotherapy, and/or radiotherapy. One hundred forty-seven patients enrolled in the study were randomly assigned to receive either 400 or 600 mg imatinib daily. These dose levels were chosen by extrapolating from the pharmacologic profile of imatinib that had been described in CML patients[24] and estimating the systemic

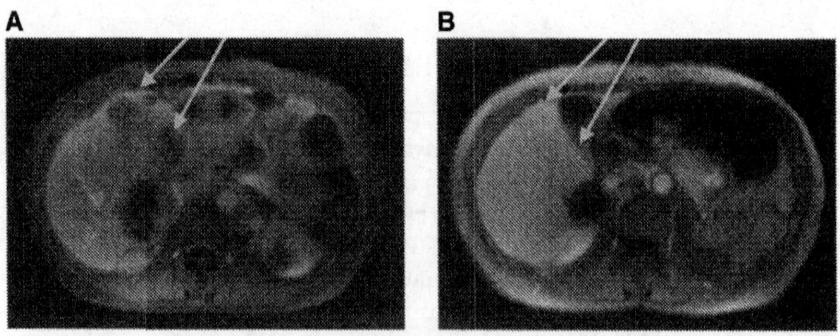

FIGURE 6.4 Serial MRI scans from a 50-year-old patient with GIST. Primary tumor regressed substantially. Panels A and B show MRI scans of the liver that demonstrate the dramatic effects of imatinib therapy (A, before therapy; B, after 4 weeks of therapy).

concentrations that would be needed to inhibit the KIT target in GIST. Early results from this trial have confirmed the overall good tolerability and efficacy of imatinib in treating patients with advanced GIST.[25] The most serious adverse event was gastrointestinal or intra-abdominal hemorrhage, which occurred in approximately 5% of patients (primarily those with large bulky tumors). This was perhaps related to the rapid anticancer effect on the tumors, with disruption of tumor-related vasculature. However, since bleeding from advanced GIST is a well-recognized complication of the natural history of this disease, it is not possible to assess what proportion of the bleeding events were due to drug therapy versus those that may have occured simply related to the natural history of such far-advanced, bulky tumors. The impact of imatinib on tumor metabolism was also demonstrated as a rapid and dramatic decrease in ^{18}FDG glycolytic activity on PET scans (Figs. 6.5 and 6.6).[26] The functional imaging with PET scans was highly predictive of subsequent anatomic response by conventional imaging with CT or MRI scanning.

The objective responses to imatinib were measured by standard oncologic criteria defining tumor regression. Specifically, partial response was defined strictly as patients who exhibited a 50% or greater decrease in the summed area of all measurable tumors. The initial presentation of this trial at the ASCO plenary session in May 2001 included only a subset of 86 patients who were evaluable for response at the time of the meeting. Objective partial responses were noted in 50 of 86 patients (59% rate of PR), while an additional 22 patients (26%) had stable disease. In a subset of patients, very rapid tumor shrinkage (within one month) was noted. However, it was not uncommon to for objective partial responses to evolve slowly in other patients (e.g., over 4 to 6 months after starting therapy with imatinib). No evidence of tumor lysis syndrome was noted in this trial. There was a small subset of patients with primary resistance to imatinib, whose disease failed to exhibit response on PET or CT scanning. This was estimated to be approximately 15% of the population in this trial

Tumor biopsies were performed before and after imatinib treatment in a subset of consenting patients. Some of the post-treatment biopsies confirmed the diffuse myxoid tumor degeneration and fibrosis, without disturbance of intratumoral vascular architecture, which had previously been noted in the first GIST patient treated with imatinib.[23]

Overall, the results of this multicenter trial indicated that imatinib was acceptably well-tolerated, with consistent bioavailability of the drug when administered orally despite the significantly compromised GI tract anatomy in many of the patients who had undergone extensive surgery in the past. Although the trial was not designed to have adequate power to assess dose-related differences, no statistically significant differences were noted between these two dose levels of imatinib. Identification of the optimally effective dose of imatinib for the treatment of GIST is the subject of much larger, appropriately powered randomized studies now ongoing.

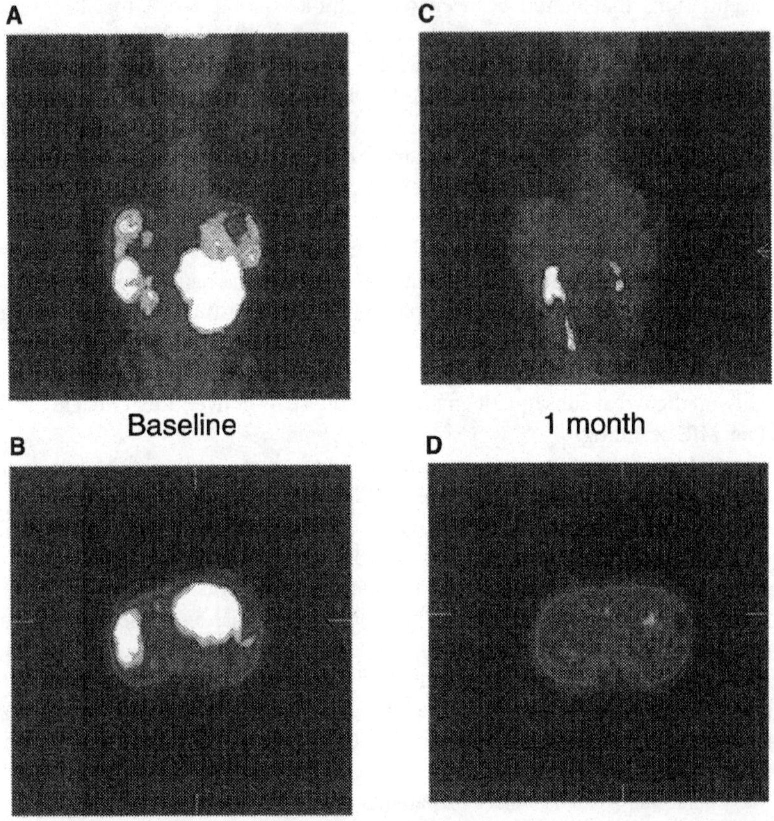

FIGURE 6.5 Impact of imatinib treatment on ^{18}FDG-PET scans of a patient with advanced GIST. Panels A and B are baseline before therapy, while Panels C and D represent scans one month after imatinib was begun. Note disappearance of abnormal tumor-associated glycolytic activity. Uptake in Panel C is physiologic (imaging of the renal collecting system).

These data were corroborated by another trial performed by a subset of the investigators from the Sarcoma Group of the European Organization for the Research and Treatment of Cancer (EORTC), also reported at the plenary session of the American Society of Clinical Oncology in 2001.[27] In this Phase I dose escalation study, 40 patients were entered, 36 of whom had GIST. Doses ranged from 400 to 1000 mg daily, with unacceptable toxicities reported at the highest dose level, consisting mainly of edema (including third-spacing of fluids with dyspnea), nausea, and vomiting. Of the 36 patients with GIST, 19 exhibited objective partial responses (53%) while another 13 had stable disease (36%). These results from the European multicenter study were remarkably consistent with the outcomes observed in the larger US-Finland trial noted above.

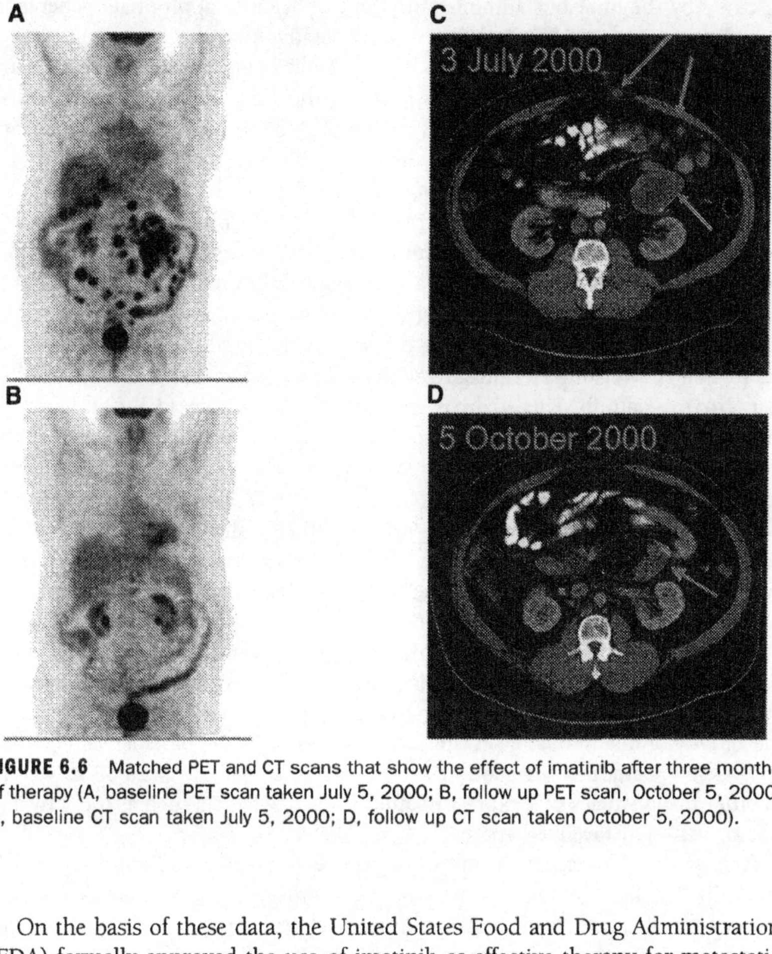

FIGURE 6.6 Matched PET and CT scans that show the effect of imatinib after three months of therapy (A, baseline PET scan taken July 5, 2000; B, follow up PET scan, October 5, 2000; C, baseline CT scan taken July 5, 2000; D, follow up CT scan taken October 5, 2000).

On the basis of these data, the United States Food and Drug Administration (FDA) formally approved the use of imatinib as effective therapy for metastatic or unresectable GIST on February 1, 2002. This approved indication makes imatinib the first systemic therapy to show consistent efficacy against this disease.

NEXT STEPS AND FUTURE DIRECTIONS

Given the extraordinary activity of imatinib in inducing objective responses and clinical benefit in patients with advanced unresectable and metastatic GIST, the logical next step is to explore the use of this active agent earlier in the course of the disease. Clinical trials have now been started to evaluate whether the use of imatinib in the post-surgical adjuvant setting will improve clinical outcomes such as disease-free survival or overall survival. It is hoped that more patients might be cured by the judicious administration of this agent to appropriate patients in the adjuvant setting. However, it is also imperative that this be evaluated in a rigorously designed, prospective, placebo-controlled clinical trial. These trials are currently in progress under the auspices of the US Sarcoma Intergroup and the Sarcoma Committee of the American College of Surgeons Oncology Group. Physicians should refer appropriately to ensure rapid accrual so that the answers may be known to these important questions.

Another question is whether the pre-operative use of imatinib might help to minimize the morbidities and maximize the effectiveness of surgery for GIST. This question is being addressed by a new trial being conducted by the Sarcoma Intergroup and the Sarcoma Working Group of the Radiation Therapy Oncology Group. The importance of this trial is that it provides an ideal chance to continue the research correlating PET imaging with molecular and clinical markers of GIST response to imatinib. This trial has an important correlative PET scan objective that is being funded by the US National Cancer Institute to explore further the use of PET scanning as an important surrogate marker of functional response to therapy in GIST (Figs. 6.5 and 6.6).

Other studies are also evaluating whether other malignancies could possibly be driven by target signaling pathways that might be sensitive to imatinib inhibition. For example, it is clear that the chromosomal translocation characterizing dermatofibrosarcoma protuberans (DFSP) leads to autocrine activation of the PDGF receptor pathway, and that this is one mechanism that stimulates the aberrant growth of this mesenchymal tumor. Since imatinib inhibits signaling through the PDGF receptor, this is an intriguing next-generation target to explore the activity of imatinib, and preclinical studies support the possible value of this approach.[28] Clinical studies are in progress to test imatinib in DFSP as well as in other malignancies that express imatinib-sensitive targets such as the activated KIT or activated PDGF receptors.

The ability of imatinib to induce objective responses that are durable and clinically beneficial for GIST patients has been proven beyond a doubt. However, the history of cancer medicine should keep us humble about the prospects for long-term cures in patients with far-advanced GIST. For most advanced or metastatic solid tumors, control of disease is transient even in patients whose disease is controlled or in complete remission due to chemotherapy. The likelihood of the emergence of acquired resistance to imatinib is very real, and GIST patients receiving this agent require vigilant follow-up. The advantage of a targeted therapy, however, is that any sort of resistance can be evaluated at a molecular level, as has already been done for CML in the laboratory of Dr. Charles Sawyers.[29] The knowledge gained from such rational analyses of any resistance will be critical to developing future effective agents targeting the fundamental signals that drive this malignancy. Additionally, the evaluation of these pathways should eventually provide us with the toolbox needed to take apart the more complex challenges of more common solid tumors such as breast cancer, prostate cancer, colorectal cancer, or lung cancer.

SUMMARY AND CONCLUSIONS

The identification and testing of imatinib as therapy for GIST represents an important and practical case study of rational drug development. It is a paradigm of how the molecular understanding of a cancer has resulted in more accurate diagnoses and, ultimately, to an effective and novel therapy that targets the critical pathway upon which the GIST cells were dependent: the uncontrollably active KIT signaling pathway. Histopathologists first noted that GISTs shared some interesting similarities with the interstitial cells of Cajal, and later Hirota and colleagues identified the frequent gain-of-function mutations in the c-*kit* gene encoding the KIT receptor tyrosine kinase.[13] Genotyping of the c-*kit* gene with a variety of highly sensitive techniques has confirmed the high prevalence of mutations in this gene and has identified mutations in the juxtamembrane domain encoded by exon 11 as the predominant sites of KIT mutation,[3,13-15] although other loci encoding the extracellular, kinase, and separate portions of the juxtamembrane domains have been reported as well.[15,30-32] All of these mutations have been associated with ligand-independent activation (phosphorylation) of the KIT tyrosine kinase, leading to subsequent uncontrolled cellular proliferation and blocking apoptosis.

Unresectable or metastatic GISTs have traditionally exhibited a rapid and inexorably fatal clinical course, with no evidence of benefit from any standard cytotoxic chemotherapy. No specific histologic criteria have been identified to predict accurately the clinical behavior of resectable primary GIST, although a subset of high-grade GISTs can be identified that are at particularly high risk for subsequent recurrence and metastasis. There is consensus that adverse prognostic features include larger tumor size (> 5 cm), higher mitotic activity (> 1-5 per 10 high-powered field), and locoregional infiltration or frank metastases at presentation.[4] The identification of KIT activation as an apparent early event in GIST pathogenesis led to the search for a new type of therapeutic compound to serve as a 'KIT inhibitor' and to interfere with the autophosphorylation related to specific activating mutations, thereby inhibiting malignant tissue growth.[33] Clarification of the molecular genetic pathophysiology of GIST and the role of KIT activation in this disease, therefore, has enabled not only improved diagnosis and differentiation of GIST from other mesenchymal neoplasms, but has also been key in identifying new targeted strategies for therapeutic intervention.

Imatinib mesylate (formerly known as STI571) is a selective inhibitor of certain tyrosine kinases that was first recognized as a potent blocker of the oncogenic Bcr-Abl kinase responsible for chronic myeloid leukemia. Subsequently, imatinib was also found to inhibit the KIT receptor tyrosine kinase. Putting this finding to clinical use, Joensuu and collaborators described the exceptional rapid and sustained response of GIST in a patient with far-advanced, rapidly progressive, chemotherapy-resistant disease.[23] Based on the strong scientific and mechanistic rationale for KIT inhibition and the promising experience in that first GIST patient, our global collaborative research team undertook a large multicenter trial to explore more fully the activity of imatinib as treatment for metastatic or unresectable GIST. Our results show that the targeted treatment of GIST with imatinib produces major objective clinical responses in the majority of patients.[24] The rapid regressions noted in many patients has been striking, in view of the traditionally chemotherapy-resistant nature of GIST. These successes were particularly exciting given that improvements have occurred even in patients with far-advanced, bulky disease as well as in patients who had previously failed multiple courses of conventional cytotoxic chemotherapies.

In summary, the improved understanding of the molecular pathophysiology of GIST, a disease which was previously untreatable with any available systemic therapy, has led to the application and testing of imatinib, a well-tolerated agent that can inhibit the dysregulated KIT signaling pathways in GIST. Molecularly-targeted therapy with imatinib—a selective inhibitor of the KIT receptor tyrosine kinase—has been shown to successfully block the proliferation and growth of GIST tumor cells in patients whose disease was uncontrollable with any standard chemotherapy. Imatinib represents the first, and currently the only, highly effective systemic therapy for patients with unresectable GIST. Imatinib therapy can induce objective responses, stabilization of disease, and clinical benefit in the majority of GIST patients treated with the drug. Furthermore, our understanding of its mechanism of action represents a model for further research on signal transduction in the pathogenesis of cancer. Although resistance to single agent therapy is distressingly common in oncology, the durability of the responses to imatinib in GIST is highly encouraging, and the analysis of potential resistance mechanisms will likely lead to even more sophisticated options for therapy in the future. Combinations utilizing targeted signaling inhibitors are clearly destined for use as alternatives or additions to standard treatment regimens in cancer medicine. Other strategies are just beginning to be explored, such as the use of imatinib earlier the in course of GIST, such as as adjuvant therapy after definitive surgical resection of early-stage disease. Integration of signal transduction inhibitors into the armamentarium of cancer therapeutics will continue based on this important paradigm of GIST. It is a model that will be informative for the development of other targeted signal transduction inhibitors in cancer.

REFERENCES

1. Perez-Atayde AR, Shamberger RC, Kozakewich HW. Neuroectodermal differentiation of the gastrointestinal tumors in the Carney triad. An ultrastructural and immunohistochemical study. Am J Surg Path 1993;17:706–714.

2. Kindblom JM. Gastrointestinal pacemaker cell tumor (GIPACT): gastrointestinal stromal tumors show phenotypic characteristics of the interstitial cells of Cajal. Am J Pathol 1998;153:2008–2011.
3. Miettinen M, Lasota J. Gastrointestinal stromal tumors: definition, clinical, histological, immunohistochemical, and molecular genetic features and differential diagnosis. Virchows Arch 2001; 438:1–12.
4. Fletcher CDM, Berman JJ, Corless C et al. Diagnosis of GISTs: A consensus approach. Human Pathol 2002 (in press).
5. Graadt van Roggen JF, van Velthuysen ML, Hogendoorn PC. The histopathological differential diagnosis of gastrointesting stromal tumours. J Clin Pathol 2001;54:96–102.
6. DeMatteo RP, Heinrich MC, El-Rifai WM, Demetri GD. Clinical management of gastrointestinal stromal tumor: Before and after STI571. Human Pathol 2002 (in press).
7. Berman J, O'Leary TJ. Gastrointestinal stromal tumor workshop. Human Pathol 2001;32:578-82
8. Goss GA, Merriam P, Manola J et al. Clinical and pathological characteristics of gastrointestinal stromal tumors (GIST) [abstract]. Proc ASCO 2000;19:559a.
9. DeMatteo RP, Lewis JJ, Leung D et al. Two hundred gastrointestinal stromal tumors: recurrence patterns and prognostic factors for survival. Ann Surg 2000;231:51–58.
10. Walker P, Dvorsk AM. Gastrointestinal autonomic nerve (GAN) tumor: ultrastructural evidence for a newly recognized entity. Arch Pathol Lab Med 1986;110:309–316.
11. Kluppel M, Huizinga JD, Malysz J, Bernstein A. Developmental origin and Kit-dependent development of the interstitial cells of Cajal in the mammalian small intestine. Dev Dyn 1998;211:60–71.
12. Sircar K, Hewlett BR, Huizinga JD et al. Interstitial cells of Cajal as precursors of gastrointestinal stromal tumors. Am J Surg Pathol 1999;23:377–389.
13. Hirota S, Isozaki K, Moriyama Y et al. Gain-of-function mutations of c-kit in human gastrointestinal stromal tumors. Science 1998;279(5350):577–580.
14. Rubin BP, Singer S, Tsao C et al. KIT activation is a ubiquitous feature of gastrointestinal stromal tumors. Cancer Res 2001;61:8118–8121.
15. Lux ML, Rubin BP, Blasé TL et al. KIT extracellular and kinase domain mutations in gastrointestinal stromal tumors. Am J Pathol 2000;156:791–795.
16. Tuveson DA, Willis NA, Jacks T et al. STI571 inactivation of the gastrointestinal stromal tumor c-KIT oncoprotein: biological and clinical implications. Oncogene 2001;20:5054–5058.
17. Nishida T, Hirota S, Taniguchi M et al. Familial gastrointestinal stromal tumours with germline mutation of the KIT gene. Nat Genet 1998;19:323–324.
18. Druker BJ, Tamura S, Buchdunger E et al. Effects of a selective inhibitor of the Abl tyrosine kinase on the growth of Bcr-Abl positive cells. Nat Med 1996;2:561–566.
19. Buchdunger E, Zimmermann J, Mett H et al. Alteration of the Abl protein-tyrosine kinase in vitro and in vivo by a 2-phenylaminopyrimidine derivative. Cancer Res 1996;56:100–104.
20. Carroll M, Ohno-Jones S, Tamura S et al. 57148, a tyrosine kinase inhibitor, inhibits the growth of cells expressing BCR-ABL, TEL-ABL, and TEL-PDGFR fusion proteins. Blood 1997;90:4947–4952.
21. Druker BJ, Talpaz M, Resta DJ et al. Efficacy and safety of a specific inhibitor of the BCR-ABL tyrosine kinase in chronic myeloid leukemia. N Engl J Med 2001;344:1031–1037.
22. Heinrich MC, Griffith DJ, Druker BJ et al. Inhibition of c-kit receptor tyrosine kinase activity by STI 571, a selective tyrosine kinase inhibitor. Blood 2000;95:925–932.
23. Joensuu H, Roberts PJ, Sarlomo-Rikala M et al Effect of the tyrosine kinase inhibitor STI571 in a patient with a metastatic gastrointestinal stromal tumor. N Engl J Med 2001;344:1052–1056.
24. Demetri GD, Von Mehren M, Blanke CD. Antitumor effects of an oral selective tyrosine kinase inhibitor, imatinib mesylate, in patients with advanced gastrointestinal stromal tumors. Manuscript submitted, 2002

25. Blanke CD, von Mehren M, Joensuu H et al. Evaluation of the safety and efficacy of an oral molecularly-targeted therapy, STI571, in patients with unresectable or metastatic gastrointestinal stromal tumors (GISTs). Proc Am Soc Clin Oncol 2001;20:1.

26. van den Abbeele AD, for the GIST Collaborative PET Study Group. F18-FDG-PET provides early evidence of biological response to STI571 in patients with malignant gastrointestinal stromal tumors (GIST). Proc Am Soc Clin Oncol 2001;20:1444.

27. van Oosterom AT, Judson I, Verweij J et al. Safety and efficacy of imatinib (STI571) in metastatic gastrointestinal stromal tumours: a phase I study. Lancet 2001;358:1421–1423.

28. Sjoblom T, Shimizu A, O'Brien KP et al. Growth inhibition of dermatofibrosarcoma protuberans tumors by the platelet-derived growth factor receptor antagonist STI571 through induction of apoptosis. Cancer Res 2001;61:5778–5783.

29. Gorre ME, Mohammed M, Ellwood K et al. Clinical resistance to STI-571 cancer therapy caused by BCR-ABL gene mutation or amplification. Science 2001;293(5531):876–880 [comment in Science 2001;293(5538):2163].

30. Nakahara M, Isozaki K, Hirota S et al. A novel gain-of-function mutation of c-kit gene in gastrointestinal stromal tumors. Gastroenterology 1998;115:1090–1095.

31. Kitamura Y, Hirota S, Nishida T. Molecular pathology of c-kit proto-oncogene and development of gastrointestinal stromal tumors. Ann Chir Gyn 1998;87:282–286.

32. Rubin BP, Singer S, Tsao C et al. KIT activation is a ubiquitous feature of gastrointestinal stromal tumors. Cancer Res 2001;61:8118–8121.

33. Longley BJ, Reguera MJ, Ma Y. Classes of cc-KIT activating mutations: proposed mechanisms of action and implications for disease classification and therapy. Leuk Res 2001;25:571–576.

Chapter 7

Epidermal Growth Factor Receptor Blockade and the Treatment of Solid Tumor Malignancies

Renier Brentjens

Leonard Saltz

The epidermal growth factor receptor (EGFr), also called *ErbB1* or *HER1*, is a member of the EGF receptor family of tyrosine kinase receptors that includes ErbB2 (HER2/neu), ErbB3 (HER3), and ErbB4 (HER4).[1,2] EGFr is a 170-kDa polypeptide composed of an extracellular ligand-binding domain, a hydrophobic membrane–anchoring region, and a cytoplasmic domain that contains a protein tyrosine kinase.[3]

EGFr was initially described by Cohen et al[4] in 1980 as the receptor for epidermal growth factor (EGF), isolated 18 years earlier.[5] To date, six ligands that have been identified bind EGFr.[2,6,7] Most prominent among these are EGF and transforming growth factor alpha (TGF-α). On binding to ligand, the EGFr molecule forms dimers, either homodimers formed by binding with other EGFr molecules or heterodimers formed by binding with other members of the EGF receptor family, most commonly ErbB2. Formation of EGFr dimers results in activation by autophosphorylation of the cytoplasmic protein tyrosine kinase.[3,8]

Activation of the EGFr protein tyrosine kinase results in the phosphorylation of downstream substrates of several mitogenic signaling pathways leading to cellular proliferation. Specifically, activation of EGFr results in signaling through the Ras-Raf-MAP-kinase pathway and through the PI-3-kinase pathway.[1,6,8,9] The latter leads to activation of Akt, resulting in antiapoptotic signaling, enhanced expression of G_1 cyclins, and down-regulation of the cyclin-dependent kinase inhibitor $p27^{Kip1}$.[2,10]

At least three significant findings have prompted researchers to investigate EGFr as a potential target for cancer therapy. First, the EGFr trans-membrane and cytoplasmic domains were found to be homologous to v-*erb-B*, a retroviral oncogene initially identified in the avian erythroblastosis virus.[11–13] The EGFr gene is, therefore, considered a cellular proto-oncogene. Second, EGFr is overexpressed in a wide variety of human cancers.[14] This overexpression is correlated to a more aggressive tumor phenotype with an overall poorer prognosis.[2,7,15] Finally, many tumors that overexpress EGFr coexpress the EGFr ligand TGF-α.[7,16–18] Coexpression of both EGFr and TGF-α obviates the requirement of tumor cells for exogenous growth factors and results in an autocrine loop of tumor cell mitogenic stimulation.

In light of these findings, it was postulated that by blocking the interaction of ligand to the EGFr receptor, one could abrogate the uncontrolled growth of malignant cells. The validity of this hypothesis has been most extensively studied using monoclonal antibodies (mAbs) targeting the extracellular ligand-binding region of EGFr. More recently, agents targeting the cytoplasmic tyrosine kinase domain have also been developed. In this chapter, we discuss preclinical studies that describe some of the mechanisms of EGFr-targeted therapy and update the current status of clinical trials of EGFr-targeted therapy in solid tumor malignancies.

PRECLINICAL STUDIES

EGFr Blockade: Monoclonal Antibodies

In 1983, Kawamoto et al[19] initially reported the development of mouse mAbs specific to human EGFr derived from the vulvar carcinoma cell line A431. Two mAbs, 225 and 528, were found to bind the EGF receptor at affinities comparable to the natural ligands EGF and TNF-α.[19–21] These mAbs block the binding of ligand to EGFr, resulting in the inhibition of receptor tyrosine kinase phosphorylation leading to a G_1 phase arrest and subsequent inhibition of tumor cell proliferation.

Van de Vijver et al[22] subsequently demonstrated that receptor blockade by these mAbs in A431 tumor cells could effectively inhibit TNF-α-dependent autocrine growth. These studies further demonstrated that complete EGFr blockade occurred at the cell surface, ruling out the possibility of significant intracellular ligand-receptor interactions.

Blocking of receptor-ligand interaction alone is not sufficient for tumor cell growth inhibition, as shown by the inability of monovalent mAb 225 Fab′ fragments to inhibit A431 tumor cell growth.[23] Rather, A431 growth inhibition is dependent on receptor dimerization though binding by bivalent mAb 225 or 225 $F(ab')_2$ fragments. EGFr dimerization in this setting results in the inhibition of tyrosine phosphorylation, receptor down-regulation, and a resulting decrease in cellular proliferation.

The mechanism of mAb-mediated growth inhibition was further elucidated when it was shown that blockade of EGFr on A431 tumor cells by mAb 225 resulted in the up-regulation of $p27^{Kip1}$ expression.[24] The $p27^{Kip1}$ protein inactivates cyclin-dependent kinase 2 activity, resulting in a G_1 arrest of A431 cells. Cell-cycle arrest after exposure to saturating levels of mAb 225 has been reported in other tumor cell lines and in nonmalignant and immortalized human cell lines.[2,25]

Although the exposure of most tumor cell lines to mAb 225 resulted in G_1 arrest associated with increased levels of $p27^{Kip1}$, studies using the DiFi human colon cancer cell line indicated that mAb 225 binding to EGFr may, in some cases, induce tumor cell apoptosis.[26] The mechanism of this apoptotic cascade is not yet fully understood. However, in these cells, mAb 225 EGFr blockade led to the activation of the caspase cascade[27] by a pathway independent of known apoptotic receptor-mediated pathways, including Fas, tumor necrosis factor receptor-1, or by way of tumor necrosis factor–related apoptosis-inducing ligand receptors.[28] Whether this novel apoptotic mechanism mediated by mAb 225 is relevant in the clinical setting or peculiar to the DiFi cell line remains to be seen.

The efficacy of mAb blockade of EGFr in vivo was first demonstrated by Masui et al.[29] In athymic mice, repeated treatment with mAbs 225 or 528 prevented the growth of A431 and epidermal carcinoma cell line T222 xenografts. Significantly, the level of EGFr expression of A431 cell is one hundredfold higher than that of T222 cells. These data suggest that the efficacy of mAb blockade is not dependent on the level of EGFr expressed by the tumor cells.

Chimerization of mAb 225 with the human IgG1 constant region enhanced the affinity of the resulting antibody (C225) to EGFr. This enhanced affinity translated in an increased inhibition of A431 tumor growth in athymic mice as compared to the native murine mAb 225.[30] The C225 antibody has subsequently been shown to inhibit the in vivo growth of several renal cell carcinoma xenografts[31] and of pancreatic carcinoma cell line BxPC-3 xenografts in athymic nude mice.[32]

The C225 mAb inhibits angiogenesis. Perrotte et al[33] reported the inhibited expression of the angiogenic factors, vascular endothelial growth factor, interleukin 8, and basic fibroblast growth factor in vitro after treatment of transition cell carcinoma cell line 253J B-V with C225. Inhibition of angiogenic factors was further demonstrated in vivo in athymic mice and correlated to a decreased neovascularization of established 253J B-V tumors, a decreased tumor growth, and a significant decrease of metastatic tumors.[33]

Although a majority of the preclinical in vivo data for mAb blockade of EGFr is derived from studies using mAbs 225 and C225, studies using other EGFr-specific mAbs have reported similar anti-tumor effects. Rodeck et al[34] reported suppression of both A431 and SW948 (a colorectal tumor cell line) xenografts in athymic mice after repeated treatments with the anti-EGFr mAb 425. In another study, the EGFr-specific mAb 108.4 was shown to suppress the growth of the epidermoid carcinoma cell line KB in nude mice.[35] Complete regression of established head and neck carcinoma HN5 and breast carcinoma MDA-MB 468 tumors in nude mice was reported after treatment with the rat mAbs ICR62 and ICR16.[36] Recently, Yang et al[37,38] reported the development of a fully humanized mAb (ABX-EGF) that specifically binds the EGFr receptor and inhibits autophosphorylation of the protein tyrosine kinase domain. Treatment of athymic mice with ABX-EGF resulted in the complete eradication of A431 tumors as large as 1.2 cm^3.

EGFr Blockade: Monoclonal Antibodies and Chemotherapy

Antibody blockade of EGFr has a synergistic anti-tumor effect when combined with chemotherapy. This finding was first reported by Aboud-Pirak et al.[35] Mice bearing KB tumor xenografts were treated with cisplatin alone, the anti-EGFr mAb 108.4 alone, or a combination of both cisplatin and mAb 108.4. Combination therapy significantly enhanced the anti-tumor effect as compared to monotherapy with either cisplatin or 108.4. Subsequent preclinical studies reported a similar anti-tumor synergy between mAbs 225 and 528 and doxorubicin against A431 and MDA-468 xenografts in mice[39] and cisplatin against A431 xenografts.[40] In vivo synergy has been reported as well with C225 and topotecan against GEO colon cancer cells,[41] with gemcitabine and 5-fluorouracil against pancreatic carcinoma cells,[32,42] and with paclitaxel against transitional cell carcinoma tumors.[43] It has been postulated that this synergy may be related to the inhibition of drug-induced damage repair through an EGFr-dependent signaling pathway. Alternatively, or in addition to this mechanism, Mendelsohn and Baselga[2] proposed that in the setting of chemotherapy-induced damage, EGFr ligands may become survival rather than mitogenic factors, with blockade of these ligands enhancing tumor cell apoptosis.

EGFr Blockade: Monoclonal Antibodies and Radiotherapy

Antibody blockade of EGFr also enhances tumor cell sensitivity to radiotherapy.[44] This effect has been demonstrated by the combined treatment with C225 and ionizing radiation in vitro against a variety of squamous cell carcinomas of the head and neck[45,46] and in vivo against established intramuscular A431 tumors in nude mice.[47] In the latter studies, researchers demonstrated enhanced tumor cell radioresponsiveness by a factor of 1.56–3.62, depending on the number of C225 treatment doses (1 dose vs 3 doses, respectively). The combination of EGFr blockade with ionizing radiation resulted in a marked increase in central tumor necrosis, tumor infiltration with granulocytes, increased tumor cell differentiation, and decreased angiogenesis within the tumor. This enhanced radiosensitivity could be further enhanced in vitro by the additional treatment with the protein kinase A antisense oligonucleotide PKAI AS.[48] This in vitro effect translated into a significantly enhanced survival of nude mice bearing GEO cell tumors. These results have prompted the initiation of clinical trials combining C225 with irradiation for head and neck cancers (see *Clinical Trials*, p. 118).

EGFr Blockade: Tyrosine Kinase Inhibitors

Most early data demonstrating the efficacy of EGFr blockade are derived from mAbs targeting the extracellular portion of EGFr. Another approach is to target the cytoplasmic EGFr tyrosine kinase domain. To this end, a variety of small molecules that have been developed bind to and inhibit the intracellular tyrosine kinase domain of EGFr.[49] Currently, the most promising and well developed of these inhibitors are quinazolin-derived molecules. Specifically, ZD1839 and OSI-774 have undergone extensive preclinical study and are being investigated in clinical trials. Both agents are reversible adenosine triphosphate–competitive inhibitors of tyrosine kinase, with relative specificity for the EGFr tyrosine kinase.

ZD 1839 is an orally active agent shown to inhibit the growth of a variety of human tumor cells, including cell lines derived from ovary (OVCAR-3), breast (ZR-75-1, MCF-10A *ras*), and colon (GEO).[50,51] Growth inhibition was cytostatic, although at higher doses, exposure to ZD 1839 resulted in tumor cell apoptosis. The addition of ZD 1839 to tumor cells treated with a variety of cytotoxic agents enhanced the inhibition of cell growth and apoptosis in a dose-dependent manner. Furthermore, ZD 1839 treatment of nude mice with well-established GEO cell tumors inhibited tumor growth during treatment, although normal tumor cell growth was reestablished after termination of treatment. The combined treatment of ZD 1839 with raltitrexed, topotecan, or paclitaxel increased the survival time of nude mice bearing GEO cell xenografts as compared to treatment with single agents alone.[50] Enhanced in vivo anti-tumor effects with combined therapy against A431 cells and a panel of lung and prostate cell lines were also reported.[52] Furthermore, recent data indicate that treatment with ZD 1839 inhibits the expression of vascular endothelial growth factor and basic fibroblast growth factor in well-established GEO cell xenografts, resulting in an inhibition of neoangiogenesis.[53] This anti-angiogenesis effect was potentiated when ZD1839 treatment was combined with paclitaxel. These findings are consistent with those reported using EGFr-targeted mAbs.

Like ZD1839, OSI-774 is an orally active quinazolin compound. Treatment of DiFi colon cancer cells with OSI-774 inhibited EGFr phosphorylation and cellular proliferation and resulted in G_1 arrest with increased tumor expression of $p27^{KIP1}$.[54] Treatment with OSI-774 also enhanced cellular apoptosis consistent with published findings using mAb EGFr blockade.

CLINICAL TRIALS

EGFr-Targeted Antibodies

The first reported clinical trial using EGFr-specific antibodies was reported in 1991.[55] In this Phase I study, Divgi et al[55] treated patients having inoperable squamous cell carcinoma of the lung with escalating doses of the murine form of mAb 225. Patients received doses of 225, ranging from 1 mg to 300 mg. Patients at the higher dose levels were also treated with 4 mg of In^{111} labeled antibody for imaging studies using single-photon emission computed tomography. Treatment in these patients was well tolerated, with no reported toxicities. Furthermore, In^{111} labeled antibody could specifically visualize tumors on single-photon emission computed tomography. However, all patients in this study developed human anti–mouse antibodies to mAb 225 as a result of treatment.

Perez-Soler et al[56] subsequently published the results of a 1994 Phase I study using the EGFr-specific murine mAb RG 83852 in patients with non-small-cell lung cancer (NSCLC) and head and neck cancers.[56] In this study, patients received escalating doses of antibody by continuous infusion over 5 days. Again, no toxicities were reported in these studies, and immunohistochemical studies verified RG 83852 localization to tumor. A Phase I study using the rat mAb ICR62 in patients with head and neck cancer also demonstrated localization of the antibody to the tumor site at higher treatment doses.[57] In this study, 4 of 20 evaluated patients developed antibodies to the unmodified ICR62 antibody.

In light of the immunogenicity of unmodified mAbs, more recent clinical trials have focused on less immunogenic mAbs (chimerized 225 [C225] or humanized ABX-EGF). In one of the first Phase I clinical trials of C225, Baselga et al[58] initially treated patients having a variety of solid tumors that overexpressed EGFr with escalating weekly doses of C225 for up to 12 weeks.[58] The maximum treatment dose in these initial phase of the study was 100 mg/m^2. Subsequently, patients with either head and neck cancer or NSCLC were treated, in combination with 60 mg/m^2 cisplatin, with escalating weekly doses of C225 to a maximum dose of 400 mg/m^2. Overall, these studies demonstrated saturation of systemic C225 clearance at dose levels between 200 and 400 mg/m^2, with minimal toxicity noted even at the higher treatment doses. Significantly, only 1 of 19 analyzed patients developed antibodies to C225. These data are consistent with a subsequent larger study that reported a 4% incidence of anti–C225 antibody in treated patients.[59] The risk for grade III and grade IV anaphylaxis to C225 was reported to be 4% in this study.

EGFr is overexpressed in 85% of renal cell carcinomas. A Phase II study investigating the efficacy of C225 as a single agent in this population was published in abstract form.[60] In this study, 53 previously untreated patients with renal cell carcinomas were treated with a loading dose of C225 at 400 mg/m^2 followed by 7 weekly treatments of 250 mg/m^2. At the time of publication, two minor recovery and one partial response (PR) were reported (in all cases, responses were seen in metastatic lung lesions), and > 25% of patients had stable disease for > 6 months.

Several trials have studied the combination of C225 with chemotherapy. The combination of cisplatin with escalating doses of C225 was studied in patients with recurrent head and neck cancers.[61] In this Phase I study, 12 patients with readily accessible tumors that overexpressed EGFr were treated with a fixed dose of cisplatin (100 mg/m^2) every 3 weeks in combination with an escalating loading dose of C225 (100 mg/m^2; 400 mg/m^2; 500 mg/m^2) followed by weekly maintenance doses (100 mg/m^2; 250 mg/m^2; 250 mg/m^2, respectively) for 6 weeks. Tumor biopsy tissue was studied before and after treatments to evaluate for EGFr antibody saturation, EGFr tyrosine kinase activity, and the presence of EGFr/C225 complexes. Of the nine evaluable patients in this study, six (67%) had major responses to treatment, with two (22%) achieving complete response (CR). Significant EGFr saturation and inhibition of EGFr activity was noted with a C225 loading dose of 400 mg/m^2 followed by a weekly maintenance dose of 250 mg/m^2. On the basis of these studies, this dosing regimen has been adopted by most investigators for subsequent Phase II and III clinical trials of C225.

In a follow-up study, the efficacy of C225 in combination with cisplatin was further evaluated in patients with recurrent squamous cell carcinomas of the head and neck.[62] Patients enrolled in this study were initially treated with two cycles of cisplatin chemotherapy. Those patients with stable disease were subsequently treated with cisplatin (at 100 mg/m^2 if treated in conjunction with paclitaxel or at 75 mg/m^2 if treated with 5-fluorouracil) in combination with weekly C225 (400 mg/m^2 loading dose followed by weekly C225 at 250 mg/m^2). Overall, 21% of the 38 patients in this study had an objective response to therapy (1 CR and 7 PR), and 58% of patients had stable disease.

In a Phase II trial reported in abstract form, the previously established C225 regimen was used in combination with gemcitabine in patients with advanced pancreatic cancer.[63] Patient tumor samples were initially screened for EGFr expression. Overall, 89% of screened patients had tumors that expressed EGFr. Selected patients with measurable disease were treated with a loading dose of C225 (400 mg/m^2) followed by weekly C225 at 250 mg/m^2 and gemcitabine at 1,000 mg/m^2 weekly for 7 weeks of an 8-week cycle. After the first cycle, patients were treated with the same dose of gemcitabine in weeks 1–3 and 5–7 with weekly C225 (250 mg/m^2). After two cycles of therapy, 12% of patients achieved a PR, and 39% had stable disease. The median time to progression was 16 weeks, which compared favorably to published reports of patients treated with gemcitabine alone, in which the median time to progression was 9 weeks. Overall, the authors of that study concluded that combination treatment with gemcitabine and C225 was well tolerated and is a promising treatment alternative for patients with advanced pancreatic cancers.

Consistent with preclinical studies, treatment with C225 appears to enhance the efficacy of radiotherapy. In one recent study, patients with advanced head and neck tumors were treated with a combination of C225 and radiotherapy.[64] Overall, of the 15 patients enrolled in the study, 13 (87%) had a CR with this combination regimen, compared to a 31%–46% CR rate reported in previous studies with radiotherapy alone.

A majority of colon carcinomas express EGFr.[65] In one early study, 77% of colonic carcinomas expressed EGFr by immunohistochemistry.[66] Although several colon cancer cell lines exhibited in vivo sensitivity to EGFr blockade in preclinical studies, Rubin et al[67] were the first to report a clinical success of EGFr blockade in a colorectal cancer (CRC) patient.[67] On a compassionate-release protocol, one patient with relapsed colorectal cancer, previously treated with surgery and radiotherapy, achieved a major response after combined treatment with C225 and irinotecan. This finding prompted a Phase II trial of C225 in combination with irinotecan in patients with irinotecan-refractory EGFr-expressing CRCs.[68,69] This study enrolled 120 patients with EGFr-expressing CRCs refractory to 5-fluorouracil and CPT-11 therapy. Patients were treated with C225 at a loading dose of 400 mg/m^2 followed by weekly doses of C225 at 250 mg/m^2 in combination with irinotecan at the same dose and schedule that had previously resulted in disease progression. (Data were reported in abstract form.) At the time of publication, 23% of treated patients with chemotherapy-refractory disease achieved a PR. The median survival of enrolled patients was 235 days. C225-related toxicities included allergic reactions (1% grade 3 and 3% grade 4) and an acneiform rash (64% grades 1–2 and 12% grade 3). Overall, the treatment was well tolerated, and the promising results from this trial have prompted the initiation of first-line combination therapies for CRC with irinotecan, 5-fluorouracil, leucovorin, and C225 and with single-agent C225 in chemotherapy-refractory CRC patients.

Another anti-EGFr mAb, the fully humanized ABX-EGF, has been studied in a Phase I trial in patients with a variety of advanced solid tumors.[70] Treatment with ABX-EGF was well tolerated, with cutaneous toxicities noted at the higher doses, similar to those seen in patients treated with C225. Significantly, no anti-ABX-EGF antibody was noted in any of the patients treated. One patient with esophageal cancer had stable disease for 6 months after the start of therapy. Further studies in patients using the higher dose levels reported in this study are currently in progress.

Although treatment with C225 and ABX-EGF was well tolerated in these Phase I and II clinical trials, skin toxicity—most commonly in the form of an acneiform rash—was consistently reported. In fact, the finding of a reversible acneiform rash was noted not only in patients treated with the C225 and ABX-EGF mAbs, but in those treated with the small-molecule tyrosine kinase inhibitors ZD 1839 and OSI-774 (see *Clinical Trials: Tyrosine Kinase Inhibitors*, p. 121). EGFr is expressed in the epidermis and therefore may be targeted by C225. Busam et al[71] recently reported the results of a histologic analysis of acneiform lesions in patients after C225 treatment. In that study, 10 patients treated with C225 monotherapy had skin biopsies analyzed before and 8 days after therapy. Histologic analysis of affected lesions found superficial dermal inflammatory infiltrates and a suppurating superficial folliculitis. An infectious etiology for these lesions was not identified. Furthermore, investigators were able to demonstrate an increased level of $p27^{Kip1}$ expression in epidermal keratinocytes of affected lesions by both immunohistochemical and in situ hybridization studies. These data suggest that reported skin toxicity is likely due to C225-mediated blockade of EGFr in the skin. Significantly, the development of an acneiform rash recently was associated with an improved response rate to C225 therapy in patients with chemotherapy-resistant CRC.[69] Publishing in abstract form, Saltz et al[69] reported an overall response rate of 4% to combined therapy with irinotecan and C225 in patients who did not develop a rash versus 28% of patients who did develop a rash ($P < 0.021$). The authors proposed that the development of skin toxicity in these patients may serve as a marker for susceptibility to EGFr blockade.

Clinical Trials: Tyrosine Kinase Inhibitors

Of the numerous EGFr tyrosine kinase inhibitors currently in development, two quinazolin-derived orally active agents, ZD1839 and OSI-774, have been studied in clinical trials. To date, several Phase I trials of ZD1839 have been reported in abstract form. Ferry et al[72] reported a dose escalation study of ZD 1839 in patients previously treated for a variety of solid tumors.[72] The treatment was well tolerated, and dose-limiting toxicity was reported as grade 3 diarrhea at the 700 mg/day dose level. An acnelike skin rash, similar to that seen with antibody-mediated EGFr blockade, and diarrhea were the most commonly observed toxicities. Response to therapy in this study was noted as stable disease in a variety of tumor cell types, with the most remarkable responses seen in patients with NSCLC. Two of 16 NSCLC patients enrolled in this study achieved PRs, 2 other patients had significant tumor regressions, and another 2 patients had stable disease.

A similar study reported at the same meeting presented combined data from two Phase I dose escalation studies of ZD 1839.[73] Overall, 127 patients with NSCLC, ovarian cancer, colon cancer, prostate cancer, or head and neck cancer were enrolled in these studies. The most common side effects once again included skin toxicities and diarrhea and nausea and vomiting. Dose-limiting toxicity had not yet been reached at a daily ZD 1839 dose of 800 mg.

Activity against NSCLC demonstrated in these early Phase I trials, prompted Miller et al[74] to perform a pilot study combining ZD 1839 therapy with carboplatin and paclitaxel in previously untreated patients with stage IIIB/IV NSCLC. In part 1 of this two-part trial, patients were treated intermittently with ZD 1839 at two different dose levels (250 mg and 500 mg daily) in combination with chemotherapy to assess the safety of this combination. In part 2 of the study, patients were treated with continuous ZD 1839 at the higher tolerated dose of 500 mg daily in combination with chemotherapy. Overall, of 20 evaluable patients, 7 (35%) achieved a PR to therapy, 10 (50%) had stable disease, and 3 (15%) had progression of disease.

A Phase I trial of OSI-774 therapy recently was published.[75] In this three-part study, investigators treated 40 patients having advanced solid tumor malignancies with escalating doses of OSI-774. In part A, patients received escalating doses of OSI-774 daily for 3 days per week for 3 weeks of a 4-week cycle to a maximum daily dose of 100 mg. In part B, patients received escalating daily doses of OSI-774 for 3 of 4 weeks to a maximum daily dose of 200 mg. A daily maximal tolerated dose of 150 mg having been established in part B, in part C patients were treated with this daily dose on an uninterrupted schedule. Dose limiting toxicities included skin toxicity (acneiform rash) and severe diarrhea. In this study, one patient with metastatic renal cell carcinoma attained complete resolution of several metastatic lymph node lesions and a pulmonary lesion. One patient with CRC had a 30% reduction in liver metastases, and another two patients with CRC had stable disease for at least 5 months. Four other patients, one each with NSCLC and prostate, cervical, and head and neck cancer, also had stable disease for at least 5 months.

In another Phase I trial, published in abstract form, Karp et al[76] studied OSI-774 on a weekly dosing schedule. In that study, the maximal tolerated dose had not yet been reached at a weekly dose of 1,000 mg. Grade 1 and grade 2 headache, nausea, diarrhea, and acneiform skin rashes were reported in this study. The final results of this trail have not yet been published in manuscript form.

To date, several Phase II trials of OSI-774 have been reported in abstract form. In one study, 114 patients with recurrent squamous cell carcinomas of the head and neck were treated with the previously established daily OSI-774 dose of 150 mg.[77] Of 78 evaluable patients, 10 (13%) achieved a PR, 23 (29%) had stable disease, and 45 (58%) had progression of disease. In this cohort, 82 patients developed an acneiform rash, requiring a dose reduction in 24 patients and discontinuation of therapy in 2 patients. Other reported toxicities included diarrhea, nausea, vomiting, and fatigue.

Finkler et al[78] treated 34 patients with chemotherapy-refractory advanced ovarian cancer with 150 mg of OSI-774 daily. Again, a large majority of patients (88%) developed skin toxicity on treatment. Three patients in this study had PRs lasting at least 2, 5, and 6 months, respectively. Fifteen other patients had stable disease lasting at least 2 months.

OSI-774 has also been studied in patients with recurrent Stage IIIB/IV NSCLC.[79] In that study, 56 patients with recurrent EGFr-expressing NSCLC tumors were treated daily with 150 mg of OSI-774. Once again, acneiform rash was seen in a majority of patients (78%), but treatment was otherwise well tolerated. Seven patients achieved a PR of at least 8 weeks, 19 patients had stable disease, and 31 patients had tumor progression.

CONCLUSIONS

With a better understanding of the molecular mechanisms involved in tumor cell growth, researchers have become increasingly capable of specifically targeting anti-cancer therapies to malignant cells. The discovery of the EGF receptor and its role in malignant cell growth serves as a prototype for this novel approach to cancer treatment. The findings that EGFr is a cellular proto-oncogene; that many different solid tumors overexpress EGFr; and, more significant, that many tumors also coexpress the EGFr ligand tumor necrosis factor-α, resulting in an autocrine mitogenic stimulus, led investigators to target EGFr for the treatment of solid tumors. The rationale of such therapy was sound. Extensive preclinical studies over the last two decades confirmed the hypothesis that the blockade of EGFr can result in the inhibition of tumor cell growth and, in some cases, tumor cell apoptosis both in vitro and in vivo. A significant anti-angiogenesis effect has been reported in in vivo models of a variety of solid tumors. Furthermore, preclinical studies demonstrate that anti-EGFr effects are synergistic with conventional therapies, including chemotherapy and radiotherapy.

With the development of humanized mAbs (C225 and ABX-EGF) and small-molecule EGFr tyrosine kinase inhibitors (ZD1839 and OSI-774), investigators are now able to test this hypothesis in human subjects. Early Phase I and Phase II studies using these agents have demonstrated promising anti-tumor effects in a variety of both pretreated and untreated malignancies, both as single agents and in combination chemotherapy and radiotherapy. To date, the most promising responses have been reported in squamous cell carcinomas of the head and neck, NSCLC, and CRC. Whether EGFr blockade in combination with standard first-line therapies will enhance the overall response and survival of patients with these and other solid tumor malignancies will be determined by current ongoing and planned future Phase III trials.

REFERENCES

1. Hackel PO, Zwick E, Prenzel N, Ullrich A. Epidermal growth factor receptors: critical mediators of multiple receptor pathways. Curr Opin Cell Biol 1999;11:184–189.
2. Mendelsohn J, Baselga J. The EGF receptor family as targets for cancer therapy. Oncogene 2000; 19:6550–6565.
3. Carpenter G, Cohen S. Epidermal growth factor. J Biol Chem 1990;265:7709–7712.
4. Cohen S, Carpenter G, King L Jr. Epidermal growth factor-receptor-protein kinase interactions. Co-purification of receptor and epidermal growth factor-enhanced phosphorylation activity. J Biol Chem 1980;255:4834–4842.
5. Cohen S. Isolation of a mouse submaxillary gland protein accelerating incisor eruption and eyelid opening in the new-born animal. J Biol Chem 1962;237:1555–1562
6. Alroy I, Yarden Y. The ErbB signaling network in embryogenesis and oncogenesis: signal diversification through combinatorial ligand-receptor interactions. FEBS Lett 1997;410:83–86.
7. Arteaga CL. The epidermal growth factor receptor: from mutant oncogene in nonhuman cancers to therapeutic target in human neoplasia. J Clin Oncol 2001;19:32S–40S.
8. Schlessinger J. Cell signaling by receptor tyrosine kinases. Cell 2000;103:211–225.
9. Yarden Y, Sliwkowski MX. Untangling the ErbB signaling network. Nat Rev Mol Cell Biol 2001; 2:127–137.

10. Chan TO, Rittenhouse SE, Tsichlis PN. AKT/PKB and other D3 phosphoinositide-regulated kinases: kinase activation by phosphoinositide-dependent phosphorylation. Annu Rev Biochem 1999;68: 965–1014.

11. Downward J, Yarden Y, Mayes E et al. Close similarity of epidermal growth factor receptor and v-erb-B oncogene protein sequences. Nature 1984;307:521–527.

12. Ullrich A, Coussens L, Hayflick JS et al. Human epidermal growth factor receptor cDNA sequence and aberrant expression of the amplified gene in A431 epidermoid carcinoma cells. Nature 1984; 309:418–425.

13. Xu YH, Ishii S, Clark AJ et al. Human epidermal growth factor receptor cDNA is homologous to a variety of RNAs overproduced in A431 carcinoma cells. Nature 1984;309:806–810.

14. Salomon DS, Brandt R, Ciardiello F, Normanno N. Epidermal growth factor–related peptides and their receptors in human malignancies. Crit Rev Oncol Hematol 1995;19:183–232.

15. Wikstrand CJ, Bigner DD. Prognostic applications of the epidermal growth factor receptor and its ligand, transforming growth factor-alpha. J Natl Cancer Inst 1998;90:799–801.

16. Markowitz SD, Molkentin K, Gerbic C et al. Growth stimulation by coexpression of transforming growth factor-alpha and epidermal growth factor-receptor in normal and adenomatous human colon epithelium. J Clin Invest 1990;86:356–362.

17. Tateishi M, Ishida T, Mitsudomi T et al. Immunohistochemical evidence of autocrine growth factors in adenocarcinoma of the human lung. Cancer Res 1990;50:7077–7080.

18. Yonemura Y, Takamura H, Ninomiya I et al. Interrelationship between transforming growth factor-alpha and epidermal growth factor receptor in advanced gastric cancer. Oncology 1992;49: 157–161.

19. Kawamoto T, Sato JD, Le A et al. Growth stimulation of A431 cells by epidermal growth factor: identification of high-affinity receptors for epidermal growth factor by an anti-receptor monoclonal antibody. Proc Natl Acad Sci USA 1983;80:1337–1341.

20. Sato JD, Kawamoto T, Le AD et al. Biological effects in vitro of monoclonal antibodies to human epidermal growth factor receptors. Mol Biol Med 1983;1:511–529.

21. Gill GN, Kawamoto T, Cochet C et al. Monoclonal anti-epidermal growth factor receptor antibodies which are inhibitors of epidermal growth factor binding and antagonists of epidermal growth factor binding and antagonists of epidermal growth factor-stimulated tyrosine protein kinase activity. J Biol Chem 1984;259:7755–7760.

22. Van de Vijver MJ, Kumar R, Mendelsohn J. Ligand-induced activation of A431 cell epidermal growth factor receptors occurs primarily by an autocrine pathway that acts upon receptors on the surface rather than intracellularly. J Biol Chem 1991;266:7503–7508.

23. Fan Z, Lu Y, Wu X, Mendelsohn J. Antibody-induced epidermal growth factor receptor dimerization mediates inhibition of autocrine proliferation of A431 squamous carcinoma cells. J Biol Chem 1994;269:27595–27602.

24. Fan Z, Shang BY, Lu Y et al. Reciprocal changes in p27(Kip1) and p21(Cip1) in growth inhibition mediated by blockade or overstimulation of epidermal growth factor receptors. Clin Cancer Res 1997;3:1943–1948.

25. Stampfer MR, Pan CH, Hosoda J et al. Blockage of EGF receptor signal transduction causes reversible arrest of normal and immortal human mammary epithelial cells with synchronous reentry into the cell cycle. Exp Cell Res 1993;208:175–188.

26. Wu X, Fan Z, Masui H et al. Apoptosis induced by an anti-epidermal growth factor receptor monoclonal antibody in a human colorectal carcinoma cell line and its delay by insulin. J Clin Invest 1995;95:1897–1905.

27. Liu B, Fang M, Schmidt M et al. Induction of apoptosis and activation of the caspase cascade by anti-EGF receptor monoclonal antibodies in DiFi human colon cancer cells do not involve the c-jun N-terminal kinase activity. Br J Cancer 2000;82:1991–1999.

28. Liu B, Fan Z. The monoclonal antibody 225 activates caspase-8 and induces apoptosis through a tumor necrosis factor receptor family-independent pathway. Oncogene 2001;20:3726–3734.

29. Masui H, Kawamoto T, Sato JD et al. Growth inhibition of human tumor cells in athymic mice by anti-epidermal growth factor receptor monoclonal antibodies. Cancer Res 1984;44:1002–1007.

30. Goldstein NI, Prewett M, Zuklys K et al. Biological efficacy of a chimeric antibody to the epidermal growth factor receptor in a human tumor xenograft model. Clin Cancer Res 1995;1:1311–1318.

31. Prewett M, Rothman M, Waksal H et al. Mouse-human chimeric anti-epidermal growth factor receptor antibody C225 inhibits the growth of human renal cell carcinoma xenografts in nude mice. Clin Cancer Res 1998;4:2957–2966.

32. Overholser JP, Prewett MC, Hooper AT et al. Epidermal growth factor receptor blockade by antibody IMC-C225 inhibits growth of a human pancreatic carcinoma xenograft in nude mice. Cancer 2000;89:74–82.

33. Perrotte P, Matsumoto T, Inoue K et al. Anti-epidermal growth factor receptor antibody C225 inhibits angiogenesis in human transitional cell carcinoma growing orthotopically in nude mice. Clin Cancer Res 1999;5:257–265.

34. Rodeck U, Herlyn M, Herlyn D et al. Tumor growth modulation by a monoclonal antibody to the epidermal growth factor receptor: immunologically mediated and effector cell-independent effects. Cancer Res 1987;47:3692–3696.

35. Aboud-Pirak E, Hurwitz E, Pirak ME et al. Efficacy of antibodies to epidermal growth factor receptor against KB carcinoma in vitro and in nude mice. J Natl Cancer Inst 1988;80:1605–1611.

36. Modjtahedi H, Eccles S, Box G et al. Immunotherapy of human tumour xenografts overexpressing the EGF receptor with rat antibodies that block growth factor-receptor interaction. Br J Cancer 1993;67:254–261.

37. Yang XD, Jia XC, Corvalan JR et al. Eradication of established tumors by a fully human monoclonal antibody to the epidermal growth factor receptor without concomitant chemotherapy. Cancer Res 1999;59:1236–1243.

38. Yang XD, Jia XC, Corvalan JR et al. Development of ABX-EGF, a fully human anti-EGF receptor monoclonal antibody, for cancer therapy. Crit Rev Oncol Hematol 2001;38:17–23.

39. Baselga J, Norton L, Masui H et al. Antitumor effects of doxorubicin in combination with anti-epidermal growth factor receptor monoclonal antibodies. J Natl Cancer Inst 1993;85:1327–1333.

40. Fan Z, Baselga J, Masui H, Mendelsohn J. Antitumor effect of anti-epidermal growth factor receptor monoclonal antibodies plus cis-diamminedichloroplatinum on well established A431 cell xenografts. Cancer Res 1993;53:4637–4642.

41. Ciardiello F, Bianco R, Damiano V et al. Antitumor activity of sequential treatment with topotecan and anti-epidermal growth factor receptor monoclonal antibody C225. Clin Cancer Res 1999;5: 909–916.

42. Bruns CJ, Harbison MT, Davis DW et al. Epidermal growth factor receptor blockade with C225 plus gemcitabine results in regression of human pancreatic carcinoma growing orthotopically in nude mice by antiangiogenic mechanisms. Clin Cancer Res 2000;6:1936–1948.

43. Inoue K, Slaton JW, Perrotte P et al. Paclitaxel enhances the effects of the anti-epidermal growth factor receptor monoclonal antibody ImClone C225 in mice with metastatic human bladder transitional cell carcinoma. Clin Cancer Res 2000;6:4874–4884.

44. Sartor CI. Biological modifiers as potential radiosensitizers: targeting the epidermal growth factor receptor family. Semin Oncol 2000;27:15–20 [discussion 92–100].

45. Huang SM, Bock JM, Harari PM. Epidermal growth factor receptor blockade with C225 modulates proliferation, apoptosis, and radiosensitivity in squamous cell carcinomas of the head and neck. Cancer Res 1999;59:1935–1940.

46. Bonner JA, Raisch KP, Trummell HQ et al. Enhanced apoptosis with combination C225/radiation treatment serves as the impetus for clinical investigation in head and neck cancers. J Clin Oncol 2000;18:47S–53S.

47. Milas L, Mason K, Hunter N et al. In vivo enhancement of tumor radioresponse by C225 antiepidermal growth factor receptor antibody. Clin Cancer Res 2000;6:701–708.

48. Bianco C, Bianco R, Tortora G et al. Antitumor activity of combined treatment of human cancer cells with ionizing radiation and anti-epidermal growth factor receptor monoclonal antibody C225 plus type I protein kinase A antisense oligonucleotide. Clin Cancer Res 2000;6:4343–4350.

49. Ciardiello F. Epidermal growth factor receptor tyrosine kinase inhibitors as anticancer agents. Drugs 2000;60:25–32 [discussion 41–22].

50. Ciardiello F, Caputo R, Bianco R et al. Antitumor effect and potentiation of cytotoxic drugs activity in human cancer cells by ZD-1839 (Iressa), an epidermal growth factor receptor-selective tyrosine kinase inhibitor. Clin Cancer Res 2000;6:2053–2063.

51. Baselga J, Averbuch SD. ZD1839 ('Iressa') as an anticancer agent. Drugs 2000;60:33–40 [discussion 41–32].

52. Sirotnak FM, Zakowski MF, Miller VA et al. Efficacy of cytotoxic agents against human tumor xenografts is markedly enhanced by coadministration of ZD1839 (Iressa), an inhibitor of EGFR tyrosine kinase. Clin Cancer Res 2000;6:4885–4892.

53. Ciardiello F, Caputo R, Bianco R et al. Inhibition of growth factor production and angiogenesis in human cancer cells by ZD1839 (Iressa), a selective epidermal growth factor receptor tyrosine kinase inhibitor. Clin Cancer Res 2001;7:1459–1465.

54. Moyer JD, Barbacci EG, Iwata KK et al. Induction of apoptosis and cell cycle arrest by CP-358,774, an inhibitor of epidermal growth factor receptor tyrosine kinase. Cancer Res 1997;57: 4838–4848.

55. Divgi CR, Welt S, Kris M et al. Phase I and imaging trial of indium 111-labeled anti-epidermal growth factor receptor monoclonal antibody 225 in patients with squamous cell lung carcinoma. J Natl Cancer Inst 1991;83:97–104.

56. Perez-Soler R, Donato NJ, Shin DM et al. Tumor epidermal growth factor receptor studies in patients with non-small-cell lung cancer or head and neck cancer treated with monoclonal antibody RG 83852. J Clin Oncol 1994;12:730–739.

57. Modjtahedi H, Hickish T, Nicolson M et al. Phase I trial and tumour localisation of the anti-EGFR monoclonal antibody ICR62 in head and neck or lung cancer. Br J Cancer 1996;73: 228–235.

58. Baselga J, Pfister D, Cooper MR et al. Phase I studies of anti-epidermal growth factor receptor chimeric antibody C225 alone and in combination with cisplatin. J Clin Oncol 2000;18:904–914.

59. Khazaeli MB, LoBuglio AF, Falcey JW et al. Low Immunogenicity of a chimeric monoclonal antibody (MoAb), IMC-C225, used to treat epidermal growth factor receptor-positive tumors. Proc Annu Meet Am Soc Clin Oncol 2000;19:207a

60. Gunnett K, Motzer R, Amato R et al. Phase II study of anti-epidermal growth factor receptor (EGFr) antibody C225 alone in patients (pts) with metastatic renal cell carcinoma (RCC). Proc Annu Meet Am Soc Clin Oncol 1999;18:340a

61. Shin DM, Donato NJ, Perez-Soler R et al. Epidermal growth factor receptor-targeted therapy with C225 and cisplatin in patients with head and neck cancer Clin Cancer Res 2001;7:1204–1213.

62. Hong WK, Arquette M, Nabell L et al. Efficacy and safety of the anti-epidermal growth factor antibody (EGFR) IMC-C225, in combination with cisplatin in patients with recurrent squamous

cell carcinoma of the head and neck (SCCHN) refractory to cisplatin containing chemotherapy. Proc Annu Meet Am Soc Clin Oncol 2001;20:224a

63. Abbruzzese JL, Rosenberg A, Xiong Q et al. Phase II study of anti-epidermal growth factor receptor (EGFR) antibody Cetuximab (IMC-C225) in combination with gemcitabine in patients with advanced pancreatic cancer. Proc Annu Meet Am Soc Clin Oncol 2001;20:130a

64. Bonner JA, Ezekiel MP, Robert F et al. Continued response following treatment with IMC-C225, an EGFr MoAb, combined with RT in advanced head and neck malignancies. Proc Annu Meet Am Soc Clin Oncol 2000;19:4a

65. Messa C, Russo F, Caruso MG, Di Leo A. EGF, TGF-alpha, and EGF-R in human colorectal adenocarcinoma. Acta Oncol 1998;37:285–289.

66. Yasui W, Sumiyoshi H, Hata J et al. Expression of epidermal growth factor receptor in human gastric and colonic carcinomas. Cancer Res 1988;48:137–141.

67. Rubin MS, Shin DM, Pasmantier M et al. Monoclonal antibody (MoAb) IMC-C225, an anti-epidermal growth factor receptor (EGFr), for patients (pts) with EGFr-positive tumors refractory to or in relapse from previous therapeutic regimens. Proc Annu Meet Am Soc Clin Oncol 2000; 19:474a

68. Saltz L, Rubin M, Hochster H et al. Cetuximab (IMC-C225) plus irinotecan (CPT-11) is active in CPT-11-refractory colorectal cancer (CRC) that expresses epidermal growth factor receptor (EGFR). Proc Annu Meet Am Soc Clin Oncol 2001;20:3a

69. Saltz L, Rubin MS, Hochster HS et al. Acne-like rash predicts response in patients treated with Cetuximab (IMC-C225) plus irinotecan (CPT-11) in CPT-11-refractory colorectal cancer (CRC) that expresses epidermal growth factor receptor (EGFR). Clin Cancer Res 2001;7:114s

70. Figlin RA, Belldegrun A, Lohner ME et al. ABX-EGF: a fully human anti-EGF receptor antibody in patients with advanced cancer. Proc Annu Meet Am Soc Clin Oncol 2001;20:276a

71. Busam KJ, Capodieci P, Motzer R et al. Cutaneous side-effects in cancer patients treated with the anti–epidermal growth factor receptor antibody C225. Br J Dermatol 2001;144:1169–1176.

72. Ferry D, Hammond L, Ranson M et al. Intermittent oral Zd1839 (Iressa), a novel epidermal growth factor inhibitor (Egfr-Tki), shows evidence of good tolerability and activity: final results from a phase I study. Proc Annu Meet Am Soc Clin Oncol 2000;19:3a

73. Baselga J, Herbst R, LoRusso P et al. Continuous administration of ZD1839 (Iressa), a novel oral epidermal growth receptor tyrosine kinase inhibitor (EGFR-TKI), in patients with five selected tumor types: evidence of activity and good tolerability. Proc Annu Meet Am Soc Clin Oncol 2000; 19:177a

74. Miller VA, Johnson D, Heelan RT et al. A pilot trial demonstrates the safety of ZD1839 ('Iressa'), an oral epidermal growth factor receptor tyrosine kinase inhibitor (EGFR-TKI), in combination with carboplatin (C) and paclitaxel (P) in previously untreated advanced non-small cell lung cancer (NSCLC). Proc Annu Meet Am Soc Clin Oncol 2001;20:326a

75. Hidalgo M, Siu LL, Nemunaitis J et al. Phase I and pharmacologic study of OSI-774, an epidermal growth factor receptor tyrosine kinase inhibitor, in patients with advanced solid malignancies. J Clin Oncol 2001;19:3267–3279.

76. Karp DD, Silberman SL, Csudae R et al. Phase I dose escalation study of epidermal growth factor receptor (EGFR) tyrosine kinase (TK) inhibitor CP-358, 774 in Patients With Advanced Solid Tumors. Proc Annu Meet Am Soc Clin Oncol 1999;18:388a

77. Senzer NN, Soulieres D, Siu L et al. Phase 2 evaluation of OSI-774, a potent oral antagonist of the EGFR-TK in patients with advanced squamous cell carcinoma of the head and neck. Proc Annu Meet Am Soc Clin Oncol 2001;20:2a

78. Finkler N, Gordon A, Crozier M et al. Phase 2 evaluation of OSI-774, a potent oral antagonist of the EGFR-TK in patients with advanced ovarian carcinoma. Proc Annu Meet Am Soc Clin Oncol 2001;20:208a

79. Perez-Soler R, Chachoua A, Huberman M et al. A phase II trial of the epidermal growth factor receptor (EGFR) tyrosine kinase inhibitor OSI-774, following platinum-based chemotherapy, in patients (pts) with advanced, EGFR-expressing, non-small cell lung cancer (NSCLC). Proc Annu Meet Am Soc Clin Oncol 2001;20:310a.

Chapter 8

The Development of Antiangiogenic Agents for the Clinic

Michael S. O'Reilly

Isaiah J. Fidler

The continuous growth of tumors and the development of metastasis are dependent on the induction of angiogenesis (i.e., the formation of an adequate vasculature).[1,2] A tumor mass smaller than 0.4 mm in diameter can receive oxygen and nutrients by diffusion, but any increase in tumor mass beyond that requires the proliferation and morphogenesis of vascular endothelial cells.[3,4] Angiogenesis consists of multiple, sequential, and interdependent steps. It begins with local degradation of the basement membrane surrounding the capillaries and is followed by invasion of the surrounding stroma by the underlying endothelial cells in the direction of the angiogenic stimulus. Endothelial cell migration is accompanied by the proliferation of endothelial cells and their organization into three-dimensional structures that join with other similar structures to form a network of new blood vessels.[5] The best treatment strategies would target each step of the angiogenic process.

In addition to providing a circulatory supply to the tumor that transports nutrients and oxygen and removes catabolites, angiogenesis can be an important source of factors that have a paracrine effect on a growing tumor. The proliferating endothelial cells within the tumor and in the adjacent stroma produce multiple growth factors that promote tumor cell growth, invasion, and survival.[6] As a result, a circuit is established in which tumor cells and endothelial cells continue to drive each other. These observations led Folkman[7] to propose a two-compartment model of malignant disease consisting of endothelial cell and tumor cell populations.

The onset of angiogenesis involves an alteration in the balance between proangiogenic and antiangiogenic molecules.[2,8,9] These molecules may mediate multiple steps in the process of angiogenesis and may affect the function of diverse cell types not involved in angiogenesis. A more refined definition of an angiogenic factor is a factor that selectively alters the characteristics of endothelial cells and associated perivascular structures (i.e., pericytes, vascular smooth-muscle cells) and their development but does not affect the function of other cell types.[8,9]

Under physiologic conditions that require neovascularization, angiogenesis is a tightly regulated process.[10] However, during tumorigenesis, the process is sustained and requires the continued tumor and stromal cell production of stimulators in excess of inhibitors. Disease states that are associated with malignant angiogenesis include cancer, ophthalmologic disorders (e.g., diabetic retinopathy or macular degeneration), arthritis, psoriasis, and arteriosclerosis.[11] In malignant angiogenesis, angiogenic vessels appear markedly disordered relative to their physiologic counterparts[12] and are characterized by the lack of pericytes and other support cells, impaired or intermittent blood flow (or both),[13] the presence of plasma proteins that function as a neostroma,[14–16] and increased vascular permeability.

A number of antiangiogenic agents have been described, and many of these are in clinical trials in cancer patients.[2,17,18] However, no angiogenesis inhibitor has yet been approved for clinical use. The successful use of antiangiogenic agents to treat cancer and other angiogenesis-dependent diseases awaits a greater understanding of the angiogenic process and of the interaction between the endothelial cell and its microenvironment. In the interim, we provide an overview of the potential benefits of antiangiogenic therapy and discuss the challenges associated with the use of antiangiogenic agents.

STRATEGIES TO CONTROL TUMOR GROWTH BY TARGETING THE ENDOTHELIAL CELL

Several angiogenesis inhibitors and antivascular agents are now in development. In this section, we discuss a few of the different strategies to inhibit angiogenesis and provide an outline of issues for consideration.

Antivascular Agents and Vascular Targeting

Although the focus of this chapter is on the use of antiangiogenic agents, it is important to distinguish between antivascular and antiangiogenic therapy. Antiangiogenic therapy is directed against the neovasculature and thus does not have a significant effect on the resting vasculature. In contrast, antivascular therapy targets existing vasculature and could well disrupt normal vessels. One strategy to target tumor vasculature selectively is to use antibodies directed against specific antigens conjugated to toxins expressed on some (but not all) endothelial cells.[19,20] Targeting of the tumor vasculature can also be achieved by using the tubulin-destabilizing agent combretastatin A4.[4] Although the precise mechanism is not yet known, combretastatin A4 can target the established tumor vasculature, leading to extensive tumor cell necrosis[21] without significant toxicity. The drug is now in clinical trial.

Recently, the heterogeneity of the endothelium was targeted. Phage display has identified specific peptide sequences that bind to receptors on the endothelial cell surface in the capillary beds of specific tissue beds.[22–24] Further, angiogenic endothelial cells can be targeted by specific peptide sequences that selectively bind to proliferating endothelial cells but not to quiescent cells. If these peptides are conjugated to the cytotoxic agent doxorubicin, the antitumor activity of the drug is enhanced severalfold in breast cancer models.[22] Whether organ-specific peptides can home to sites of angiogenesis in selected tissues remains to be determined, but targeting the tumor vasculature is an attractive approach.

Given that in normal tissues endothelial cells generally remain quiescent for months or years,[25] antiangiogenic strategies are not associated with significant toxicity; however, many agents will have both antivascular and antiangiogenic effects.

Agents That Decrease the Expression of Proangiogenic Molecules

Angiogenesis is controlled by the balance between stimulators and inhibitors.[9,26] For angiogenesis to proceed, there must be a shift in the balance of angiogenic factors in favor of stimulation. Tumors can achieve this by increasing the expression of proangiogenic molecules, such as basic fibroblast growth factor (bFGF),[26,27] vascular endothelial growth factor–vascular permeability factor (VEGF/VPF),[28,29] interleukin-8,[30] hepatocyte growth factor,[31] or others, or by decreasing the expression of antiangiogenic molecules, such as thrombospondin.[32,33] It is important to note that both tumor cells and host cells can be the source of angiogenic factors.[34] Enzymes produced by tumor cells or stromal cells can mobilize proangiogenic molecules that can induce tumor angiogenesis. These enzymes can also mobilize antiangiogenic molecules.[35,36] Alternatively, tumor-derived growth factors can induce stromal cells to produce proangiogenic molecules. For example, the colonic mucosa adjacent to the colonic adenocarcinoma is responsible for the production of proangiogenic molecules that support tumor angiogenesis.[34] Thus, strategies to block the expression of angiogenic molecules offer great potential. One excellent example is the interferons.

Antiangiogenic Activity of Interferon The interferon (IFN) family consists of three major glycoproteins that exhibit species specificity: leukocyte-derived IFN-α, fibroblast-derived IFN-β, and immune cell-produced IFN-γ. Although IFN-α and IFN-β share a common receptor (the type I IFN receptor) and induce a similar pattern of cellular responses, certain cellular reactions can be stimulated only by IFN-β, probably by the phosphorylation of a receptor-associated protein that is uniquely responsive to IFN-β.[37] In addition to their well-recognized activity as antiviral agents, IFNs regulate multiple biological activities, such as cell growth,[38] differentiation,[39] oncogene expression,[40] host immunity,[41] and tumorigenicity.[42–44] IFNs can also inhibit a number of steps in the angiogenic process. IFN has antiproliferative properties, especially on tumor cells,[45,46] an effect that has also been demonstrated on endothelial cells in vitro. IFN-α can inhibit fibroblast growth factor–induced endothelial proliferation, and IFN-γ can inhibit endothelial proliferation.[47,48] IFN-α and IFN-γ have been shown to be cytostatic to human dermal microvascular endothelial cells[49] and human capillary endothelial cells.[50]

Systemic therapy using recombinant IFNs produces antiangiogenic effects in vascular tumors, including life-threatening infantile hemangioma,[51–53] Kaposi's sarcoma,[54] giant-cell tumor of the mandible,[55] and bladder carcinoma.[56] These tumors have also been documented as producing the high levels of bFGF often detectable in the urine or serum of these patients.[57,58] IFN-α and IFN-β (but not IFN-γ) down-regulate the expression of bFGF mRNA and protein in human carcinoma cells.[3] Indeed, systemic administration of human IFN-α decreased the in vivo expression of bFGF, decreased blood vessel density, and inhibited tumor growth of a human bladder carcinoma implanted orthotopically in nude mice.[59]

In the original studies of the antiangiogenic effects of IFN-α, the relative activity was thought to be low.[60] However, by administering IFN at lower doses given more frequently, its antiangiogenic activity can be significantly enhanced and its toxicity diminished.[61] Studies of the effects of antiangiogenic IFN doses, both alone and in combination with other modalities, are now under way or will commence shortly at several centers throughout the world.

Endogenous Inhibitors of Angiogenesis

As stated, to promote angiogenesis, tumor cells produce a number of stimulatory factors and down-regulate the production of angiogenesis inhibitors, such as troponin I[62] and thrombospondin, which is under the regulation of the wild-type *p53* tumor suppressor gene.[32] As thrombospondin also contains a domain that can stimulate angiogenesis and is up-regulated in many tumors,[63] it may be prudent to use fragments of thrombospondin from the antiangiogenic domains of the molecule rather than the intact molecule for cancer treatment. Indeed, several peptide fragments of thrombospondin that have been generated can effectively inhibit angiogenesis and are being developed for clinical use.[64]

Several experimental rodent models suggest that the growth of a primary tumor can inhibit the production of distant metastases (reviewed by Gorelik[65] and by Prehn[66]). In one model, a variant of Lewis lung carcinoma that completely suppresses the growth of its metastases—angiostatin, a fragment of plasminogen—was purified from the urine of tumor-bearing mice.[67,68] Angiostatin potently inhibits endothelial cell proliferation[69] and migration in vitro, induces endothelial cell apoptosis[70] in a variety of endothelial cell types, and induces the activation of focal adhesion kinase.[71] Angiostatin has also been shown to interfere with several proteinases that are important in endothelial cell migration.[72] Adenosine triphosphate synthase[73] and angiomotin[74] on the surface of endothelial cells recently were described as receptors for angiostatin. Fragments of plasminogen that include the first three, four, or five kringles have angiostatin activity. Larger fragments do not have that activity.

Endostatin,[75,76] a 20-kDa carboxyl-terminal fragment of collagen XVIII, is a specific inhibitor of endothelial cell proliferation and migration[77] and has no obvious effect on resting endothelial cells[78] or on a variety of nonendothelial cells.[75] The crystal structures of human and mouse endostatin have now been determined, allowing for development of analogs.[79,80] Recently, endostatin was shown to induce endothelial cell apoptosis[81] and a marked reduction in Bcl-2 and Bcl-Xl antiapoptotic protein, to inhibit migration and proliferation, and to cause G_1 arrest of endothelial cells stimulated with bFGF or VEGF. It has also been shown to bind tropomyosin[82] on the surface of endothelial cells and to interact with endothelial integrins[83] and proteases that are important in endothelial cell shape[84] and motility.[85]

Endostatin is derived from the NC1 domain on collagen XVIII. Recently, several groups described fragments from the NC1 domain of other collagens that can also inhibit angiogenesis. Restin, a C-terminal fragment of collagen XV that is homologous to collagen XVIII, has also been shown to be antiangiogenic.[86] As with endostatin, restin potently inhibits the growth of human renal cell carcinoma xenografts. Further, fragments from the NC1 domain of collagen IV, which can regulate endothelial cell migration,[87] have also been shown to be antiangiogenic.[88,89] Several groups are studying fragments derived from other collagens to elucidate their role in angiogenesis.

It has been determined that several other endogenous angiogenesis inhibitors are fragments of proteins with distinct functions. One of the first such fragments to be described is a 16-kDa prolactin fragment produced in the pituitary.[90] Native and recombinant 16-kDa prolactins maintain biological activity as prolactin agonists but, unlike intact prolactin, also inhibit endothelial proliferation and capillary tube formation in vitro and angiogenesis in vivo; they also have a potent antitumor effect.[91] Recently, both the N-terminal fragments and intact versions of the human prolactin–growth hormone family were found to have opposing effects on angiogenesis.[92] Recombinant N-terminal fragments of prolactin, growth hormone, placental lactogen, and growth hormone variant all inhibit angiogenesis, possibly by blocking the activation of mitogen activated protein (MAP) kinase downstream of bFGF and VEGF or by increased expression of plasminogen activator inhibitor-1 in capillary endothelial cells.[93] A dual role in angiogenesis has also been described for proliferin, which is angiogenic, and proliferin-related peptide, which is antiangiogenic, in the placenta.[94] The existence of both stimulatory and inhibitory angiogenic activities within the same molecules may provide an efficient means of regulating physiologic angiogenesis. Further, a plasmin-derived internal fragment of the angiogenesis inhibitor platelet factor 4[95] is up to fiftyfold more potent[96] than is the intact molecule. Synthetic fragments of murine epidermal growth factor[97] and fragments of laminin[98] all inhibit endothelial cell proliferation and angiogenesis. Vasostatin,[99–101] a potent and specific angiogenesis inhibitor, is an N-terminal fragment of calreticulin that was purified from the supernatant of Epstein-Barr virus–immortalized cell lines. The generation of vasostatin, along with IP-10 and Mig, is in part responsible for angiogenesis suppression and tumor regression induced by Epstein-Barr virus-immortalized cells.[102]

While studying the inhibition by a human small-cell lung cancer model in a model system to screen human tumors for the production of angiogenesis inhibitors, we discovered that the cleaved conformation of antithrombin has potent antiangiogenic and antitumor activity.[103] The intact native molecule did not have this effect. As with angiostatin and endostatin, the inhibitory activity was specific for endothelial cells. However, in the case of antithrombin, it is the change in conformation of the molecule, and not the cleavage per se, that accounts for the antiangiogenic activity.[103–105]

When this is taken together with the discovery of angiostatin and endostatin, a theme has emerged in which endogenous inhibitors of angiogenesis arise from larger proteins with distinct and varied functions. If common proteases or similar cleavage patterns (or both) are found, a new general mechanism of proteolytic events regulating the vascular system may be revealed.

Targeted Therapy

Many angiogenesis regulators interact with growth factor receptors.[106,107] Many of these, such as VEGF/VPF and FGF, are receptor tyrosine kinases. Recently, a new class of ligands for the receptor tyrosine kinase Tie2, which is expressed almost exclusively by endothelial cells, was described.[108,109] These molecules—angiopoietin-1 and angiopoietin-2—regulate angiogenesis and vascular development. Angiopoietin-1 recruits pericytes to newly formed capillary sprouts and may help to stabilize newly formed capillaries, whereas angiopoietin-2 may antagonize the process. Strategies that target receptor tyrosine kinases that are involved in angiogenesis are being developed for use in the treatment of cancer, and several are in clinical trial. Through the use of these agents, angiogenesis can be targeted directly or indirectly.[2,110] One strategy involves directly blocking the binding of the growth factor to its target receptor using antibodies or small molecule inhibitors. Monoclonal antibodies to such angiogenic factors as bFGF, VEGF/VPF,[111] epidermal growth factor (EGF),[112,113] and Tie2 can potently inhibit angiogenesis tumor growth for a wide variety of tumors. Alternatively, the signaling of the growth factor receptor can be blocked using antibodies or small-molecule receptor tyrosine kinase antagonists.[114–117] A variety of agents that have also been produced target autophosphorylation or the downstream signals of receptor tyrosine kinase activity. By selectively targeting the endothelial cell, these strategies have shown significant anti-tumor efficacy.

Soluble receptors for angiogenic factors may play a role in the systemic regulation of angiogenesis and can be used to inhibit the activity of proangiogenic molecules. Circulating soluble receptors for flt-1, a receptor for VEGF/VPF, and binding proteins for FGFs have been described.[118,119] Their physiologic function is not known, but they may limit the levels of angiogenic factors in the circulation, reducing the levels typically seen in cancer patients. When delivered regionally using adenovirus-mediated gene therapy, a secreted form of the soluble flt-1 VEGF/VPF receptor inhibited tumor growth in murine metastasis models of colon cancer.[120] Similar strategies using locoregional or systemic therapy with soluble receptors for VEGF/VPF and other growth factors may provide a means to control angiogenesis and tumor growth. Antisense targeting of angiogenic factors or their receptors, such as the VEGF/VPF receptor, can be used to inhibit angiogenesis and tumor growth.[121,122]

Many receptor tyrosine kinases are important for both tumor cells and endothelial cells. For example, blockade of the EGF receptor targets both the tumor cell and tumor-associated endothelial cells,[116] leading to apoptosis and regression of pancreatic cancer in mice. The blockade of these receptors works in part by causing the down-regulation of expression of proangiogenic factors by tumor cells but may also have direct effects on the endothelial cells in some cases.[123] Thus, these agents offer the potential for both indirect and direct effects on both the tumor and endothelial cell compartments. Recently, it was shown that the expression of EGF or transforming growth factor alpha (TGF-α) by tumor cells increases expression of the EGF receptor by endothelial cells in vivo.[123] Platelet-derived growth factor (PDGF) may also have both indirect effects on the tumor vasculature by increasing expression of such proangiogenic molecules as VEGF/VPF[124,125] and direct effects on endothelial cells that increase their expression of PDGF receptor in response to PDGF production by tumor cells.[126]

Although strategies to target angiogenesis by blocking the proangiogenic molecules offer great promise, they are also associated with several potential limitations. The expression of receptor tyrosine kinases varies markedly between different tumor types, and not all tumor cells will express each receptor. It will, therefore, be critical to first screen tumor specimens for both the ligand and its receptor before initiating therapy with a specific protein tyrosine kinase inhibitor. However, even tumors that express the targeted growth factor receptor could eventually become resistant to the agents by expressing different growth factors or their receptors (or both). In addition, most advanced malignant tumors produce multiple angiogenic factors, so targeting only one may not be adequate for complete tumor control. For example, PTK787, an inhibitor of VEGF/VPF receptor tyrosine kinase phosphorylation, significantly reduced the malignant pleural effusion associated with lung adenocarcinoma in mice but did not reduce the lung tumor burden.[127] One strategy to overcome the limitations of targeting individual growth factors is to design small molecules that can target multiple factors. SU6668, for example, is a small-molecule synthetic tyrosine kinase inhibitor of the receptors for VEGF/VPF (flk-1), FGF, and PDGF.[128] In vivo, SU6668 is a potent inhibitor of angiogenesis and tumor growth; in some cases, it induces tumor regression when used alone in mice. As an alternative to using a single agent, such as SU6668, it may also be possible to combine individual drugs that target different growth factors so that antiangiogenic therapy can be optimized on an individual basis.

Many receptor tyrosine kinases can affect the survival of both proliferating and quiescent endothelial cells. As a result, some of these agents could be associated with toxicity due to effects on or disruption of the normal vasculature. VEGF, for example, is critical not only for angiogenesis but for endothelial cell integrity and function.[129–131] In clinical trials with agents that target VEGF, hemorrhagic and thrombotic complications may result from disruption of the normal vascular integrity. Thus, therapy with these agents will have to be monitored closely and optimized for each patient.

Antiangiogenic Scheduling of Chemotherapy

Endothelial cell proliferation is an important component of angiogenesis, and dividing endothelial cells are highly sensitive to most chemotherapeutics in vitro. However, cytotoxic chemotherapy is typically administered at high doses relatively infrequently, allowing for repopulation of endothelial cells between doses. Thus, current strategies used to administer chemotherapy have only a limited effect on angiogenesis. By increasing the frequency of administration of these agents and by giving them over prolonged periods, the antiangiogenic activity of cytotoxic agents can be enhanced. For example, cyclophosphamide at low dose given every 6 days for prolonged periods can produce an antiangiogenic effect greater than that of higher doses given every 21 days.[132] It is important to note that it is not the low dose of the chemotherapeutic agent that is responsible for the observed antiangiogenic effects. Instead, it is the more frequent and prolonged administration of the drug that results in the those effects. The lower doses are used to minimize the toxicity and mortality that would normally be associated with the frequent administration and prolonged course of chemotherapy.

Antiangiogenic scheduling of chemotherapeutic agents was effective at controlling the growth of tumors that were almost completely resistant to the conventional scheduling. However, tumor growth resumed in many cases despite the continued administration of the antiangiogenic chemotherapy[132] when it was used alone. The mechanism of this apparent resistance is an increase in the production of proangiogenic molecules by the tumor cells in the treated mice, leading to an enhanced survival of endothelial cells.[133] The treatment of neuroblastomas in mice with an antiangiogenic schedule of vinblastine was associated with an increased expression of VEGF/VPF and, hence, increased survival of endothelial cells.[133] By combining the vinblastine therapy with VEGF/VPF blockade, an almost complete and durable tumor control was achieved. A similar enhancement of the anti-tumor effects of antiangiogenic scheduling have been reported for cyclophosphamide combined with TNP-470[132] and of carboplatinum and etoposide combined with the angiogenesis inhibitor PEX, a fragment of matrix metalloproteinase-2 (MMP-2).[134] The various combinations of cytotoxic agents with antiangiogenic agents provided a means of overcoming the resistance to therapy encountered with cytotoxic agents administered alone.

Given that cytotoxic drugs at conventional doses can produce rapid anti-tumor effects, an effective and rapid anticancer strategy might be to administer cytotoxic agents at conventional does but to continue therapy using antiangiogenic doses of chemotherapeutics given chronically. Because the use of antiangiogenic schedules of chemotherapy can still be associated with toxicity to normal tissues, this strategy may be useful only until more specific antiangiogenic agents become available.

Antiangiogenic Therapy-Induced Tumor Dormancy

Prior to the discovery of angiostatin, it had been generally assumed that antiangiogenic therapy would produce cytostasis in tumors but not tumor regression. Studies with angiostatin, however, demonstrated that tumors can be induced to regress.[67,135] Indeed, tumor dormancy was characterized by a balance of tumor cell proliferation and apoptosis and a virtually complete suppression of angiogenesis.[67,68,135] Nevertheless, this antiangiogenic monotherapy was unable to eradicate the disease completely. Since the discovery of angiostatin, several antiangiogenic agents, including endostatin,[75] an antiangiogenic form of antithrombin,[103] and SU6668,[136,137] an inhibitor of VEGF, bFGF, and PDGF receptor tyrosine kinase signaling, have been shown to induce regression of tumors. These agents and other angiogenesis inhibitors offer great potential but present a number of unique challenges. Before these agents can be integrated into clinical research, a better understanding of their mechanism of action and their interaction with conventional modalities is required, and surrogates with which to monitor response to therapy must be developed.

Antiangiogenic Therapy to Control Metastasis

The mobilization of angiogenesis inhibitors,[67] such as angiostatin, by enzymes produced by tumor cells or tumor-associated host cells[35,36] can inhibit the growth of distant metastases. Curative radiotherapy of primary tumors in rodents can be followed by the rapid growth of previously dormant metastases that kill the animal within 18 days after the completion of radiotherapy.[138] Systemic administration of recombinant angiostatin, however, prevents the growth of the metastases, suggesting that a population of patients may benefit from the addition of antiangiogenic therapy during or after radiotherapy to prevent the expansion of distant metastases.

DUAL ROLES OF PROTEINASES AND THEIR INHIBITORS IN THE REGULATION OF ANGIOGENESIS

Proangiogenic Effects of Proteases

Increased protease activity is a critical step in angiogenesis because it contributes to the invasive phenotype of endothelial cells. Indeed, the extracellular matrix and its components play a critical role in angiogenesis (reviewed by Liotta[139] and Stetler-Stevenson[140,141]). Plasmin is also important in the outgrowth of capillaries in the angiogenic response. The serpin plasminogen activator inhibitor-1 has been shown to inhibit angiogenesis, possibly by blocking the interaction of $\alpha v\beta 3$ with vitronectin.[142,143] Taken together with the discovery that antithrombin, another serpin, can also inhibit angiogenesis, these findings suggest that other serpins involved in the coagulation system may have effects on the endothelial cell. Further, the degradation of plasminogen by plasminogen activators in the presence of sulfhydryl donors can mobilize angiostatin.[144,145] Thus, the regulation of plasminogen activation has both a stimulatory and an inhibitory role in angiogenesis.

Inhibitors of Metalloproteinases

A family of endogenous proteins, the tissue inhibitors of the metalloproteinase family, has been shown to inhibit angiogenesis. The presence of MMP inhibitors in cartilage may in part explain its resistance to angiogenesis,[146,147] and cartilage also contains other factors, such as troponin I, that can inhibit angiogenesis.[62] Small molecules that can inhibit MMP activity have been described, including minocycline and other tetracyclines[148,149] and COL-3.[150] More recently, inhibitors that target the incorporation of zinc into the catalytic site of MMPs, such as marimistat and batimistat or the selective inhibitors BAY 12-9566[151,152] and AG3340,[153] have been developed to target only those MMPs that are important for tumor growth and angiogenesis. However, advanced clinical trials with many of these agents used alone or in combination with chemotherapeutics in cancer patients have been disappointing,[152] suggesting that a better understanding of their role in angiogenesis is needed.

Possible Decrease in Mobilization of Endogenous Angiogenesis Inhibitors by Proteinase Inhibitors

Although the inhibition of protease activity may offer both a direct antitumor effect and an antiangiogenic effect, there may be a disadvantage to administering a metalloproteinase inhibitor in some patients. As was described, many of the endogenous inhibitors of angiogenesis are generated by the cleavage of other proteins by metalloproteinases and other enzymes. In our original studies of the suppression of tumor growth by tumor mass,[67] we developed a variant of Lewis lung carcinoma (LLC-LM) in which a primary tumor could completely suppress the growth of its metastases by generating the angiogenesis inhibitor angiostatin from plasminogen. At the time of the initial discovery of angiostatin, the source of the protein was unclear. Northern analysis of the LLC-LM cells revealed no evidence that the tumor cells expressed angiostatin or other fragments of plasminogen, suggesting that angiostatin was derived from proteolysis of plasminogen.[36,67]

In a series of studies of a variant of LLC-LM lung carcinomas in mice, tumors that suppressed the growth of their metastases were found to express high levels of granulocyte macrophage colony-stimulating factor.[35] In response, granulocyte macrophage colony-stimulating factor[154] tumor-infiltrating macrophages were induced to increase their expression of MMP-12. Once activated, this MMP-12 then mobilized angiostatin from plasma-derived plasminogen and plasmin that was part of the tumor's neostroma. Thus, the production of angiostatin was dependent on the interaction of the tumor cells with their microenvironment and infiltrating stromal cells. Stromal cells have also been shown to be a critical source for stimulators of angiogenesis in colon and other malignancies.[34]

In a separate series of studies designed to determine whether LLC-LM cells secrete metalloproteinase activity, active gelatinase A (MMP-2) was identified in the conditioned medium of the tumor cells. MMP-2 could process plasminogen into angiostatin and, by specifically neutralizing the enzymatic activity, the mobilization of angiostatin from plasminogen by the tumor cells in an in vitro system could be blocked. Metalloproteinases can process other precursor or parent proteins into their bioactive form. For example, MMPs are involved in the processing of the TNF-α precursor protein,[155,156] TGF-α,[157] the β-amyloid precursor protein,[158] the lymphocyte L–selectin adhesion molecule,[159-161] the interleukin-6 receptor ectodomain,[162] the human thyrotropin receptor ectodomain,[163] the fibroblast growth factor receptor 1 ectodomain,[164] and EGF-like growth factor.[165] Taken together, these studies show that metalloproteinases can process a wide range of substrates, many of which play a role in angiogenesis.

Subsequent work has demonstrated that a variety of metalloproteinases and other enzymes important in tumor progression can cleave angiostatin from plasminogen.[144,166–168] An increasing number of studies now demonstrate that most angiogenesis inhibitors are fragments of larger parental molecules.[2] For example, an internal 16-kDa fragment of prolactin inhibits angiogenesis, whereas the parent molecule—intact prolactin—does not.[90,92,93,169] Other inhibitors of EC proliferation that are fragments of larger molecules include fragments of platelet factor 4,[95] which has greater antiangiogenic activity than does the intact molecule,[96] and thrombospondin,[64] EGF,[97] laminin,[170] fibronectin,[171] and endostatin.[75,76] Thus, metalloproteinases and other enzymes can play a central role in the regulation of tumor angiogenesis and potentially act in an inhibitory[146,147] or a stimulatory capacity. Further, the finding that angiogenesis inhibitors can be mobilized or activated by metalloproteinases suggests that therapeutic strategies for using inhibitors of metalloproteinase and other enzymatic activities must be carefully designed to consider both the clinical setting and the net effect on angiogenesis. Diagnostic and clinical strategies[138,172] for these inhibitors will have to be developed before they can be successfully incorporated into clinical practice.

The production of angiostatin by gelatinase A, metalloelastase, and other proteinases from the tumor or stromal cells helps to resolve the question as to why a primary tumor might produce angiostatin. By increased production of gelatinase A, the tumor may become more locally invasive but might also mobilize more angiostatin.[36] It may, therefore, be prudent to consider gelatinase A and other metalloproteinase inhibitors and metalloproteinases themselves as angiogenesis modulators instead of as merely inhibitors or stimulators. Angiogenesis may, therefore, depend not only on the balance of endothelial stimulators and inhibitors but on the balance of matrix-degrading proteases and their endogenous inhibitors. In addition, the increased permeability of the tumor vessels may lead to the sequestration of circulating plasminogen into the tumor's neostroma[15,173] that could then be cleaved into active angiostatin.

It has been widely suggested that the limited clinical success of broad-spectrum MMP inhibitors is due, at least in part, to their lack of specificity and associated side effects. However, an alternate explanation is that the regulation of MMP activity may, in some cases, decrease the release of angiogenesis inhibitors. This possibility suggests that it will be important to define, for each different tumor type, the precise roles of MMPs and their inhibitors in the modulation of angiogenesis and malignancy. In affected patients, the level of endogenous angiogenesis inhibitors could potentially decrease and would, therefore, need to be replaced.

LIMITATIONS OF ANTIANGIOGENIC MONOTHERAPY

Although antiangiogenic agents show great promise in preclinical cancer models, their use, particularly when administered as monotherapy, has been associated with a number of potential limits and problems in the clinic. In this section, we outline some of these limitations.

Heterogeneity of the Endothelium

Recent work shows that endothelial cells in different organs express different surface receptors[22] and have different patterns of gene expression.[174] Angiogenic endothelial cells also express discrete surface receptors that were used effectively to target the tumor vasculature with Adriamycin and other drugs. More recently, organ microenvironment has been shown to regulate the expression for the growth factors EGF and PDGF in mice.[123,126] These data suggest that endothelial cells in different tissue beds may respond differentially to antiangiogenic therapy. Thus, antiangiogenic agents may have to be used in combination with each other, and therapy may have to be optimized on an organ- and tissue-specific, and perhaps patient-specific, basis.

Potential for Undesirable Toxicity with Some Antiangiogenic Agents

In adults, endothelial cells typically maintain a state of prolonged quiescence in most tissues.[25] The female menstrual cycle is an exception to this pattern. In addition, wound healing requires angiogenesis. It had been assumed that antiangiogenic therapy would, therefore, impair wound healing. TNP-470 treatment of mice led to a decrease in the tensile strength of cutaneous wound repair. However, this decrease occurred only if the drug was administered within 24 hours of the wounding.[175] TNP-470 has also been shown to impair fracture healing in the bones of rats.[176] Although TNP-470 is a selective angiogenesis inhibitor, it has effects on other tissues, and it is unclear whether the effects on wound and fracture healing were due to its antiangiogenic effect. More recently, endostatin was tested for its effect on wound healing in mice. In one study, no effect was seen in mice receiving doses of endostatin that could completely suppress tumor and ocular angiogenesis.[177] In another study, only subtle histologic changes were seen in healing wounds of mice treated with endostatin.[178] Indeed, the decreased fibrosis observed in this model could be beneficial. In clinical trials of endostatin, no effect on wound healing has been observed.[179]

Factors that target the growth factor VEGF may disrupt endothelial integrity. Although VEGF is a stimulator of angiogenesis, an equally important role for the molecule is to maintain endothelial cell survival.[130] Thus, these factors may lead to a disruption of the normal vasculature architecture. Indeed, VEGF is critical for normal vascular development and, indeed, VEGF knockout was lethal to mouse embryos.[180] In clinical trials, VEGF inhibitors that target the protein directly or target its receptor have been associated with thrombotic or hemorrhagic complications. Although observed only in a small percentage of patients, these data suggest that anti-VEGF strategies will have to be monitored closely, particularly if the agents are given at high doses for prolonged periods.

Delay in Tumor Response After Initiation of Antiangiogenic Therapy

Angiostatin,[67] endostatin,[75] and antiangiogenic antithrombin[103] are endogenous angiogenesis inhibitors that are mobilized by proteolytic cleavage[35,36,181,182] of their parent proteins: plasminogen, collagen XVIII, and antithrombin, respectively. All three are highly specific for microvascular endothelial cells, can induce a blockade of tumor angiogenesis, and have not caused any significant toxicity in preclinical and clinical use even after prolonged therapy. However, preclinical studies with all these agents have demonstrated a number of potential therapeutic limitations that could arise with their use as monotherapy in the treatment of cancer. In several in vivo models, all these agents inhibited tumor growth but were associated with a delayed onset of activity.[76,135] In many of the animal models, tumors progressed by as much as 400% in the first several days after initiation of therapy. All these models used rapidly growing tumors. Given that the doubling time of murine tumors is severalfold higher than that observed in the presentation of human cancer, this delay in the onset of activity could translate to several months in patients. For example, antiangiogenic therapy with IFN-α for the treatment of life-threatening pediatric hemangiomas[51] or giant-cell tumors[55] required several months of continued therapy before a significant clinical response was observed. For patients with advanced metastatic or locally advanced disease, this delay in onset of activity may render the use of these agents impractical.

Another potential limit for the use of antiangiogenic agents is the high dose over the prolonged treatment course that is required to obtain maximal efficacy. As a result, it may not be feasible or practical to produce the amount of material that would be required for widespread clinical use. For angiostatin protein, a dose of up to 100 mg/kg/day[135] was required to reduce tumor size in mice, and treatment had to be continued for several months to prevent tumor recurrence. Although recent work suggests that the delivery of antiangiogenic agents via continuous infusion[183,184] or sustained release[75,76] may allow for a reduction of the bolus dose, the amount of protein needed for widespread use may restrict the utility of this therapeutic approach. By combining antiangiogenic agents with one another and conventional agents, it may be possible to reduce the dose required and frequency of administration and render their use more practical.

Persistence of Microscopic Residual Disease After Antiangiogenic Therapy

Perhaps the most significant limitation of antiangiogenic monotherapy is the inability of these agents to eradicate disease completely even after prolonged administration at high doses. For most angiogenesis inhibitors, tumor growth generally resumes within a short time[135] after cessation of therapy. Although prolonged therapy with endostatin, either by cycled administration of the drug[76] or by prolonged administration at high dose (M.S. O'Reilly, unpublished data), did induce a self-sustained dormancy for a wide variety of tumors that persisted off therapy, residual microscopic disease was still present in all the treated mice. Immunohistochemistry of the residual microscopic tumor revealed little or no evidence of angiogenesis but also revealed a high proliferative index of the tumor cells that was offset by a high apoptotic index. Repeated injury of the site of residual disease or the administration of a combination of TGF-β1 and bFGF in these mice resulted in rapid locoregional recurrence (M.S. O'Reilly, unpublished data). If these same results are observed in patients treated with antiangiogenic agents, they might then require prolonged antiangiogenic therapy. Although little or no toxicity has been observed to date for angiostatin or endostatin, their prolonged use could result in late effects. Endothelial cells normally exist in a quiescent state with a turnover rate of months to years.[25] The prevention of this turnover by prolonged therapy could lead to potential normal organ toxicities. Further, it would obviously be preferable to develop strategies using angiogenesis inhibitors in combination with more traditional modalities to eradicate the disease at the time of initial treatment in as many patients as possible.

ANTIANGIOGENIC AGENTS AS PART OF COMBINED-MODALITY THERAPY

To overcome the limitations of antiangiogenic monotherapy, it will be necessary to combine antiangiogenic agents with one another and with existing and emerging modalities. In this section, we discuss the combination of antiangiogenic agents with chemotherapy and radiotherapy in the treatment of cancer.

Combination of Antiangiogenic Therapy with Chemotherapy

Teicher et al[185] were among the first to show a synergistic effect between cytotoxic agents, such as tetrahydrocortisol, β-cyclodextrin tetradecasulfate, minocycline, and antiangiogenic agents for treatment of transplantable murine tumors.[185] In a similar set of experiments, a combination of the angiogenesis inhibitor TNP-470 (AGM-1470) and minocycline given alone or in combination with cytotoxic agents was administered to mice bearing Lewis lung carcinoma.[186] The angiogenesis inhibitor cortisone acetate has also been shown to enhance the activity of chemotherapy in a model of transitional cell carcinoma.[187] In a model of non-Hodgkin's lymphoma, the sequential administration of cytotoxic therapy followed by endostatin therapy stabilized disease in mice.[188] Clinical trials are now being designed using antiangiogenic schedules of cytotoxic agents in patients with advanced malignancy that is resistant to conventional regimens of cytotoxic agents. It may be prudent to combine conventional doses of chemotherapy (i.e., maximum tolerated dose) with antiangiogenic doses to achieve rapid and durable control of primary and metastatic disease.

Effects of Radiotherapy on Angiogenesis

Radiochemotherapy may have a systemic or local effect on angiogenesis. Studies by Canney and Dean[189] demonstrated an increase in the level of TGF-β1, which is a potent stimulator of angiogenesis in vivo, after radiochemotherapy to the liver. More recently, Gorski et al[190] demonstrated that the expression of VEGF, detected within tumors by both immunohistochemistry and Northern analysis, was increased after local irradiation. The increased expression of VEGF was associated with a decreased efficacy of the irradiation against the primary tumor. Radiotherapy may, in some cases, inhibit systemic angiogenesis. In a recent study by Hartford et al,[191] radiotherapy of a primary tumor in rodents was associated with an inhibition of angiogenesis seen in a cranial window at a distant site. This apparent inhibition of systemic angiogenesis after radiotherapy was in contrast to the effect seen after surgery, in which the net result was stimulation of angiogenesis in the cranial window. An interesting finding was that the plasma levels of endostatin, an endogenous angiogenesis inhibitor, in the irradiated mice were twice those found in the nonirradiated mice. When taken together with prior studies,[138] these findings strongly suggest that radiotherapy may have a proangiogenic effect at a remote site by increasing the levels of angiogenesis stimulators, such as VEGF or TGB-β, or by decreasing the mobilization of angiogenesis inhibitors, such as angiostatin. Therefore, the addition of antiangiogenic therapy to radiotherapy may restore the delicate balance of angiogenic factors and thereby control locoregional and metastatic tumor growth.

Combination of Antiangiogenic Agents with Radiotherapy

It had long been assumed that an angiogenesis inhibitor would impair the effect of ionizing radiation by inducing hypoxia in the tumor bed. Teicher et al.,[192] however, observed that antiangiogenic therapy given in combination with the angiogenesis inhibitors TNP-470 and minocycline, a weak inhibitor of metalloproteinase activity, improved tumor oxygenation and the anti-tumor effect of radiotherapy. To understand better the benefits of combining antiangiogenic agents with radiotherapy, Hansen-Algenstaedt and colleagues[193] examined intratumoral Po_2 during antiangiogenic therapy with anti-VEGF-R-2 antibodies. They observed that Po_2 initially decreased with therapy but then subsequently increased.[193]

The antitumor effect of hypothermia is also enhanced by the combination with antiangiogenic therapy of TNP-470.[194–196] Murata et al,[197] however, observed that the concurrent treatment of mouse breast carcinoma xenografts with TNP-470 and fractionated radiotherapy decreased tumor oxygenation and decreased therapeutic response. The enhancement of the effect of radiotherapy by antiangiogenic therapy may also be dependent on the tumor microenvironment. Lund et al[198] treated mice bearing xenografts of glioblastoma multiforme (growing in the muscle or the cranium) with TNP-470 alone, radiotherapy alone, or their combination. Tumors growing at different sites responded differently. Specifically, tumors in the muscle regressed in mice given combination therapy, whereas tumors in the cranium did not. It is tempting to speculate that differences in the capillary beds and the microenvironment of the brain and the musculature of the thigh may have contributed to the differences in response. In the first study of the combination of a specific inhibitor of angiogenesis with radiotherapy, Mauceri et al[199] demonstrated a synergistic effect when angiostatin and ionizing radiation were combined to treat a variety of transplantable tumors in mice.

More recently, a number of antiangiogenic agents in combination with concurrent radiotherapy for cancer have been tested in preclinical models. Milas and colleagues[200] observed an enhancement of the response to radiotherapy when it was combined with a selective inhibitor of the cyclooxygenase-2 enzyme or with antibodies directed against the EGF receptor.[201] An increase in tumor growth delay and an augmentation of tumor curability was observed in the combined modality groups. A similar enhancement of the response to radiotherapy occurred when it is combined with anti-VEGF agents. For example, Gorski et al[190] showed that treatment of tumor-bearing mice with radiotherapy and antibodies against VEGF had a synergistic effect against the primary tumor. More recently, it was shown that the combination of agents that prevent VEGF signaling plus radiotherapy reduces tumor resistance to irradiation and improves response to therapy.[202] Kozin et al[203] treated mice implanted with human small-cell lung cancer or glioblastoma multiforme with fractionated radiotherapy combined with antibodies directed against the VEGF receptor 2 and followed up the surviving mice for at least 6 months. The dose of radiation required to control 50% of tumors was diminished by at least 1.3-fold by the concurrent addition of the antiangiogenic agent.

In most of the studies to date, radiotherapy has been administered concurrent with the antiangiogenic agents. In the only published study to date comparing different sequencing of radiotherapy and antiangiogenic therapy,[204] the concurrent administration of irradiation with antiangiogenic therapies produced the best therapy. However, determining the optimal strategies for combining antiangiogenic therapy with radiotherapy or other modalities will require extensive preclinical and clinical testing.

MONITORING ANTIANGIOGENIC THERAPY

Antiangiogenic agents, as with many other biological therapies, may not result in the same pattern of regressions and responses that are seen with effective chemotherapeutic agents. As described, tumor progression over a period of several weeks or months may occur when antiangiogenic agents are used to treat advanced malignancy. Thus, conventional strategies for monitoring anticancer therapies may not apply for antiangiogenic agents. Instead, novel surrogates must be developed and validated.

Circulating levels of angiogenic factors have been used to determine prognosis for a wide variety of cancers in patients. In patients with early stages of disease, elevated levels of circulating proangiogenic factors are associated with an increased risk of locoregional failure and metastatic disease for a broad range of malignancies for VEGF/VPF,[205,206] bFGF,[207] and other proangiogenic molecules.[208] These strategies were based on the prognostic value to tumor microvessel density that was initially demonstrated for breast cancer[209,210] and has since been demonstrated for many malignancies.[211] However, the use of circulating levels of these factors as surrogates for responses is not as clear. Levels of bFGF and VEGF have been measured in clinical trials of several different angiogenesis inhibitors and, in most cases, have shown no definitive correlation to response. In many cases, there is a marked variability in the levels of these factors prior to therapy. Thus, circulating levels of individual factors may not be adequate, and angiogenic profiles that include both stimulators and inhibitors of angiogenesis may have to be developed.

Tumor biopsies may also provide information that can be used as surrogate markers for angiogenesis,[212–216] as can determinations of tissue expression of both pro- and antiangiogenic factors. Tissues can also be studied for evidence of tumor and endothelial cell proliferation, apoptosis, and microvessel density. However, these strategies have yet to be validated as surrogates for response to antiangiogenic therapy, are impractical for many patients, and are invasive.

As an alternative to invasive strategies, imaging of tumor blood flow and tumor blood volume has been proposed to monitor angiogenesis. Ultrasonography, magnetic resonance imaging, computed tomography, and positron emission tomography are all being studied in clinical trials of angiogenesis inhibitors. However, whether blood flow per se is a direct measure of decreased angiogenesis is unclear. Carmeliet and Jain[217] and Boucher et al[218] proposed that the inhibition of angiogenesis may lead to tumor growth inhibition that would then result in a decrease in interstitial pressure and an apparent increase in blood flow. As with the use of tumor biopsies and bodily fluids, however, imaging modalities have not yet been validated as surrogates for response to antiangiogenic therapy. Thus, clinical trials of antiangiogenic agents have to be designed not only to determine whether the agents are safe and effective but to validate both invasive and noninvasive surrogates of response.

CONCLUSION

Since its beginning in the early 1970s, the field of angiogenesis research has grown and has broadened the understanding of a number of biological processes. It is now apparent that angiogenesis is a complex process that involves the interaction of endothelial cells with host stromal cells and the organ microenvironment. Many endothelial targets have now been identified, and many antiangiogenic agents are being evaluated for clinical efficacy. These agents should have far-reaching applications in a variety of clinical settings and have the potential to improve efficacy and diminish toxicity in treatment of a variety of diseases. However, a better understanding of the process of angiogenesis is still needed before these agents can be successfully incorporated into clinical practice. To target the tumor vasculature effectively, therapies will have to be individualized and customized. Antiangiogenic therapy is likely to evolve on an organ- and tissue-specific basis and integrated with existing and emerging therapies for treating cancer.

ACKNOWLEDGMENTS

The authors thank Walter Pagel for critical editorial comments and Lola López for expert assistance with the preparation of this chapter. This work was supported in part by Cancer Center Support Core Grant CA16672 from the National Cancer Institute, National Institutes of Health.

REFERENCES

1. Folkman J. What is the evidence that tumors are angiogenesis dependent? J Natl Cancer Inst 1990;82:4–6.
2. O'Reilly MS. Antiangiogenesis: basic principles. In: Rosenberg SA, ed. Principles and Practice of the Biologic Therapy of Cancer, 3rd ed. Philadelphia: Lippincott Williams & Wilkins, 2000: 827–843.
3. Singh RK, Gutman M, Bucana CD et al. Interferons alpha and beta downregulate the expression of basic fibroblast growth factor in human carcinomas. Proc Natl Acad Sci USA 1995;92: 4562–4566.
4. Dark GG, Hill SA, Prise VE et al. Combretastatin A-4, an agent that displays potent and selective toxicity toward tumor vasculature, Cancer Res 1997;57:1829–1834.
5. Fidler IJ, Kerbel RS, Ellis LM. Biology of cancer: angiogenesis. In: DeVita VT, Hellman S, Rosenberg SA, eds. Cancer Principles and Practice of Oncology, 6th ed. Philadelphia: Lippincott Williams & Wilkins, 2001:137–147.
6. Rak J, Filmus J, Kerbel RS. Reciprocal paracrine interactions between tumour cells and endothelial cells: the 'angiogenesis progression' hypothesis. Eur J Cancer 1996;32A:2438–2450.
7. Folkman J. Tumor angiogenesis and tissue factor. Nat Med 1996;2:167–168.
8. Fidler IJ, Ellis LM. The implications of angiogenesis to the biology and therapy of cancer metastasis. Cell 1994;79:185–188.
9. Hanahan D, Folkman J. Patterns and emerging mechanisms of the angiogenic switch during tumorigenesis. Cell 1996; 86:353–364.
10. Folkman J. Angiogenesis in cancer, vascular, rheumatoid and other disease. Nat Med 1995;1: 27–31.
11. Moulton KS, Heller E, Konerding MA et al. Angiogenesis inhibitors endostatin or TNP-470 reduce intimal neovascularization and plaque growth in apolipoprotein E–deficient mice. Circulation 1999;99:1726–1732.
12. Jain RK. Normalizing tumor vasculature with anti-angiogenic therapy: a new paradigm for combination therapy. Nat Med 2001;7:987–989.
13. Konerding MA, Malkusch W, Klapthor B et al. Evidence for characteristic vascular patterns in solid tumours: quantitative studies using corrosion casts. Br J Cancer 1999;80:724–732.
14. Brown LF, Guidi AJ, Schnitt SJ et al. Vascular stroma formation in carcinoma *in situ*, invasive carcinoma, and metastatic carcinoma of the breast. Clin Cancer Res 1999;5:1041–1056.
15. Dvorak HF. Tumors: wounds that do not heal. N Engl J Med 1986;315:1650–1659.
16. Nagy JA, Brown LF, Senger DR et al. Pathogenesis of tumor stroma generation: a critical role for leaky blood vessels and fibrin deposition. Biochim Biophys Acta 1989;948:305–326.
17. Libutti SK, Pluda JM. Antiangiogenesis: clinical applications. In: Rosenberg SA, ed. Principles and Practice of the Biologic Therapy of Cancer, 3rd ed. Philadelphia: Lippincott Williams & Wilkins, 2000:844–864.
18. Folkman J. Clinical applications of angiogenesis research. N Engl J Med 1995;333:1757–1763.
19. Burrows FJ, Thorpe PE. Eradication of large solid tumors in mice with an immunotoxin directed against tumor vasculature. Proc Natl Acad Sci USA 1993;90:8996–9000.

20. Huang X, Molema G, King S et al. Tumor infarction in mice by antibody-directed targeting of tissue factor to tumor vasculature. Science 1997;275:547–550.

21. Tozer GM, Prise VE, Wilson J et al. Combretastatin A-4 phosphate as a tumor vascular-targeting agent: early effects in tumors and normal tissues. Cancer Res 1999;59:1626–1634.

22. Arap W, Pasqualini R, Ruoslahti E. Cancer treatment by targeted drug delivery to tumor vasculature in a mouse model. Science 1998;279:377–380.

23. Ellerby HM, Arap W, Ellerby LM et al. Anti-cancer activity of targeted pro-apoptotic peptides. Nat Med 1999; 5:1032–1038.

24. Pasqualini R, Koivunen E, Kain R et al. Aminopeptidase N is a receptor for tumor-homing peptides and a target for inhibiting angiogenesis. Cancer Res 2000;60:722–727.

25. Hobson B, Denekamp J. Endothelial proliferation in tumors and normal tissues: continuous labeling studies. Br J Cancer 1984;49:405–413.

26. Kandel J, Bossy-Wetzel E, Radvany F et al. Neovascularization is associated with a switch to the export of bFGF in the multistep development of fibrosarcoma. Cell 1991;66:1095–1104.

27. Shing Y, Folkman J, Sullivan R et al. Heparin-affinity: purification of a tumor-derived capillary endothelial cell growth factor. Science 1984;223:1296–1299.

28. Senger DR, Galli SJ, Dvorak AM et al. Tumor cells secrete a vascular permeability factor that promotes accumulation of ascites fluid. Science 1983;219:983–985.

29. Ferrara N, Henzel WJ. Pituitary follicular cells secrete a novel heparin-binding growth factor specific for vascular endothelial cells. Biochem Biophys Res Commun 1989;161:851–858.

30. Koch AE, Polverini PJ, Kunkel SL et al. Interleukin-8 as a macrophage-derived mediator of angiogenesis. Science 1992;258:1798–1801.

31. Grant DS, Kleinman HK, Goldberg ID et al. Scatter factor induces blood vessel formation *in vivo*. Proc Natl Acad Sci USA 1993;90:1937–1941.

32. Dameron KM, Volpert OV, Tainsky MA, Bouck N. Control of angiogenesis in fibroblasts by p53 regulation of thrombospondin-1. Science 1994;265:1582–1584.

33. Nickoloff BJ, Mitra RS, Varani J et al. Aberrant production of interleukin-8 and thrombospondin-1 by psoriatic keratinocytes mediates angiogenesis. Am J Pathol 1994;144:820–828.

34. Kuniyasu H, Yasui W, Shinohara H et al. Induction of angiogenesis by hyperplastic colonic mucosa adjacent to colon cancer. Am J Pathol 2000;157:1523–1535.

35. Dong Z, Kumar R, Yang X, Fidler IJ. Macrophage-derived metalloelastase is responsible for the generation of angiostatin in Lewis lung carcinoma. Cell 1997;88:801–810.

36. O'Reilly MS, Wiederschain D, Stetler-Stevenson WG et al. Regulation of angiostatin production by matrix metalloproteinase-2 in a model of concomitant resistance. J Biol Chem 1999;274: 29568–29571.

37. Uze G, Lutfalla G, Mogensen KE. Alpha and beta interferons and their receptor and their friends and relations. J Interferon Cytokine Res 1995;15:3–26.

38. Tamm I, Lin SL, Pfeffer LM, Sehgal PB. Interferons alpha and beta as cellular regulatory molecules. Interferon 1987;9:13–74.

39. Rossi G. Interferons and cell differentiation. Interferon 1985;6:31–68.

40. Resnitzky D, Yarden A, Zipori D, Kimchi A. Autocrine beta-related interferon controls c-myc suppression and growth arrest during hematopoietic cell differentiation. Cell 1986;46:31–40.

41. Strander H. Interferon treatment of human neoplasia. Adv Cancer Res 1986;46:1–265.

42. Ferrantini M, Proietti E, Santodonato L et al. Alpha 1-interferon gene transfer into metastatic Friend leukemia cells abrogated tumorigenicity in immunocompetent mice: antitumor therapy by means of interferon-producing cells. Cancer Res 1993;53:1107–1112.

43. Gresser I, Belardelli F, Maury C, et al. Injection of mice with antibody to interferon enhances the growth of transplantable murine tumors. J Exp Med 1983;158:2095–2107.

44. Gutterman JU. Cytokine therapeutics: lessons from interferon alpha. Proc Natl Acad Sci USA 1994;91:1198–1205.

45. Johns TG, Mackay IR, Callister KA et al. Antiproliferative potencies of interferons on melanoma cell lines and xenografts: higher efficacy of interferon beta. J Natl Cancer Inst 1992;84:1185–1190.

46. Sica G, Fabbroni L, Castagnetta L et al. Antiproliferative effect of interferons on human prostate carcinoma cell lines. Urol Res 1989;17:111–115.

47. Heyns AD, Eldor A, Vlodavsky I et al. The antiproliferative effect of interferon and the mitogenic activity of growth factors are independent cell cycle events. Studies with vascular smooth muscle cells and endothelial cells. Exp Cell Res 1985;161:297–306.

48. Friesel R, Komoriya A, Maciag T. Inhibition of endothelial cell proliferation by gamma-interferon. J Cell Biol 1987;104:689–696.

49. Ruszczak Z, Detmar M, Imcke E, Orfanos CE. Effects of rIFN alpha, beta, and gamma on the morphology, proliferation, and cell surface antigen expression of human dermal microvascular endothelial cells *in vitro*. J Invest Dermatol 1990;95:693–699.

50. Hicks C, Breit SN, Penny R. Response of microvascular endothelial cells to biological response modifiers. Immunol Cell Biol 1989;67:271–277.

51. Ezekowitz RAB, Mulliken JB, Folkman J. Interferon alpha-2a therapy for life-threatening hemangiomas of infancy. N Engl J Med 1992;326:1456–1463.

52. Orchard P, Smith C, Woods W et al. Treatment of hemangioendotheliomas with alpha interferon. Lancet 1989;2:565–567.

53. White CM, Sondheimer HM, Crouch EC et al. Treatment of pulmonary hemangiomatosis with recombinant interferon alfa-2a. N Engl J Med 1989;320:1197–1200.

54. Mitsuyasu RT. Interferon alpha in the treatment of AIDS-related Kaposi's sarcoma. Br J Haematol 1991;7:69–73.

55. Kaban LB, Mulliken JB, Ezekowitz RA et al. Antiangiogenic therapy of a recurrent giant cell tumor of the mandible with interferon alfa-2a. Pediatrics 1999;103:1145–1149.

56. Stadler WM, Kuzel TM, Raghavan D et al. Metastatic bladder cancer: advances in treatment. Eur J Cancer 1997;33:S23–S26.

57. Nanus DM, Schmitz-Drager BJ, Motzer RJ et al. Expression of basic fibroblast growth factor in primary human renal tumors: correlation with poor survival. J Natl Cancer Inst 1993;85: 1597–1599.

58. Nguyen M, Watanabe H, Budson AE et al. Elevated levels of the angiogenic peptide basic fibroblast growth factor in urine of bladder cancer patients. J Natl Cancer Inst 1993;85:241–242.

59. Dinney CP, Bielenberg DR, Perrotte P et al. Inhibition of basic fibroblast growth factor expression, angiogenesis, and growth of human bladder carcinoma in mice by systemic interferon-alpha administration. Cancer Res 1998;58:808–814.

60. Brouty-Boye D, Zetter BR. Inhibition of cell motility by interferon. Science 1980;206:516–518.

61. Slaton JW, Perrotte P, Inoue K et al. Interferon-α-mediated down-regulation of angiogenesis-related genes and therapy of bladder cancer are dependent on optimization of biological dose and schedule. Clin Cancer Res 1999;5:2726–2734.

62. Moses MA, Wiederschain D, Wu I et al. Troponin I is present in human cartilage and inhibits angiogenesis. Proc Natl Acad Sci USA 1999;96:2645–2650.

63. Taraboletti G, Morbidelli L, Donnini S et al. The heparin binding 25 kDa fragment of thrombospondin-1 promotes angiogenesis and modulates gelatinase and TIMP-2 production in endothelial cells. FASEB J 2000;14:1674–1676.

64. Tolsma SS, Volpert OV, Good DJ et al. Peptides derived from two separate domains of the matrix protein thrombospondin-1 have antiangiogenic activity. J Cell Biol 1993;122:497–511.

65. Gorelik E. Concomitant tumor immunity and the resistance to a second tumor challenge. Adv Cancer Res 1983;39:71–120.

66. Prehn RT. The inhibition of tumor growth by tumor mass. Cancer Res 1991;51:2–4.

67. O'Reilly MS, Holmgren L, Shing Y et al. Angiostatin: a novel angiogenesis inhibitor that mediates the suppression of metastases by a Lewis lung carcinoma. Cell 1994;79:315–328.

68. Holmgren L, O'Reilly MS, Folkman J. Dormancy of micrometastases: balanced proliferation and apoptosis in the presence of angiogenesis suppression. Nature Med 1995;1:149–153.

69. Hari D, Beckett MA, Sukhatme VP et al. Angiostatin induces mitotic cell death of proliferating endothelial cells. Mol Cell Biol Res Comm 2000;3:277–282.

70. Lucas R, Holmgren L, Garcia I et al. Multiple forms of angiostatin induce apoptosis in endothelial cells. Blood 1998;92:4730–4741.

71. Claesson-Welsh L, Welsh M, Ito N et al. Angiostatin induces endothelial cell apoptosis and activation of focal adhesion kinase independently of the integrin-binding motif RGD. Proc Natl Acad Sci USA 1998;95:5579–5583.

72. Stack MS, Gately S, Bafetti LM et al. Angiostatin inhibits endothelial and melanoma cellular invasion by blocking matrix-enhanced plasminogen activation. Biochem J 1999;340:77–84.

73. Moser TL, Stack MS, Asplin I et al. Angiostatin binds ATP synthase on the surface of human endothelial cells. Proc Natl Acad Sci USA 1999;96:2811–2816.

74. Troyanovsky B, Levchenko T, Mansson G et al. Angiomotin: an angiostatin binding protein that regulates endothelial cell migration and tube formation. Cell Biol 2001;152:1247–1254.

75. O'Reilly MS, Boehm T, Shing Y et al. Endostatin: an endogenous inhibitor of angiogenesis and tumor growth. Cell 1997;88:277–285.

76. Boehm T, Folkman J, Browder T, O'Reilly MS. Antiangiogenic therapy of experimental cancer does not induce acquired drug resistance. Nature 1997;390:404–407.

77. Yamaguchi N, Anand-Apte B, Lee M et al. Endostatin inhibits VEGF-induced endothelial cell migration and tumor growth independently of zinc binding. EMBO J 1999;18:4414–4423.

78. Read TA, Farhadi M, Bjerkvig R et al. Intravital microscopy reveals novel antivascular and antitumor effects of endostatin delivered locally by alginate-encapsulated cells. Cancer Res 2001; 61:6830–6837.

79. Hohenester E, Sasaki T, Olsen BR, Timpl R. Crystal structure of the angiogenesis inhibitor endostatin at 1.5 A resolution. EMBO J 1998;17:1656–1664.

80. Ding YH, Javaherian K, Lo KM et al. Zinc-dependent dimers observed in crystals of human endostatin. Proc Natl Acad Sci USA 1998;95:10443–10448.

81. Dhanabal M, Ramchandran R, Waterman MJF et al. Endostatin induces endothelial cell apoptosis. J Biol Chem 1999;274:11721–11726.

82. MacDonald NJ, Shivers WY, Narum DL et al. Endostatin binds tropomyosin. A potential modulator of the antitumor activity of endostatin. J Biol Chem 2001;276:25190–25196.

83. Rehn M, Veikkola T, Kukk-Valdre E et al. Interaction of endostatin with integrins implicated in angiogenesis. Proc Natl Acad Sci USA 2001;98:1024–1029.

84. Wickstrom SA, Veikkola T, Rehn M et al. Endostatin-induced modulation of plasminogen activation with concomitant loss of focal adhesions and actin stress fibers in cultured human endothelial cells. Cancer Res 2001;61:6511–6516.

85. Huang X, Wong MK, Zhao Q et al. Soluble recombinant endostatin purified from *Escherichia coli*: antiangiogenic activity and antitumor effect. Cancer Res 2001;61:478–481.

86. Ramchandran R, Dhanabal M, Volk R et al. Antiangiogenic activity of restin, NC10 domain of human collagen XV: comparison to endostatin. Biochem Biophys Res Commun 1999;255: 735–739.

87. Xu J, Rodriguez D, Petitclerc E et al. Proteolytic exposure of a cryptic site within collagen type IV is required for angiogenesis and tumor growth *in vivo*. J Cell Biol 2001;154:1069–1079.

88. Petitclerc E, Boutaud A, Prestayko A et al. New functions for non-collagenous domains of human collagen type IV. Novel integrin ligands inhibiting angiogenesis and tumor growth *in vivo*. J Biol Chem 2000;275:8051–8061.

89. Colorado PC, Torre A, Kamphaus G et al. Anti-angiogenic cues from vascular basement membrane collagen. Cancer Res 2000;60:2520–2526.

90. Ferrara N, Clapp C, Weiner RI. The 16K fragment of prolactin specifically inhibits basal or FGF stimulated growth of capillary endothelial cells. Endocrinology 1991;129:896–900.

91. Bentzien F, Struman I, Martini JF et al. Expression of the antiangiogenic factor 16K hPRL in human HCT116 colon cancer cells inhibits tumor growth in Rag1(-/-) mice. Cancer Res 2001; 61:7356–7362.

92. Struman I, Bentzien F, Lee H et al. Opposing actions of intact and N-terminal fragments of human prolactin/growth hormone family members on agniogenesis: an efficient mechanism for the regulation of angiogenesis. Proc Natl Acad Sci USA 1999;96:1246–1251.

93. D'Angelo G, Struman I, Martial J, Weiner RI. Activation of mitogen-activated protein kinases by vascular endothelial growth factor and basic fibroblast growth factor in capillary endothelial cells is inhibited by the antiangiogenic factor 16-kDa N-terminal fragment of prolactin. Proc Natl Acad Sci USA 1995;92:6374–6378.

94. Jackson D, Volpert O, Bouck N, Linzer D. Stimulation and inhibition of angiogenesis by placental proliferin and proliferin-related protein. Science 1994;266:1581–1585.

95. Maione TE, Gray GS, Petro et al. Inhibition of angiogenesis by recombinant human platelet factor-4 and related peptides. Science 1990;247:77–79.

96. Gupta SK, Hassel T, Singh JP. A potent inhibitor of endothelial cell proliferation is generated by proteolytic cleavage of the chemokine platelet factor 4. Proc Natl Acad Sci USA 1995; 92: 7799–7803.

97. Nelson J, Allen WE, Scott WN et al. Murine epidermal growth factor (EGF) fragment (33-42) inhibits both EGF- and laminin-dependent endothelial cell motility and angiogenesis. Cancer Res 1995;55:3772–3776.

98. Sakamato N, Iwahana M, Tanaka NG, Osaka Y. Inhibition of angiogenesis and tumor growth by a synthetic laminin peptide, CDPGYIGSR-NH_2. Cancer Res 1991;51:903–906.

99. Pike SE, Yao L, Jones KD et al. Vasostatin, a calreticulin fragment, inhibits angiogenesis and suppresses tumor growth. J Exp Med 1998;188:2349–2356.

100. Pike SE, Yao L, Setsuda J et al. Calreticulin and calreticulin fragments are endothelial cell inhibitors that suppress tumor growth. Blood 1999;94:2461–2468.

101. Yao L, Pike SE, Setsuda J et al. Effective targeting of tumor vasculature by the angiogenesis inhibitors vasostatin and interleukin-12. Blood 2000;96:1900–1905.

102. Angiolillo AL, Sgadari C, Taub DD et al. Human interferon-inducible protein 10 is a potent inhibitor of angiogenesis *in vivo*. J Exp Med 1995;182:155–162.

103. O'Reilly MS, Pirie-Shepherd S, Lane WS, Folkman J. Antiangiogenic activity of the cleaved conformation of the serpin antithrombin. Science 1999;285:1926–1928.

104. Larsson H, Sjoblom T, Dixelius J et al. Antiangiogenic effects of latent antithrombin through perturbed cell-matrix interactions and apoptosis of endothelial cells. Cancer Res 2000;60: 6723–6729.

105. Larsson H, Akerud P, Nordling K et al. A novel antiangiogenic form of antithrombin with retained proteinase binding ability and heparin affinity. J Biol Chem 2001;276:11996–2002.

106. Gale NW, Yancopoulos GD. Growth factors acting via endothelial cell-specific receptor tyrosine kinases: VEGFs, angiopoietins, and ephrins in vascular development. Genes Dev 1999;13: 1055–1066.

107. Klint P, Claesson-Welsh L. Signal transduction by fibroblast growth factor receptors. Front Biosci 1999;4:D165–D177.

108. Davis S, Aldrich TH, Jones PF et al. Isolation of angiopoietin-1, a ligand for the TIE2 receptor, by secretion-trap expression cloning. Cell 1996;87:1153–1155.

109. Maisonpierre PC, Suri C, Jones PF et al. Angiopoietin-2, a natural antagonist for tie2 that disrupts in vivo angiogenesis. Science 1997;277:55–60.

110. Baker CH, Solorzano CC, Fidler IJ. Angiogenesis and cancer metastasis: antiangiogenic therapy of human pancreatic adenocarcinoma. Int J Clin Oncol 2001;6:59–65.

111. Yuan F, Chen Y, Dellian M et al. Time-dependent vascular regression and permeability changes in established human tumor xenografts induced by an anti-VEGF/VPF antibody. Proc Natl Acad Sci USA 1996;93:14765–14770.

112. Perrotte P, Matsumoto T, Inoue K et al. Anti-epidermal growth factor receptor antibody C225 inhibits angiogenesis in human transitional cell carcinoma growing orthotopically in nude mice. Clin Cancer Res 1999;5:257–265.

113. Petit AM, Rak J, Hung MC et al. Neutralizing antibodies against epidermal growth factor and ErbB-2/neu receptor tyrosine kinases down-regulate vascular endothelial growth factor production by tumor cells *in vitro* and *in vivo*: angiogenic implications for signal transduction therapy of solid tumors. Am J Path 1997;151:1523–1530.

114. Sirotnak FM, Zakowski MF, Miller VA et al. Efficacy of cytotoxic agents against human tumor xenografts is markedly enhanced by coadministration of ZD1839 (Iressa), an inhibitor of EGFR tyrosine kinase. Clin Cancer Res 2000;6:4885–4892.

115. Drevs J, Hofmann I, Hugenschmidt H et al. Effects of PTK787/ZK 222584, a specific inhibitor of vascular endothelial growth factor receptor tyrosine kinases, on primary tumor, metastasis, vessel density, and blood flow in a murine renal cell carcinoma model. Cancer Res 2000;60: 4819–4824.

116. Solorzano CC, Baker CH, Tsan R et al. Optimization for the blockade of epidermal growth factor receptor signaling for therapy of human pancreatic carcinoma. Clin Cancer Res 2001;7: 2563–2572.

117. Wood JM, Bold G, Buchdunger E et al. PTK787/ZK 222584, a novel and potent inhibitor of vascular endothelial growth factor receptor tyrosine kinases, impairs vascular endothelial growth factor-induced responses and tumor growth after oral administration. Cancer Res 2000;60: 2178–2189.

118. Kendall RL, Thomas KA. Inhibition of vascular endothelial cell growth factor activity by an endogenously encoded soluble receptor. Proc Natl Acad Sci USA 1993;90:10705–10709.

119. Kendall RL, Wang G, Thomas KA. Identification of a natural soluble form of the vascular endothelial growth factor receptor, FLT-1, and its heterodimerization with KDR. Biochem Biophys Res Commun 1996;226:324–328.

120. Kong HL, Hecht D, Song W et al. Regional suppression of tumor growth by in vivo transfer of a cDNA encoding a secreted form of the extracellular domain of the flt-1 vascular endothelial growth factor receptor. Hum Gene Ther 1998;9:823–833.

121. Pavco PA, Bouhana KS, Gallegos AM et al. Antitumor and antimetastatic activity of ribozymes targeting the messenger RNA of vascular endothelial growth factor receptors. Clin Cancer Res 2000;6:2094–2103.

122. Parry TJ, Cushman C, Gallegos AM et al. Bioactivity of anti-angiogenic ribozymes targeting Flt-1 and KDR mRNA. Nucleic Acids Res 1999;27:2569–2577.

123. Baker CH, McCarty MF, Tsan R, Fidler IJ. Phenotypic diversity of organ-specific endothelial cells [abstract]. Proc Am Assoc Cancer Res 2001;42:2186.

124. Tsai JC, Goldman CK, Gillespie GY. Vascular endothelial growth factor in human glioma cell lines: induced secretion by EGF, PDGF-BB, and bFGF. J Neurosurg 1995;82:864–873.

125. Brogi E, Wu T, Namiki A, Isner JM. Indirect angiogenic cytokines upregulate VEGF and bFGF gene expression in vascular smooth muscle cells, whereas hypoxia upregulates VEGF expression only. Circulation 1994;90:649–652.

126. Uehara H, Kim SJ, Karashima T et al. Blockade of the PDGF-R signaling by STI571 inhibits angiogenesis and growth of human prostate cancer cells in the bone of nude mice [abstract]. Proc Am Assoc Cancer Res 2001;42:2192.

127. Yano S, Herbst RS, Shinohara H et al. Treatment for malignant pleural effusion of human lung adenocarcinoma by inhibition of vascular endothelial growth factor receptor tyrosine kinase phosphorylation. Clin Cancer Res 2000;6:957–965.

128. Laird AD, Vajkoczy P, Shawver LK et al. SU6668 is a potent antiangiogenic and antitumor agent that induces regression of established tumors. Cancer Res 2000;60:4152–4160.

129. Jakkula M, Le Cras TD, Gebb S et al. Inhibition of angiogenesis decreases alveolarization in the developing rat lung. Am J Phys Lung Cell Mol Phys 2000;279:L600–L607.

130. Alon T, Hemo I, Itin A et al. VEGF acts as a survival factor for newly formed retinal vessels and has implications for retinopathy of prematurity. Nat Med 1995;1:1024–1028.

131. Verheul HM, Hoekman K, Lupu F et al. Platelet and coagulation activation with vascular endothelial growth factor generation in soft tissue sarcomas. Clin Cancer Res 2000;6:166–171.

132. Browder T, Butterfield CE, Kraling BM et al. Antiangiogenic scheduling of chemotherapy improves efficacy against experimental drug-resistant cancer. Cancer Res 2000;60:1878–1886.

133. Klement G, Baruchel S, Rak J et al. Continuous low-dose therapy with vinblastine and VEGF receptor-2 antibody induces sustained tumor regression without overt toxicity. J Clin Invest 2000;105:R15–R24.

134. Bello L, Carrabba G, Giussani C et al. Low-dose chemotherapy combined with an antiangiogenic drug reduces human glioma growth *in vivo*. Cancer Res 2001;61:7501–7506.

135. O'Reilly MS, Holmgren L, Chen C, Folkman J. Angiostatin induces and sustains dormancy of human primary tumors in mice. Nat Med 1996;2:689–692.

136. Laird AD, Vajkoczy P, Shawver LK et al. SU6668 is a potent antiangiogenic and antitumor agent that induces regression of established tumors. Cancer Res 60:4152–4160.

137. Shaheen RM, Davis DW, Liu W et al. Antiangiogenic therapy targeting the tyrosine kinase receptor for vascular endothelial growth factor receptor inhibits the growth of colon cancer liver metastasis and induces tumor and endothelial cell apoptosis. Cancer Res 1999;59:5412–5416.

138. Camphausen K, Moses MA, Beecken W et al. Radiation therapy to a primary tumor accelerates metastatic growth in mice, Cancer Res 2001;61:2207–2211.

139. Liotta LA, Stetler-Stevenson WG, Steeg PS. Cancer invasion and metastasis: positive and negative regulatory elements. Cancer Invest 1991;9:543–551.

140. Stetler-Stevenson WG. Matrix metalloproteinases in angiogenesis: a moving target for therapeutic intervention. J Clin Invest 1999;103:1237–1241.

141. Kleiner DE, Stetler-Stevenson WG. Matrix metalloproteinases and metastasis. Cancer Chem Pharm 1999;43:S42–S51.

142. Stefansson S, Petitclerc E, Wong MK et al. Inhibition of angiogenesis *in vivo* by plasminogen activator inhibitor-1. J Biol Chem 2001;276:8135–8141.

143. Stefansson S, Lawrence DA. The serpin PAI-1 inhibits cell migration by blocking integrin αvβ3 binding to vitronectin. Nature 1996;383:441–443.

144. Stathakis P, Fitzgerald M, Matthias LJ et al. Generation of angiostatin by reduction and proteolysis of plasmin. J Biol Chem 1997;272:20641–20645.

145. Gately S, Twardowski P, Stack MS et al. The mechanism of cancer-mediated conversion of plasminogen to the angiogenesis inhibitor angiostatin. Proc Natl Acad Sci USA 1997;94: 10868–10872.

146. Moses MA, Sudhalter J, Langer R. Identification of an inhibitor of neovascularization from cartilage. Science 1990;248:1408–1410.

147. Moses MA. The regulation of neovascularization by matrix metalloproteinases and their inhibitors. Stem Cells 1997;15:180–189.

148. Tamargo RJ, Bok RA, Brem H. Angiogenesis inhibition by minocycline. Cancer Res 1991;51: 672–675.

149. Guerin C, Laterra J, Masnyk T et al. Selective endothelial growth inhibition by tetracyclines that inhibit collagenase. Biochem Biophys Res Commun 1992;188:740–745.

150. Rudek MA, Figg WD, Dyer V et al. Phase I clinical trial of oral COL-3, a matrix metalloproteinase inhibitor, in patients with refractory metastatic cancer. J Clin Oncol 2001;19:584–590.

151. Gatto C, Rieppi M, Borsotti P et al. BAY 12-9566, a novel inhibitor of matrix metalloproteinases with antiangiogenic activity. Clin Cancer Res 1999;5:3603–3607.

152. Zucker S, Cao J, Chen WT. Critical appraisal of the use of matrix metalloproteinase inhibitors in cancer treatment. Oncogene 2000;19:6642–6650.

153. Shalinsky DR, Brekken J, Zou H et al. Marked antiangiogenic and antitumor efficacy of AG3340 in chemoresistant human non–small cell lung cancer tumors: single agent and combination chemotherapy studies. Clin Cancer Res 1999;5:1905–1917.

154. Dong Z, Yoneda J, Kumar R, Fidler IJ. Angiostatin-mediated suppression of cancer metastases by primary neoplasms engineered to produce granulocyte/macrophage colony-stimulating factor. J Exp Med 1998;188:755–763.

155. McGeehan GM, Becherer JD, Bast RC Jr et al. Regulation of tumour necrosis factor-alpha processing by a metalloproteinase inhibitor. Nature 1994;370:558–561.

156. Gearing AJ, Beckett P, Christodoulou M et al. Processing of tumour necrosis factor-α precursor by metalloproteinases. Nature 1994;370:555–557.

157. Arribas J, Coodly L, Vollmer P et al. Diverse cell surface protein ectodomains are shed by a system sensitive to metalloprotease inhibitors. J Biol Chem 1996;271:11376–11382.

158. Arribas J, Massague J. Transforming growth factor-alpha and beta-amyloid precursor protein share a secretory mechanism. J Cell Biol 1995;128:433–441.

159. Walcheck B, Kahn J, Fisher JM et al. Neutrophil rolling altered by inhibition of L-selectin shedding *in vitro*. Nature 1996;380:720–723.

160. Feehan C, Darlak K, Kahn J et al. Shedding of the lymphocyte L-selectin adhesion molecule is inhibited by a hydroxamic acid-based protease inhibitor. Identification with an L-selectin-alkaline phosphatase reporter. J Biol Chem 1996;271:7019–7024.

161. Bennett TA, Lynam EB, Sklar LA, Rogelj S. Hydroxamate-based metalloprotease inhibitor blocks shedding of L-selectin adhesion molecule from leukocytes: functional consequences for neutrophil aggregation. J Immunol 1996;156:3093–3097.

162. Mullberg J, Durie FH, Otten-Evans C et al. A metalloprotease inhibitor blocks shedding of the IL-6 receptor and the p60 TNF receptor. J Immunol 1995;155:5198–5205.

163. Couet J, Sar S, Jolivet A, et al. Shedding of human thyrotropin receptor ectodomain: involvement of a matrix metalloprotease. J Biol Chem 1996;271:4545–4552.

164. Levi E, Fridman R, Miao HQ et al. Matrix metalloproteinase 2 releases active soluble ectodomain of fibroblast growth factor receptor 1. Proc Natl Acad Sci USA 1996;93:7069–7074.

165. Suzuki M, Raab G, Moses MA et al. Matrix metalloproteinase-3 releases active heparin-binding EGF-like growth factor by cleavage at a specific juxtamembrane site. J Biol Chem 272: 31730–31737, 1997.

166. Gately S, Twardowski P, Stack MS et al. Human prostate carcinoma cells express enzymatic activity that converts human plasminogen to the angiogenesis inhibitor, angiostatin. Cancer Res 1996;56:4887–4890.

167. Patterson BC, Sang QXA. Angiostatin-converting enzyme activities of MMP-7 and MMP-9. J Biol Chem 1997;272:28823–28830.

168. Falcone D, Khan MF, Layne T, Fernandes L. Macrophage formation of angiostatin during inflammation. J Biol Chem 1998;273:31480–31485.

169. Clapp C, Martial JA, Guzman RC et al. The 16-kilodalton N-terminal fragment of human prolactin is a potent inhibitor of angiogenesis. Endocrinology 1993;133:1292–1299.

170. Grant DS, Tashiro K-I, Sequi-Real B et al. Two different laminin domains mediate the differentiation of human endothelial cells into capillary-like structures *in vitro*. Cell 1989;58:933–943.

171. Homandberg GA, Williams JE, Grant DBS, Eisenstein R. Heparin-binding fragments of fibronectin are potent inhibitors of endothelial cell growth. Am J Pathol 1985;120:327–332.

172. Moses MA, Wiederschain D, Loughlin KR et al. Increased incidence of matrix metalloproteinases in urine of cancer patients. Cancer Res 1998;58:1395–1399.

173. Dvorak HF, Nagy JA, Dvorak JT, Dvorak AM. Identification and characterization of the blood vessels of solid tumors that are leaky to circulating macromolecules. Am J Pathol 1988;133: 95–109.

174. St Croix B, Rago C, Velculescu V et al. Genes expressed in human tumor endothelium. Science 2000;289:1197–2202.

175. Brem H, Goto F, Budson A et al. Minimal drug resistance after prolonged antiangiogenic therapy with AGM-1470. Surg Forum 1994;XLV:674–677.

176. Hausman MR, Schaffler MB, Majeska RJ. Prevention of fracture healing in rats by an inhibitor of angiogenesis. Bone 2001;29:560–564.

177. Berger AC, Feldman AL, Gnant MF et al. The angiogenesis inhibitor, endostatin, does not affect murine cutaneous wound healing. J Surg Res 2000;91:26–31.

178. Bloch W, Huggel K, Sasaki T et al. The angiogenesis inhibitor endostatin impairs blood vessel maturation during wound healing. FASEB J 2000;14:2373–2376.

179. Mundhenke C, Thomas JP, Wilding G et al. Tissue examination to monitor antiangiogenic therapy a phase I clinical trial with endostatin. Clin Cancer Res 2001;7:3366–3374.

180. Gerber HP, Hillan KJ, Ryan AM et al. VEGF is required for growth and survival in neonatal mice. Development (Suppl) 1999;126:1149–1159.

181. Felbor U, Dreier L, Bryant RA et al. Secreted cathepsin L generates endostatin from collagen XVIII. EMBO J 2000;19:1187–1194.

182. Wen W, Moses MA, Wiederschain D et al. The generation of endostatin is mediated by elastase. Cancer Res 1999;59:6052–6056.

183. Drixler TA, Rinkes IH, Ritchie ED et al. Continuous administration of angiostatin inhibits accelerated growth of colorectal liver metastases after partial hepatectomy. Cancer Res 2000;60: 1761–1765.

184. Kisker O, Becker CM, Prox D et al. Continuous administration of endostatin by intraperitoneally implanted osmotic pump improves the efficacy and potency of therapy in a mouse xenograft tumor model. Cancer Res 2001;61:7669–7674.

185. Teicher BA, Sotomayor EA, Huang ZD. Antiangiogenic agents potentiate cytotoxic cancer therapies against primary and metastatic disease. Cancer Res 1992;52:6702–6704.

186. Teicher BA, Holden SA, Dupuis NP et al. Potentiation of cytotoxic therapies by TNP-470 and minocycline in mice bearing EMT-6 mammary carcinoma. Breast Cancer Res Treat 1995;36: 227–236.

187. Lee K, Erturk E, Mayer R, Cockett AT. Efficacy of antitumor chemotherapy in C3H mice enhanced by the antiangiogenesis steroid, cortisone acetate. Cancer Res 1987;47:5021–5024.

188. Bertolini F, Fusetti L, Mancuso P et al. Endostatin, an antiangiogenic drug, induces tumor stabilization after chemotherapy or anti-CD20 therapy in a NOD/SCID mouse model of human high-grade non-Hodgkin lymphoma. Blood 2000;96:282–287.

189. Canney P, Dean S. Transforming growth factor beta: a promoter of late connective tissue injury following radiotherapy? Br J Radiol 1990;63:620–623.

190. Gorski DH, Beckett MA, Jaskowiak NT et al. Blockage of the vascular endothelial growth factor stress response increases the antitumor effects of ionizing radiation. Cancer Res 1999;59: 3374–3378.

191. Hartford AC, Gohongi T, Fukumura D, Jain RK. Irradiation of a primary tumor, unlike surgical removal, enhances angiogenesis suppression at a distal site: potential role of host-tumor interaction. Cancer Res 2000;60:2128–2131.

192. Teicher BA, Dupuis N, Kusomoto T et al. Antiangiogenic agents can increase tumor oxygenation and response to radiation therapy. Rad Oncol Invest 1995;2:269–276.

193. Hansen-Algenstaedt N, Stoll BR, Padera TP et al. Tumor oxygenation in hormone-dependent tumors during vascular endothelial growth factor receptor-2 blockade, hormone ablation, and chemotherapy. Cancer Res 2000;60:4556–4560.

194. Ikeda S, Akagi K, Shiraishi T, Tanaka Y. Enhancement of the effect of an angiogenesis inhibitor on murine tumors by hyperthermia. Oncol Rep 1998;5:181–184.

195. Masunaga S, Ono K, Nishimura Y et al. Combined effects of tirapazamine and mild hyperthermia on anti-angiogenic agent (TNP-470) treated tumors-reference to the effect on intratumor quiescent cells. Int J Radiat Oncol Biol Phys 2000;47:799–807.

196. Nishimura Y, Murata R, Hiraoka M. Combined effects of angiogenesis inhibitor (TNP-470) and hyperthermia. Br J Cancer 1996;73:270–274.

197. Murata R, Nishimura Y, Hiraoka M. An antiangiogenic agent (TNP-470) inhibited reoxygenation during fractionated radiotherapy of murine mammary carcinoma. Int J Radiat Oncol Biol Phys 1997;37:1107–1113.

198. Lund EL, Bastholm L, Kristjansen PE. Therapeutic synergy of TNP-470 and ionizing radiation: effects on tumor growth, vessel morphology, and angiogenesis in human glioblastoma multiforme xenografts. Clin Cancer Res 2000;6:971–978.

199. Mauceri HJ, Hanna NN, Beckett MA et al. Combined effects of angiostatin and ionizing radiation in antitumour therapy. Nature 1998;394:287–291.

200. Milas L, Kishi K, Hunter N et al. Enhancement of tumor response to gamma-radiation by an inhibitor of cyclooxygenase-2 enzyme. J Natl Cancer Inst 1999;91:1501–1504.

201. Milas L, Mason K, Hunter N et al. *In vivo* enhancement of tumor radioresponse by C225 antiepidermal growth factor receptor antibody. Clin Cancer Res 2000;6:701–708.

202. Geng L, Donnelly E, McMahon G et al. Inhibition of vascular endothelial growth factor receptor signaling leads to reversal of tumor resistance to radiotherapy. Cancer Res 2001;61:2413–2419.

203. Kozin S, Boucher Y, Hicklin DJ et al. Vascular endothelial growth factor receptor-2-blocking antibody potentiates radiation-induced long-term control of human tumor xenografts. Cancer Res 2001;61:39–44.

204. Gorski DH, Mauceri HJ, Salloum RM et al. Potentiation of the antitumor effect of ionizing radiation by brief concomitant exposures to angiostatin. Cancer Res 1998;58:5686–5689.

205. Salven P, Orpana A, Teerenhovi L, Joensuu H. Simultaneous elevation in the serum concentrations of the angiogenic growth factors VEGF and bFGF is an independent predictor of poor prognosis in non-Hodgkin lymphoma: a single-institution study of 200 patients. Blood 2000;96:3712–3718.

206. Fontanini G, Boldrini L, Chine S et al. Expression of vascular endothelial growth factor mRNA in non-small-cell lung carcinomas. Br J Cancer 1999;79:363–369.

207. Watanabe H, Nguyen M, Schizer M et al. Basic fibroblast growth factor in human serum-a prognostic test for breast cancer. Mol Biol Cell 1992;3:234a.

208. Poon RT, Fan ST, Wong J. Clinical implications of circulating angiogenic factors in cancer patients. J Clin Oncol 2001;19:1207–1225.

209. Weidner N, Semple JP, Welch WR, Folkman J. Tumor angiogenesis and metastasis—correlation in invasive breast carcinoma. N Engl J Med 1991;324:1–8.

210. Gasparini G. Clinical significance of determination of surrogate markers of angiogenesis in breast cancer. Crit Rev Oncol Hematol 2001;37:97–114.

211. Fox SB, Harris AL. Markers of tumor angiogenesis: clinical applications in prognosis and anti-angiogenic therapy. Invest New Drugs 1997;15:15–28.

212. Yano S, Shinohara H, Herbst RS et al. Expression of vascular endothelial growth factor is necessary but not sufficient for production and growth of brain metastasis. Cancer Res 2000;60:4959–4967.

213. Bruns CJ, Solorzano CC, Harbison MT et al. Blockade of the epidermal growth factor receptor signaling by a novel tyrosine kinase inhibitor leads to apoptosis of endothelial cells and therapy of human pancreatic carcinoma. Cancer Res 2000;60:2926–2035.

214. Herbst RS, Yano S, Kuniyasu H et al. Differential expression of E-cadherin and type IV collagenase genes predicts outcome in patients with stage I non–small cell lung carcinoma. Clin Cancer Res 2000;6:790–797.

215. Kuniyasu H, Troncosco P, Johnston D et al. Relative expression of type IV collagenase, E-cadherin, and vascular endothelial growth factor/vascular permeability factor in prostatectomy specimens distinguishes organ-confined from pathologically advanced prostate cancers. Clin Cancer Res 2000;6:2295–2308.

216. Kuniyasu H, Ellis LM, Evans DB et al. Relative expression of E-cadherin and type IV collagenase genes predicts disease outcome in patients with resectable pancreatic carcinoma. Clin Cancer Res 1999;5:25–33.

217. Carmeliet P, Jain RK. Angiogenesis in cancer and other diseases. Nature 2000;407:249–257.

218. Boucher Y, Leunig M, Jain RK. Tumor angiogenesis and interstitial hypertension. Cancer Res 1996;56:4264–4266.

Chapter 9

Cyclooxygenase-2 Inhibitors in Colorectal Cancer

Rajnish A. Gupta

Raymond N. DuBois

Colorectal cancer (CRC) leads annually to approximately 550,000 deaths worldwide and is thus a major public health concern.[1] By the time CRC is diagnosed in an individual, the disease is often advanced, and current treatment regimens are ineffective and highly toxic. Recently, cyclooxygenase-2 (COX-2) inhibitor therapy has emerged as a promising novel therapy for CRC prevention or treatment (or both). As currently available treatment regimens for CRC are not effective, there is renewed interest in the area of cancer prevention. This chapter reviews some of the key findings from both clinical and laboratory settings that have led to the hypothesis that COX-2 inhibitors may be useful in reducing morbidity and mortality due to CRC.

BASIC SCIENCE STUDIES OF NONSTEROIDAL ANTI-INFLAMMATORY DRUGS AND CRC

Function of the COX Enzymes

The COX enzymes catalyze the enzymatic conversion of the endoperoxide intermediate PGH_2 from arachidonic acid.[2] PGH_2 is then converted to one of several

This chapter is a modification of a review entitled "Colorectal cancer prevention and treatment by inhibition of cyclooxygenase-2," published in *Nat Revs Cancer* 2001;1:11–21.

structurally related prostaglandins (PGs), including PGE_2, PGD_2, $PGF_2\alpha$, PGI_2, and thromboxane A_2, by the enzymatic activity of specific PG synthases. PGs play roles in a broad number of physiologic processes, including blood clotting, ovulation, initiation of labor, bone metabolism, nerve growth and development, wound healing, kidney function, blood vessel tone, and immune responses.[3] The importance of the COX pathway in human disease became obvious with the discovery that nonsteroidal anti-inflammatory drugs (NSAIDs), a group of compounds that have been used for more than a century in the treatment of various inflammatory disorders, were shown in the 1970s to inhibit the activity of COX.

Discovery of COX-2 and the Biochemistry of COX-2 Selective Inhibitors

Until recently, only one isoform of COX (now known as *COX-1*) had been cloned and identified. However, approximately 10 years ago, two independent groups identified and cloned a second COX isoform, COX-2. Subsequent research has suggested a paradigm in which COX-1 is responsible for "housekeeping" PG biosynthesis and is constitutively expressed in many tissues in the body.[4] COX-2, conversely, is not normally expressed in most tissues but is induced by a wide spectrum of growth factors and proinflammatory cytokines in specific pathophysiological conditions. It was thus hypothesized that the anti-inflammatory and analgesic properties of traditional NSAIDs, which inhibit both COX-1 and COX-2, are most likely due to their ability to inhibit COX-2.[5] In contrast, the erosion and ulceration of the gastric mucosa seen with chronic NSAID therapy may be due, in large measure, to inhibition of PG production mediated by COX-1.

To test the foregoing hypothesis, compounds that selectively inhibit the COX-2 isoform were developed. The most well-known nonselective COX inhibitor, aspirin, inactivates COX enzymatic activity by covalent modification via acetylation of serine residue 530 in COX-1 and serine residue 516 in COX-2. In contrast, most other nonselective NSAIDs are competitive inhibitors that compete with the substrate arachidonic acid for active site binding in both COX-1 and COX-1. On the basis of the availability of the three-dimensional structure of both COX-1 and COX-2, compounds that preferentially bind to the active site of COX-2 were synthesized.[6] Currently available clinical evidence suggests that these COX-2 specific inhibitors ("Coxib" drugs) offer the therapeutic benefits of traditional NSAIDs with reduced toxicity to the gastrointestinal mucosa.[7] Finally, a new aspirin-like COX-2 inhibitor, APHS (o-(acetoxypheny)hept-2-ynyl sulfide), that has been developed is twenty-one times more selective for COX-2 than is COX-1.[8] Although this level of selectivity is not as significant as that of some other COX-2 inhibitors, APHS offers a unique advantage in that it covalently modifies the enzyme, thus ensuring permanent inactivation of COX-2.

Effects of NSAIDs on Tumor Growth in Animals

Early observational studies in the clinical setting suggested that NSAIDs might restrict the growth of CRC (see the section *Clinical Studies of NSAIDs and CRC,*

p. 164). These observations prompted a number of follow-up studies that examined the chemopreventive properties of these drugs in animal models of intestinal neoplasia (Table 9.1; reviewed in Ref. 9). One well-known murine model of colon cancer is the Min/+ mouse, which represents the murine homolog of the polyposis syndrome familial adenomatous polyposis (FAP) in humans. Multiple investigators have examined the ability of both nonselective and COX-2 selective NSAIDs to inhibit polyposis using this model. Without exception, either nonselective or COX-2 selective inhibitors have proven to be potent suppressors of polyp formation in these mice. Another widely used animal model for colon cancer is the rat treated with azoxymethane (AOM), in which the chemical carcinogen AOM induces preneoplastic colonic lesions, *termed aberrant crypt foci*, which later progress to carcinomas. Both nonselective and COX-2 selective NSAIDs reduce the incidence, multiplicity, and size of colonic carcinomas in the AOM rat model.

Role of Cyclooxygenase-2 in CRC Growth

The findings in animal models served as a stimulus for basic science investigations into the mechanism by which NSAIDs inhibit CRC growth. Because the COX enzymes are the most well-defined pharmacological targets of NSAIDs, one of the first ideas to emerge was the hypothesis that these drugs were inhibiting the presumed protumorigenic activity of either COX-1 or COX-2. This reasoning was strengthened by studies that demonstrated increased levels of PGs in human colorectal tumors as compared to normal adjacent colon[10] and by in vitro experiments showing that some PGs can increase the proliferation rate of human CRC cells.[11] In early attempts to examine the role of COX in CRC, several groups determined the levels of COX-1 and COX-2 in adenomas in human colorectal adenomas and adenocarcinomas.[12,13] These results point to essentially the same

TABLE 9.1 Effects of NSAID Treatment in Animal Models of Colorectal Cancer

Animal Model	NSAID Treatment	Outcome
Min/+ mouse		
	Sulindac[a]	↓ Polyp multiplicity
	Piroxicam[a]	↓ Polyp multiplicity
	Celecoxib[b]	↓ Polyp multiplicity
	Aspirin[a]	↓ Tumor incidence and multiplicity
Azoxymethane rat		
	Celecoxib[b]	↓ Tumor incidence and multiplicity
	NS-398[b]	↓ Tumor incidence and multiplicity
	Nimesulide[b]	↓ Tumor incidence and multiplicity

NSAID, nonsteroidal antiinflammatory drug.
[a]Nonselective NSAID.
[b]COX-2-selective NSAID.
Note: Reviewed in Ref. 9.

conclusion: Comparison of neoplastic and adjacent normal tissue finds little change in COX-1 expression but increased levels of COX-2 in adenoma and adenocarcinoma tissue as compared to the normal colonic mucosa.

These expression data were suggestive that NSAIDs could be suppressing tumor growth via inhibition of COX-2. However, it could still be argued that elevated levels of COX-2 are simply a consequence of the carcinogenic process and that the enzyme has no direct role in promoting CRC growth. One way to determine the role of COX-2 in intestinal neoplasia is to use a genetic approach. Oshima et al[14] did this by assessing the development of intestinal polyposis in $Apc^{\Delta716}$ mice (a model similar to the Min/+ mouse) in a wild-type and homozygous null COX-2 genetic background.[14] The number and size of polyps was reduced dramatically in the COX-2 null mice as compared to COX-2 wild-type mice. In addition, treatment of the $Apc^{\Delta716}$ COX-2 wild-type mice with a novel COX-2 selective inhibitor, MF tricyclic, reduced polyp number more significantly than did sulindac. This experiment was one of the first to offer rigorous evidence in support of the hypothesis that NSAIDs inhibit tumor growth via inhibition of COX-2.

More recent studies have confirmed a pro-oncogenic role for COX-2. For example, Liu et al[15] demonstrated that overexpression of COX-2 alone is sufficient to induce cellular transformation. This group developed transgenic mice in which the murine mammary tumor virus promoter-enhancer directs COX-2 expression. Although virgin mice overexpressing COX-2 did not develop mammary tumors, multiparous mice showed significant increases in mammary gland carcinomas as compared with age-matched controls. A related study by Neufang et al[16] reported that transgenic expression of COX-2 in basal keratinocytes results in epidermal hyperplasia and dysplasia, suggesting a causal association between COX-2 expression and the development of preneoplastic lesions in the skin.

COX-Independent Effects of NSAIDS

Multiple groups have now documented that high doses of NSAIDs can modify the biology of cultured cells independently of their ability to bind and inhibit COX-1 or COX-2. For example, transformed fibroblast cell lines derived from wild-type, COX-1-/-, COX-2-/-, or COX-1-/-/COX-2-/- mice all show comparable sensitivity to NSAID-induced cell death.[17] Such results are not surprising, as any xenobiotic agent is likely to have multiple targets, depending on the dose of the drug used. Non-COX cellular targets that have been proposed include IkB kinase b,[18] the peroxisome proliferator–activated receptor family of nuclear hormone receptors,[19,20] and the proapoptotic gene BAX.[21] However, in all instances, "COX-independent" effects are seen at drug concentrations in the 50- to 1000-mM range. This is ten to two hundredfold higher than the serum concentration of celecoxib (approximately 2–5 mM) required to inhibit tumor growth in animal models of CRC.[22] At these low concentrations, the best characterized biochemical target of NSAIDs remains the COX enzymes, although it is likely that other unknown "high-affinity" targets could be affected as well.

Mechanisms Involved in COX-2-Mediated Promotion of CRC

COX-2 has been localized to both tumor epithelial cells and adjacent stromal cells. Thus, COX-2-derived PGs may be acting on the malignant epithelial cells (a cell autonomous effect) or on the surrounding stroma (cell nonautonomous or "landscaping" effect) to promote tumor development (Fig. 9.1). There is evidence to support both theories.

If COX-2 inhibitors reduce tumor growth only though blockade of COX-2-derived PGs within the stromal compartment, one would predict that most CRC cell lines, irrespective of their level of COX-2 expression, would be sensitive to therapy with COX-2 inhibitors. This does not appear to be the case: In the nude mouse xenograft model, tumor cells that express COX-2 are more sensitive to

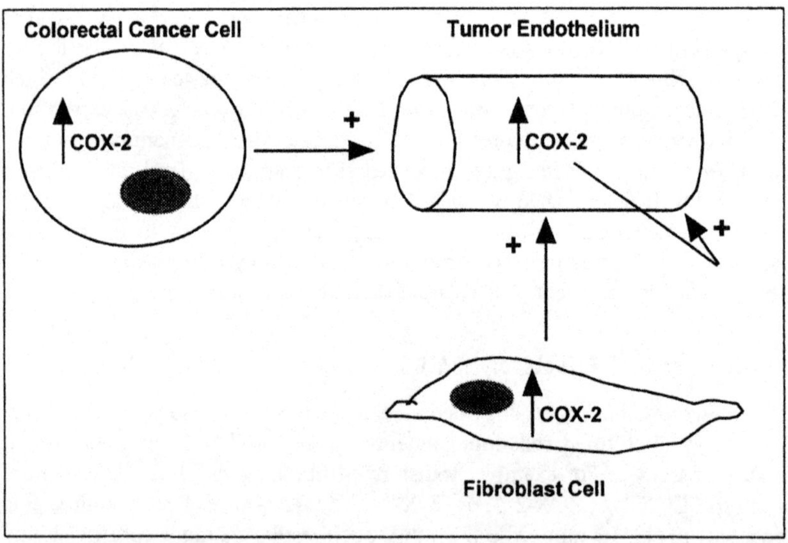

FIGURE 9.1 Mechanisms by which elevated COX-2 promotes colorectal cancer (CRC) growth. Forced expression of COX-2 in CRC cell lines leads to changes in key regulatory genes that promote blood vessel growth (angiogenesis). In other model systems, cultured skin fibroblasts from COX-2-/- mice exhibit defects in the basal secretion of several angiogenic growth factors, arguing that COX-2 may modify tumor growth by limiting the ability of fibroblasts to support neovascularization within the microenvironment of a tumor. COX-2 has also been localized to the tumor endothelial cells, and several groups have demonstrated that COX-2 inhibitors can block both the migration of endothelial cells. (COX-2, cyclooxygenase-2.)

treatment with selective COX-2 inhibitors.[23] Consistent with this, several studies suggest that forced expression of COX-2 in intestinal epithelial cell lines leads to changes in cellular pathways linked to carcinogenesis. For example, rat intestinal epithelial cells engineered to overexpress COX-2 have elevated levels of the antiapoptotic protein Bcl-2 and exhibit increased resistance to apoptosis induced by sodium butyrate.[24] In the Caco-2 cancer cell line, overexpression of COX-2 leads to an increase in cell migration and invasion that is associated with elevated levels of several members of the matrix metalloprotease family.[25] This same cell line also secretes higher levels of several angiogenic factors as compared with vector-transfected control cells and promotes the formation of endothelial cell tubes when cocultured with human umbilical vein endothelial cells.[26] The in vivo relevance of these findings has not yet been determined.

Several reports have suggested that COX-2 can also promote tumorigenesis through direct actions on the stromal compartment. These studies have largely centered on the ability of COX-2-derived PGs to stimulate tumor-associated angiogenesis. Using a model in which angiogenesis is assessed in sponge implants injected with various growth factors, Majima et al[27,28] were one of the first groups to demonstrate that COX-2 inhibitors could block neovascularization. COX-2 inhibitors also blocked the migration of human microvascular endothelial cells and growth factor–induced corneal angiogenesis, effects that could be reconstituted with a TXA_2 agonist.[29] A related study reported strong COX-2 immunoreactivity in tumor neovasculature in human colon, breast, prostate, and lung cancer biopsy tissue.[30] In addition, corneal blood vessel formation in rats was potently suppressed by selective COX-2 (but not COX-1) inhibitors. Jones et al[31] reported that both nonselective and COX-2–selective NSAIDs inhibit angiogenesis through direct actions on endothelial cells through both COX and non-COX mechanisms. Finally, a recent study provided genetic evidence that stroma-derived COX-2 can promote tumor growth by a landscaping mechanism.[32] In this study, the growth of a lung cancer cell line was attenuated if engrafted onto COX-2-/- versus wild-type control mice. COX-2 expression within the stroma surrounding the tumor was localized primarily to fibroblasts, and cultured skin fibroblasts from the COX-2-/- mice exhibited defects in the basal secretion of several angiogenic growth factors.

Collectively, this last set of experiments argues that COX-2 may modify tumor growth by limiting the ability of fibroblasts to support neovascularization within the microenvironment of a tumor. Recent experiments by Dormond et al[33] helped to clarify the mechanism by which COX-2-derived PGs promote angiogenesis. These authors' studies demonstrated that COX-2-derived PGE_2 and PGI_2 play essential roles in $\alpha V\beta 3$ integrin–mediated endothelial cell spreading and migration. Specifically, both PGs appear to be important in the activation of the small GTPases Cdc42/Rac that occurs after engagement of $\alpha V\beta 3$ integrin with its substrate.[33]

Prostaglandin Receptors in CRC

The different classes of PGs exert their effects by binding to a G protein–coupled cell- surface receptor that then leads to changes in the cellular levels of cAMP and Ca2+ (reviewed in Ref. 34). In addition, increasing evidence points to the possibility that PGs can also modulate cellular pathways by directly acting within the nucleus. For example, COX-2 has been localized to the perinuclear envelope,[35] the PGE_2 receptor EP1 has been localized to the nuclear envelope in certain cell types, and activation of the receptor led to changes in nuclear levels of Ca2+.[36]

Studies of the role of specific PGs and PG receptors that act downstream of COX-2 during the progression of CRC have been limited. Several groups have reported elevated levels of the PG subtype PGE_2 in CRC biopsies as compared with normal colonic mucosa.[10,37] However, because many PGs are highly unstable, the physiologic relevance of these studies is not known. Furthermore, there have been no systematic surveys documenting the expression of the known PG synthases and PG receptors in CRC.

Several studies have reported a procarcinogenic effect of PGE_2 in cultured CRC cells. For example, Sheng et al[38] reported a reduction in the basal apoptotic rate and increased levels of Bcl-2 after treatment of a human CRC cell line with PGE_2. Exposure of a different colorectal cell line to PGE_2 led to an increase in cell proliferation and motility associated with activation of the phosphatidylinositol 3-kinase-Akt pathway, an effect likely to be due to activation of the PGE_2 receptor subtype EP4.[39] A related study implicated PGE_2 in the ability of heregulin-β1 to induce colon cancer cell migration and invasion.[40] Genetic studies in mice suggest that PGE_2 promotes tumorigenesis at least in part by activating the EP1 receptor subtype. Mice with homozygous deletions in the EP1 (but not EP3) gene were partially resistant to AOM-mediated induction of aberrant crypt foci.[41,42] Moreover, in AOM-treated wild-type mice, an EP1 receptor antagonist also decreased the incidence of aberrant crypt foci. Finally, Apc^{Min} mice treated with the same EP1 receptor antagonist had 57% fewer intestinal polyps than did untreated mice. In contrast, Sonoshita[43] identified an important role for the EP2 receptor in CRC development. They examined the genetic role of all four PGE_2 receptors in the development of intestinal polyposis in $Apc^{\Delta 716}$ mice. The number and size of intestinal polyps was significantly reduced only in mice also harboring a homozygous deletion of the EP2 receptor.

CLINICAL STUDIES OF NSAIDs AND CRC

Observational Studies

There are more than 13 published observational studies of the relationship between NSAID use and CRC incidence or mortality (reviewed in Ref. 44). This group of studies is remarkable for its consistency in demonstrating a protective effect of NSAIDs against the development of CRC. Only one of the studies failed to demonstrate a protective effect, and this study did not offer any methodological advantage over other studies in the group.[45] The studies were carried out in three countries in a variety of settings (hospital-based, population-based, national surveys) using various measures of aspirin and nonaspirin NSAID use (questionnaire and computerized pharmacy records). History suggests that it is unusual for a putative chemopreventive factor to have such a consistent effect across several different studies.

Observational studies have demonstrated a protective effect for both aspirin and nonaspirin NSAIDs. Because each study had a distinct method of measuring and categorizing NSAID exposure, making comparisons across studies is difficult. However, the dominant theme to emerge from a comparison of the different studies is that consistent use of drug is important to see statistically meaningful effects in cancer risk reduction.[46–50] A second theme that emerges is that continual use of drug is also important because attenuation of the chemopreventive effect is seen with as little as 1 year of nonexposure.[49,51] Most studies that have examined duration of NSAID use have demonstrated increased protection with more years of exposure. Three studies indicated that at least 5–10 years of use was required for a protective benefit,[49,50,52] whereas a fourth study indicated that some protection could be acquired with as little as 4 years of use.[47] Higher doses seemed to provide more protection in two studies[48,52] but not in a third.[47] Finally, it should be noted that no large-scale observational studies have examined how the exposure to the new "Coxib" drugs affects CRC incidence.

Polyp Prevention in FAP Syndrome by Nonselective and COX-2-Selective NSAIDs

The first clinical observations of the effect of NSAIDs (sulindac) on adenoma formation occurred in groups of patients who had FAP syndrome. This disease is an autosomal dominant inherited condition marked by the development of hundreds to thousands of adenomatous polyps in the colon during early adulthood. Without colectomy, the vast majority of these patients will develop cancer in their thirties or forties. In most centers, the standard of care is a "subtotal colectomy," an operation that leaves behind the most distal colonic segment (rectum) to preserve normal bowel function. Because cancer may occur in this segment, these patients are usually followed up with surveillance sigmoidoscopies during which polyps are identified and removed.

Waddell et al[53] noted a paucity of polyps on a routine sigmoidoscopic surveillance examination in a single FAP patient who had received sulindac for other reasons.[53] Because of this observation, subsequent randomized controlled trials of polyp prevention in patients with FAP were carried out. The trial reported by Giardiello and colleagues[54] is the most notable and served as a paradigm for subsequent studies. In this trial, sulindac or placebo was given to FAP patients who had previously undergone subtotal colectomy and were engaged in a rectal screening program. Patients receiving sulindac had a decrease in both the number and average size of their rectal polyps on examinations at 3 and 6 months. When the drug was stopped, the polyps increased in size and started to recur at the pretreatment rate. There were no such effects among those treated with placebo.

Recently, the COX-2-selective drug celecoxib was tested as a potential chemopreventive agent in patients with FAP.[55] This drug offers a potential advantage because it causes fewer serious gastrointestinal tract side effects than do traditional NSAIDs, such as sulindac. The trial used celecoxib at two doses, compared to placebo in cohorts of patients with FAP who were engaged in screening regimens. There was a 28% reduction in polyp formation among those who took celecoxib at the higher dose (400 mg twice daily). Those receiving celecoxib at the lower dose (100 mg twice daily) had a smaller (11%) nonsignificant decrease in the number of polyps at the follow-up endoscopy.

Thus, both traditional NSAIDs and at least one of the newer COXIB drugs decrease polyp formation in patients with FAP. It should be noted that authorities have recommended that NSAID therapy be considered only as a possible adjunct to established screening practices. The absolute decrease in polyps in the treatment groups is modest and is not sufficient to replace standard screening practices and surgical intervention in FAP. Alarmingly, there are case reports of cancer of the rectum occurring in FAP patients who were receiving sulindac therapy.[56]

Future Clinical Studies of COX-2 Inhibitors and CRC

The CRC chemoprevention trials under way are designed to test the efficacy of selective COX-2 inhibitors in preventing adenoma recurrence after polypectomy. These studies are not yet completed, and their design is similar to previously published studies of calcium carbonate in preventing polyp recurrence.[57] In these studies, patients with sporadic polyps removed at an index colonoscopy are recruited from practices that provide screening colonoscopic examinations. The standard practice for most patients with adenomatous polyps would be to have a repeat colonoscopy in 3 years. Many of the chemoprevention studies incorporate a colonoscopy at 1 year after the index examination to ensure that the colon has been "cleared" of polyps and that any polyps found on subsequent examinations are "incident" polyps. Thus, the endpoint of interest is the recurrence rate of polyps at 3 or 4 years after the index date. The agents currently being tested in polyp prevention trials include aspirin and two of the Coxib drugs, celecoxib and rofecoxib.

No clinical data exist regarding the efficacy of COX-2 blockade therapy in the treatment of established CRCs. However, a number of clinical experiments that are under way test the ability of COX-2 inhibitors to potentiate the effects of traditional anti-cancer regimens. There is emerging evidence from preclinical studies that combination therapy with COX-2 inhibitors and drugs that target other oncogenic pathways can lead to improved clinical outcomes. For example, two studies recently reported enhanced anti-tumor efficacy in combination regimens consisting of an NSAID and an inhibitor that targets the ErbB/HER family of growth factor receptors.[58,59]

SUMMARY

Although there is now compelling evidence from both animal and cell culture systems to suggest that targeted inhibition of COX-2 is a viable approach for CRC prevention or treatment (or both), many questions remain unanswered. Future studies examining intestinal polyp susceptibility in mice with targeted deletions in specific PG synthases and receptors should help to clarify the mechanisms by which COX-2 promotes tumorigenesis. The precise signaling pathways and direct target genes that COX-2-derived PGs modulate in CRC cells are also largely unknown and must be identified. Collectively, these experiments may lead to the discovery of novel and more potent inhibitors of CRC cell growth.

ACKNOWLEDGMENTS

This work is supported in part by United States Public Health Services Grants RO1DK 47279 (RND), P030 ES-00267-29 (RND), and P01CA-77839 (RND). RND is a recipient of a VA Research Merit Grant and is the Mina C. Wallace Professor of Cancer Prevention. We also thank the T.J. Martell Foundation and the NCCRA for generous support.

REFERENCES

1. Greenlee RT, Murray T, Bolden S, Wingo PA. Cancer statistics, 2000. CA Cancer J Clin 2000; 50(1):7–33.
2. Smith WL, DeWitt DL, Garavito RM. Cyclooxygenases: structural, cellular, and molecular biology. Annu Rev Biochem 2000;69:145–182.
3. DuBois RN, Abramson SB, Crofford L et al. Cyclooxygenase in biology and disease. FASEB J 1998;12(12):1063–1073.
4. Isakson P, Seibert K, Masferrer J et al. Discovery of a better aspirin. Adv Prostaglandin Thromboxane Leukot Res 1995;23:49–54.
5. Masferrer JL, Zweifel BS, Manning PT et al. Selective inhibition of inducible cyclooxygenase 2 in vivo is antiinflammatory and nonulcerogenic. Proc Natl Acad Sci USA 1994;91(8):3228–3232.
6. Kurumbail RG, Stevens AM, Gierse JK et al. Structural basis for selective inhibition of cyclooxygenase-2 by anti-inflammatory agents. Nature 1996;384(6610):644–648.
7. Silverstein FE, Faich G, Goldstein JL et al. Gastrointestinal toxicity with celecoxib vs nonsteroidal anti-inflammatory drugs for osteoarthritis and rheumatoid arthritis: the CLASS study: a randomized controlled trial. Celecoxib Long-term Arthritis Safety Study. JAMA 2000;284(10):1247–1255.
8. Kalgutkar AS, Crews BC, Rowlinson SW et al. Aspirin-like molecules that covalently inactivate cyclooxygenase-2. Science 1998;280(5367):1268–1270.

9. Williams C, Shattuck-Brandt RL, DuBois RN. The role of COX-2 in intestinal cancer. Ann NY Acad Sci 1999;889:72–83.

10. Rigas B, Goldman IS, Levine L. Altered eicosanoid levels in human colon cancer. J Lab Clin Med 1993;122(5):518–523.

11. Qiao L, Kozoni V, Tsioulias GJ et al. Selected eicosanoids increase the proliferation rate of human colon carcinoma cell lines and mouse colonocytes in vivo. Biochim Biophys Acta 1995;1258(2): 215–223.

12. Eberhart CE, Coffey RJ, Radhika A et al. Up-regulation of cyclooxygenase 2 gene expression in human colorectal adenomas and adenocarcinomas. Gastroenterology 1994;107(4):1183–1188.

13. Sano H, Kawahito Y, Wilder RL et al. Expression of cyclooxygenase-1 and -2 in human colorectal cancer. Cancer Res 1995;55(17):3785–3789.

14. Oshima M, Dinchuk JE, Kargman SL et al. Suppression of intestinal polyposis in Apc delta716 knockout mice by inhibition of cyclooxygenase 2 (COX-2). Cell 1996;87(5):803–809.

15. Liu CH, Chang SH, Narko K et al. Overexpression of cyclooxygenase-2 is sufficient to induce tumorigenesis in transgenic mice. J Biol Chem 2001;276(21):18563–18569.

16. Neufang G, Furstenberger G, Heidt M et al. Abnormal differentiation of epidermis in transgenic mice constitutively expressing cyclooxygenase-2 in skin. Proc Natl Acad Sci USA 2001;98(13): 7629–7634.

17. Zhang X, Morham SG, Langenbach R, Young DA. Malignant transformation and antineoplastic actions of nonsteroidal antiinflammatory drugs (NSAIDs) on cyclooxygenase-null embryo fibroblasts. J Exp Med 1999;190(4):451–459.

18. Yin MJ, Yamamoto Y, Gaynor RB. The anti-inflammatory agents aspirin and salicylate inhibit the activity of I(kappa)B kinase-beta. Nature 1998;396(6706):77–80.

19. Lehmann JM, Lenhard JM, Oliver BB et al. Peroxisome proliferator-activated receptors alpha and gamma are activated by indomethacin and other non-steroidal anti-inflammatory drugs. J Biol Chem 1997;272(6):3406–3410.

20. Yamamoto Y, Yin MJ, Lin KM, Gaynor RB. Sulindac inhibits activation of the NF-kappaB pathway. J Biol Chem 1999;274(38):27307–27314.

21. Zhang L, Yu J, Park BH et al. Role of BAX in the apoptotic response to anticancer agents. Science 2000;290(5493):989–992.

22. Williams CS, Watson AJ, Sheng H et al. Celecoxib prevents tumor growth in vivo without toxicity to normal gut: lack of correlation between in vitro and in vivo models. Cancer Res 2000;60(21): 6045–6051.

23. Sheng H, Shao J, Kirkland SC et al. Inhibition of human colon cancer cell growth by selective inhibition of cyclooxygenase-2. J Clin Invest 1997;99(9):2254–2259.

24. Tsujii M, DuBois RN. Alterations in cellular adhesion and apoptosis in epithelial cells overexpressing prostaglandin endoperoxide synthase 2. Cell 1995;83(3):493–501.

25. Tsujii M, Kuwano S, DuBois RN. Cyclooxygenase-2 expression in human colon cancer cells increases metastatic potential. Proc Natl Acad Sci USA 1997;94(7):3336–3340.

26. Tsujii M, Kawano S, Tsuji S et al. Cyclooxygenase regulates angiogenesis induced by colon cancer cells. Cell 1998;93(5):705–716.

27. Majima M, Isono M, Ikeda Y et al. Significant roles of inducible cyclooxygenase (COX)-2 in angiogenesis in rat sponge implants. Jpn J Pharmacol 1997;75(2):105–114.

28. Majima M, Hayashi I, Muramatsu M et al. Cyclo-oxygenase-2 enhances basic fibroblast growth factor-induced angiogenesis through induction of vascular endothelial growth factor in rat sponge implants. Br J Pharmacol 2000;130(3):641–649.

29. Daniel TO, Liu H, Morrow JD et al. Thromboxane A2 is a mediator of cyclooxygenase-2-dependent endothelial migration and angiogenesis. Cancer Res 1999;59(18):4574–4577.

30. Masferrer JL, Leahy KM, Koki AT et al. Antiangiogenic and antitumor activities of cyclooxygenase-2 inhibitors. Cancer Res 2000;60(5):1306–1311.

31. Jones MK, Wang H, Peskar BM et al. Inhibition of angiogenesis by nonsteroidal anti-inflammatory drugs: insight into mechanisms and implications for cancer growth and ulcer healing. Nature Med 1999;5(12):1418–1423.

32. Williams CS, Tsujii M, Reese J et al. Host cyclooxygenase-2 modulates carcinoma growth. J Clin Invest 2000;105(11):1589–1594.

33. Dormond O, Foletti A, Paroz C, Ruegg C. NSAIDs inhibit alpha V beta 3 integrin-mediated and Cdc42/Rac-dependent endothelial-cell spreading, migration and angiogenesis. Nature Med 2001; 7(9):1041–1047.

34. Sugimoto Y, Narumiya S, Ichikawa A. Distribution and function of prostanoid receptors: studies from knockout mice. Prog Lipid Res 2000;39(4):289–314.

35. Morita I, Schindler M, Regier MK et al. Different intracellular locations for prostaglandin endoperoxide H synthase-1 and -2. J Biol Chem 1995;270(18):10902–10908.

36. Bhattacharya M, Peri KG, Almazan G et al. Nuclear localization of prostaglandin E2 receptors. Proc Natl Acad Sci USA 1998;95(26):15792–15797.

37. Giardiello FM, Spannhake EW, DuBois RN et al. Prostaglandin levels in human colorectal mucosa: Effects of sulindac in patients with familial adenatomous polyposis (FAP). Gastroenterology 1997; 112:A568.

38. Sheng H, Shao J, Morrow J et al. Modulation of apoptosis and Bcl-2 expression by prostaglandin E2 in human colon cancer cells. Cancer Res 1998;58(2):362–366.

39. Sheng H, Shao J, Washington MK, DuBois RN. Prostaglandin E2 increases growth and motility of colorectal carcinoma cells. J Biol Chem 2001;276(21):18075–18081.

40. Adam L, Mazumdar A, Sharma T et al. A three-dimensional and temporo-spatial model to study invasiveness of cancer cells by heregulin and prostaglandin E2. Cancer Res 2001;61(1):81–87.

41. Watanabe K, Kawamori T, Nakatsugi S et al. Role of the prostaglandin E receptor subtype EP1 in colon carcinogenesis. Cancer Res 1999;59(20):5093–5096.

42. Watanabe K, Kawamori T, Nakatsugi S et al. Inhibitory effect of a prostaglandin E receptor subtype EP(1) selective antagonist, ONO-8713, on development of azoxymethane-induced aberrant crypt foci in mice. Cancer Lett 2000;156(1):57–61.

43. Sonoshita M, Takaku K, Sasaki N et al. Acceleration of intestinal polyposis through prostaglandin receptor EP2 in Apc(Delta 716) knockout mice. Nature Med 2001;7(9):1048–1051.

44. DuBois RN, Giardiello FM, Smalley WE. Nonsteroidal anti-inflammatory drugs, eicosanoids, and colorectal cancer prevention. Gastroenterol Clin North Am 1996;25(4):773–791.

45. Paganini-Hill A, Hsu G, Ross RK, Henderson BE. Aspirin use and incidence of large-bowel cancer in a California retirement community. J Natl Cancer Inst 1991;83(16):1182–1183.

46. Thun MJ, Namboodiri MM, Heath CWJ. Aspirin use and reduced risk of fatal colon cancer. N Engl J Med 1991;325(23):1593–1596.

47. Smalley W, Ray WA, Daugherty J, Griffin MR. Use of nonsteroidal anti-inflammatory drugs and incidence of colorectal cancer: a population-based study. Arch Intern Med 1999;159(2):161–166.

48. Peleg II, Maibach HT, Brown SH, Wilcox CM. Aspirin and nonsteroidal anti-inflammatory drug use and the risk of subsequent colorectal cancer. Arch Intern Med 1994;154(4):394–399.

49. Rosenberg L, Palmer J, Zauber A et al. A hypothesis: nonsteroidal anti-inflammatory drugs reduce the incidence of large-bowel cancer. J Natl Cancer Inst 1991;83(5):355–358.

50. Giovannucci E, Egan KM, Hunter DJ et al. Aspirin and the risk of colorectal cancer in women. N Engl J Med 1995;333(10):609–614.

51. Williams CS, Smalley W, DuBois RN. Aspirin use and potential mechanisms for colorectal cancer prevention. J Clin Invest 1997;100(6):1–5.

52. Collet JP, Sharpe C, Belzile E et al. Colorectal cancer prevention by non-steroidal anti-inflammatory drugs: effects of dosage and timing. Br J Cancer 1999;81(1):62–68.

53. Waddell WR, Gasner GF, Cerise EJ, Loughry RW. Sulindac for polyposis of the colon. Am J Surg 1989;157(1):175–179.

54. Giardiello FM, Hamilton SR, Krush AJ et al. Treatment of colonic and rectal adenomas with sulindac in familial adenomatous polyposis. N Engl J Med 1993;328(18):1313–1316.

55. Steinbach G, Lynch PM, Phillips RKS et al. The effect of celecoxib, a cyclooxygenase-2 inhibitor, in familial adenomatous polyposis. N Engl J Med 2000;342(26):1946–1952.

56. Matsuhashi N, Nakajima A, Shinohara K et al. Rectal cancer after sulindac therapy for a sporadic adenomatous colonic polyp. Am J Gastroenterol 1998;93(11):2261–2266.

57. Baron JA, Beach M, Mandel JS et al. Calcium supplements for the prevention of colorectal adenomas. Calcium Polyp Prevention Study Group. N Engl J Med 1999;340(2):101–107.

58. Torrance CJ, Jackson PE, Montgomery E et al. Combinatorial chemoprevention of intestinal neoplasia. Nature Med 2000;6(9):1024–1028.

59. Mann M, Sheng H, Shao J et al. Targeting cyclooxygenase 2 and HER-2/neu pathways inhibits colorectal carcinoma growth. Gastroenterology 2001;120(7):1713–1719.

Chapter 10

Late Effects of Childhood Cancer Therapy

Smita Bhatia

Wendy Landier

Leslie L. Robison

The undisputed progress in pediatric oncology over the past few decades, as evidenced by cure rates now approaching 80%, underscores the need to screen survivors of childhood cancer for late effects of therapy. Approximately 50% of these survivors are likely to develop complications that alter quality of life. Unlike the adult, the growing child tolerates the acute side effects of therapy relatively well. However, the use of cancer therapy at an early age can produce complications that may not become apparent until years later as the child matures. Therefore, ongoing evaluation of childhood cancer survivors is an essential component of follow up. The resulting complications may be related to myriad factors, most notably specific therapy employed and the age of the child at the time the therapy was administered. This article discusses the long-term complications that can occur among pediatric patients treated for cancer, along with recommendations for follow up.

NEUROLOGIC FUNCTION

Neurocognitive Complications

Neurocognitive sequelae of treatment for childhood cancer are most often the result of radiation to the whole brain or of therapy with high-dose or intrathecal methotrexate or cytarabine. Children with a history of brain tumors, acute lymphoblastic leukemia (ALL), or non-Hodgkin's lymphoma (NHL) are most likely to be affected. Risk factors include increasing radiation dose, young age at the time of treatment, treatment with both cranial irradiation and systemic or intrathecal chemotherapy, and female gender.[1,2] Severe deficits are more frequently noted in children with brain tumors, especially those who were treated with radiotherapy, and in children who were younger than 5 years at the time of treatment.[3] The pathogenesis of central nervous system damage is only partially understood, and evidence suggests that direct effects on intracranial endothelial cells and brain white matter and from immunologic mechanisms play a role. A spectrum of clinical syndromes may occur, including radionecrosis, necrotizing leukoencephalopathy, mineralizing microangiopathy with dystrophic calcification, cerebellar sclerosis, and spinal cord dysfunction.[4]

Neurocognitive deficits usually become evident within 1–2 years after irradiation[5] and are progressive in nature. Affected children may experience information-processing deficits resulting in academic difficulties. These children are particularly prone to problems with receptive and expressive language, attention span, and visual and perceptual motor skills, most often manifested in academic difficulties in the areas of reading, language, and mathematics. Children in the younger age groups and those treated for brain tumors may experience significant drops in intelligence quotient scores,[3,6,7] with irradiation- or chemotherapy-induced destruction in normal white matter partially explaining intellectual and academic achievement deficits.[8] A better understanding of chemotherapy use and the development of newer agents may increase efficacy, reduce side effects, and allow deferral of radiotherapy in a greater percentage of patients.

Children who have received therapy with the potential to cause neurocognitive deficits should receive close monitoring of academic performance. Referral for neuropsychiatric evaluation should be initiated if any deficits are noted, and affected children's teachers should be kept closely informed regarding any special learning needs. When necessary, curricular modifications and special services, such as speech and language therapy or social skills training, should be implemented to foster attainment of children's greatest potential.[5]

Auditory Complications

Several potentially ototoxic agents are commonly used in the treatment of children with malignancies, including platinum-based chemotherapy, aminoglycoside antibiotics, loop diuretics, and radiotherapy. All these agents are capable of causing sensorineural hearing loss. Significant risk factors for hearing loss include age younger than 4 years at the time of treatment, diagnosis of central nervous system neoplasm, treatment with platinum-based chemotherapy in combination with cranial irradiation, and treatment involving multiple ototoxic agents.[9] Children whose renal function was diminished at the time of treatment, often as a result of treatment with nephrotoxic chemotherapeutic agents, are also at increased risk for ototoxicity.[10] Diagnoses commonly associated with hearing loss include brain and germ cell tumors, neuroblastoma, and osteosarcoma. Hearing loss associated with ototoxic chemotherapy generally begins in the high frequency ranges (> 2000 Hz) with progression to the lower frequencies with additional therapy. Schell et al[9] found that 50% of 146 nonirradiated children receiving ≥ 450 mg/m² of cisplatin developed substantial (> 50 decibels) hearing loss at 6000–8000 Hz and that 25% of children receiving ≥ 720 mg/m² developed significant hearing loss in the more critical 500- to 3000-Hz range. Children who also received cranial irradiation developed high-frequency hearing loss with three fewer cisplatin courses than those not receiving irradiation.[9]

Children who received ototoxic agents during their cancer treatment should undergo yearly audiological evaluations. Interventions to assist children experiencing hearing loss as a result of cancer treatment include the use of hearing aids and other assistive devices, along with preferential seating in the front of the classroom. For more severely affected children, placement in special educational environments for the hearing-impaired may be required. Affected patients should be counseled to avoid exposure to loud noise, to use ear protection in noisy environments, and to avoid exposure to ototoxic medications (e.g., aminoglycosides, loop diuretics) to prevent further hearing loss. All children with hearing loss related to cancer treatment should receive an evaluation and ongoing follow up from a pediatric audiologist or otologist.[11]

OCULAR FUNCTION

Children at risk for cataract formation related to cancer treatment include those who received treatment with busulfan or long-term corticosteroids, total body irradiation (TBI), or irradiation to the brain, head, or orbit.[12,13] Surgical removal of cataracts is indicated when visual impairment interferes with the child's ability to carry out normal activities.[14] Systemic corticosteroid therapy also places children at risk for glaucoma and uveitis. TBI and cranial irradiation may result in dry eyes (Sjögren's syndrome) related to decreased lacrimation. A history of orbital irradiation also places children at risk for corneal ulceration, dry eyes, optic nerve damage, retinitis, iritis, glaucoma, blepharitis, and orbital hypoplasia.[14] Children who received radiotherapy to the orbit should be evaluated by an ophthalmologist at least yearly, and children with other risk factors should be seen by an ophthalmologist at least once within 5 years of completing therapy.[15] Management of ocular sequelae of cancer therapy should be accomplished collaboratively with an ophthalmologist. Surgical interventions, including cataract extraction and photocoagulation, and use of ophthalmic drops and ointments may be indicated,[14] with preservation of the child's sight being the overall goal.

CARDIOVASCULAR FUNCTION

Chronic cardiotoxicity usually manifests itself as cardiomyopathy, pericarditis, and congestive heart failure. The anthracyclines doxorubicin and daunorubicin are well-known causes of cardiomyopathy.[16–19] Cardiomyopathy can occur many years after completion of therapy, and the onset may be spontaneous or coincide with exertion or pregnancy. The incidence of cardiomyopathy is dose-dependent and may exceed 30% among patients who received cumulative doses of anthracyclines in excess of 600 mg/m^2.[20–22] Kremer et al[23] evaluated the cumulative incidence of anthracycline-induced clinical heart failure in a cohort of 607 children who had been treated with anthracyclines to a mean cumulative dose of 301 mg/m^2 and followed up for a median of 6.3 years. A cumulative dose of anthracyclines > 300 mg/m^2 was associated with an increased risk of clinical heart failure (relative risk, 11.8), compared with a cumulative dose < 300 mg/m^2. The estimated risk of clinical heart failure increased with time and approached 5% after 15 years.[23]

The incidence of subclinical anthracycline myocardial damage is the subject of much interest recently. Steinherz et al[24] found 23% of 201 patients to have echocardiographic abnormalities a median of 7 years after therapy. The median cumulative dose of doxorubicin received by these patients was 450 mg/m^2 (range, 200–1275 mg/m^2). Lipshultz and colleagues[25] evaluated survivors of childhood cancer who had received a median doxorubicin dose of 334 mg/m^2 (range, 12–550 mg/m^2). They concluded that doxorubicin causes progressive elevation of afterload or depression of left ventricular contractility in approximately 75% of the patients. Pathologic specimens in seven patients showed myocyte hypertrophy, and the investigators speculated that doxorubicin administered in childhood results in acute asymptomatic loss of myocytes, which, in turn, results in hypertrophy of the remaining myocytes, with inadequate left ventricular mass and secondary heart disease later in life.

Risk factors known to be associated with anthracycline-related cardiac toxicity include mediastinal irradiation,[26] uncontrolled hypertension,[19,20] underlying cardiac abnormalities (including involvement by tumor),[20,27] exposure to other chemotherapeutic agents (especially cyclophosphamide,[20] dactinomycin,[28] mitomycin,[20] dacarbazine,[29] vincristine, bleomycin, and methotrexate),[30] female gender,[31] younger age,[19,32,33] and such electrolyte imbalances as hypokalemia and hypomagnesemia.[18] The pattern of anthracycline administration is also important, with lesser toxicity associated with continuous infusions or with weekly doxorubicin as compared to boluses every 3 weeks.[21,34,35]

Chronic cardiac toxicity associated with irradiation alone most commonly involves pericardial effusions or constrictive pericarditis, sometimes in association with pancarditis. Although 4000 cGy of total-heart radiation dose appears to be the usual threshold, pericarditis has been reported after as little as 1500 cGy, even in the absence of radiomimetic chemotherapy.[36,37] Recent studies of patients in whom combined anterior and posterior ports were used found asymptomatic pericardial effusions in 5%–30% shortly after therapy, with one-half of these resolving over 1 year.[36,38] Symptomatic pericarditis, which usually develops 10–30 months after irradiation, is found in 2%–10% of patients.[36,37,39] Subclinical pericardial and myocardial damage as well as valvular thickening may be common in this population,[40,41] and symptomatic pericarditis may first appear as late as 45 years after therapy.[42,43] Coronary artery disease has been reported after irradiation to the mediastinum, although the mortality rate was not significantly higher in patients who had Hodgkin's disease and received mediastinal irradiation than in the general population.[44,45]

Prevention of cardiotoxicity is a primary focus of investigation. Certain analogs of doxorubicin and daunorubicin, with decreased cardiotoxicity but equivalent antitumor activity, are being explored. In addition, the liposomal anthracyclines are being explored to reduce cardiotoxicity. The anthracyclines chelate iron, and the anthracycline-iron complex catalyzes the formation of extremely hydroxyl radicals. Agents such as dexrazoxane, which are able to remove iron from the anthracyclines, have been investigated as cardioprotectants. Clinical trials of dexrazoxane have been conducted in children, with encouraging evidence of short-term cardioprotection.[46,47] The long-term avoidance of cardiotoxicity with the use of this agent has to be determined.[48] Smaller doses and reduced radiotherapy port sizes may also help in decreasing the incidence of carditis.

Diagnosis of cardiovascular disease requires a high index of suspicion, an understanding of the natural course of disease, and an awareness of the potential risk factors that could accentuate the risk in patients who have received anthracyclines or irradiation to the mediastinum. Owing to the known long latency of cardiac complications, a yearly standard history and physical examination for life is recommended for high-risk patients, and an echocardiogram or gated radionuclide angiography and electrocardiogram are recommended every 2–3 years for patients who have received any anthracyclines.[49] In addition, patients at high risk for development of cardiac abnormalities should be cautioned to refrain from participating in strenuous activities, such as weightlifting. Moreover, pregnant women should be cautioned about the risk of development of congestive heart failure during labor. In patients with severe anthracycline-induced cardiomyopathy refractory to medical management, cardiac transplantation may be an option.

PULMONARY FUNCTION

Radiation-induced restrictive lung disease is seen in patients who received whole-lung irradiation at a dose of 1100–1400 cGy and is consistent with a proportionate interference with the growth of both the lung and the chest wall.[50–52] Children younger than 3 years at time of therapy seem to be more susceptible to chronic toxicity.[52] Obstructive changes are also reported after conventional radiotherapy and have been reported after 1000 cGy TBI for bone marrow transplantation (BMT).[53]

Several chemotherapeutic agents have been associated with pulmonary disease in long-term survivors. Bleomycin toxicity is the prototype for chemotherapy-related lung injury. The chronic lung toxicity is dose-dependent past a threshold cumulative dose of 400 units and is exacerbated by previous or concurrent radiotherapy,[54] cyclophosphamide,[55] or subsequent oxygen therapy.[56] At doses exceeding 400 units, 10% of the patients experience fibrosis, and 35%–55% suffer severe symptoms in the face of combinations of other injuries.[57] Other chemotherapeutic agents associated with chronic lung injury include carmustine,[58] busulfan, melphalan, cyclophosphamide, vinblastine, and prolonged low-dose methotrexate therapy.

A population-based cohort of survivors of ALL in first remission, with no BMT or spinal irradiation and followed up for a median of 8 years revealed slight pulmonary restrictive disease in the absence of pulmonary symptoms.[59] Conversely, assessment of pulmonary function in survivors of Wilms' tumor revealed that patients receiving any form of radiotherapy were at risk of developing abnormalities in pulmonary function.[60] Survivors of Hodgkin's disease and NHL similarly revealed lung volumes and diffusion capacity to be reduced several years after childhood Hodgkin's disease or NHL, and the risk factor identified was irradiation at a young age.[61]

Symptoms of pulmonary dysfunction include chronic cough or dyspnea, and close evaluation should be performed during yearly follow up. All patients must understand the risks of smoking. The best possible approach to chronic pulmonary toxicity of anticancer therapy is preventive and includes careful monitoring of pulmonary function and chest radiographs before and during bleomycin and irradiation, respecting cumulative dose restrictions on bleomycin administration, and limiting radiation dosage and port sizes.

ENDOCRINE FUNCTION

Thyroid

Hypothyroidism is the most common nonmalignant late effect involving the thyroid gland and almost always is due to irradiation of the neck for a nonthyroid malignancy. After radiation doses exceeding 1500 cGy, laboratory evidence of primary hypothyroidism is evident in 40%–90% of patients with Hodgkin's disease, NHL, and primary intracranial or head and neck tumors.[62–64] In some instances, hypothyroidism is reversible after as long as 3 years, even without replacement therapy.[65] The actuarial risk of clinical hypothyroidism for subjects treated with 4500 cGy or more is 50% at 20 years from diagnosis of Hodgkin's disease. Risk factors associated with the development of hypothyroidism include increasing dose of radiation, thyroidectomy, use of iodide-containing contrast material (as in lymphangiography), older age at irradiation, and female gender.[66] Use of hyperfractionated radiotherapy has been associated with a lower risk of hypothyroidism as compared to that of conventionally fractionated radiotherapy used in the treatment of patients with medulloblastoma or primitive neuroectodermal tumors.[67]

Hyperthyroidism has been reported in up to 5% of the survivors of Hodgkin's disease and is associated with radiation doses exceeding 3500 cGy.[66] Thyroid nodules are observed among patients exposed to irradiation; female gender and radiation doses exceeding 2500 cGy have been identified as risk factors.[66] The actuarial risk of female survivors of Hodgkin's disease developing a thyroid nodule is 20% at 20 years from diagnosis. Hodgkin's disease patients receiving irradiation to the thyroid gland have been reported to be at an eighteenfold increased risk of developing thyroid cancer, compared to the general population.

Careful shielding of the thyroid during irradiation, elimination of irradiation or the use of lower doses, and avoidance of concurrent use of iodide-containing contrast material should help to decrease the incidence of thyroid abnormalities. Routine annual screening for thyroid abnormalities by physical examination and biochemical measures for patients who have received 1000 cGy or more to the neck is advised. If any abnormalities are detected, evaluation and treatment by an endocrinologist is recommended.

Growth

Poor linear growth and short adult stature are common complications after successful treatment of childhood cancer.[68] Although catch-up growth may occur in some children, in others short stature may be permanent or even progressive. Severe growth retardation, defined as a standing height below the fifth percentile, has been observed in as many as 30%–35% of survivors of childhood brain tumors[69–71] and in 10%–15% of patients treated for leukemia.[72,73] In children treated for ALL, whole-brain irradiation has been identified as the principal cause of short stature.[72] The effects of cranial irradiation appear to be related to age and gender, with children younger than 5 years at time of therapy and females being more susceptible to the radiation effect.[74–76] The effects of radiation are also dose-dependent, with doses exceeding 3000 cGy being associated with growth retardation in 50% of the patients.[70,71] The growth retardation after 1800 or 2400 cGy, as used in children with ALL, is less frequent and is generally milder, although patients treated with 2400 cGy of cranial radiation have a greater decrease in final height as compared with those receiving 1800 cGy.[76–78] The mechanism by which cranial irradiation induces short stature is not clear. Growth hormone deficiency and early onset of puberty in girls may contribute to loss of final height.[79] Direct inhibition of vertebral growth by spinal irradiation often contributes to short stature.

Standardized growth curves should be used to monitor sequential growth in survivors of childhood cancer. Frequent measurements of sitting and standing heights are essential to establish trends. Children experiencing abnormal growth patterns should be referred to an endocrinologist for evaluation and management. Early diagnosis and timely therapy of the endocrine sequelae of cancer treatment (i.e., growth hormone deficiency, hypothyroidism, and precocious puberty) ensures that these individuals will reach their optimal growth potential.

Body Mass Index

An increased prevalence of obesity has been reported among survivors of childhood ALL. The risk factors responsible for the increased prevalence have remained controversial. A recent investigation reported that the percentage of subjects who were overweight at attainment of final height was 10.5%, 40%, and 38% for subjects treated with no cranial radiation, 1800 cGy of cranial radiation, and 2400 cGy of cranial radiation, respectively.[80] This study documented that children with ALL given cranial radiation develop increases in their body mass index early on during their treatment and remain at significant risk for becoming overweight as young adults.

GONADAL FUNCTION

Males

Male survivors of childhood cancer may experience germ cell depletion and abnormalities of gonadal endocrine function. These abnormalities may be secondary to irradiation, chemotherapy, or surgery, with the effects of therapy varying depending on age at treatment. At doses of 400–600 cGy, azoospermia may persist for 3–5 years; at doses in excess of 600 cGy, germinal loss with resulting increases in follicle-stimulating hormone (FSH) and decreases in testicular volume usually appears irreversible.[81,82] Prepubertal testicular germ cells also appear to be radiosensitive, although tubular damage may be difficult to assess until the patient has gone through puberty. Radiotherapy also is toxic to Leydig's cells, with resulting inadequate production of testosterone.[83,84]

Chemotherapy can also interfere with testicular function. Alkylating agents decrease spermatogenesis in long-term survivors of cancer. The effects of cyclophosphamide and chlorambucil are dose-dependent but reversible in up to 70% of patients after several years.[85] Among pubertal males treated for Hodgkin's disease with six cycles of mechlorethamine, vincristine, prednisone, and procarbazine, azoospermia is found in 80%–100%, and is reversible in only 20% of cases.[86] After doxorubicin, bleomycin, vinblastine, and dacarbazine, the incidence of azoospermia is 36%, with 100% recovery.[87] The effect of mechlorethamine, vincristine, prednisone, and procarbazine on Leydig's cell function appears to be age-related, with normal pubertal progression after therapy before puberty, gynecomastia with low testosterone and increased luteinizing hormone (LH) in patients treated during adolescence, and compensated Leydig's cell failure without gynecomastia in adults.[85]

Screening for gonadal dysfunction should be included in routine evaluation, with specific attention paid to problems with impotence, fertility, or libido and examination for gynecomastia and Tanner staging. Pubertal boys and boys with delayed puberty should undergo hormonal evaluation, including measurement of serum FSH, LH, and testosterone levels. If abnormalities are detected, collaborative management with an endocrinologist is essential in planning hormone replacement therapy or monitoring for spontaneous recovery.

Females

Radiotherapy effects on the ovary are both age- and dose-dependent. Irreversible ovarian failure is seen in 100% of women older than 40 years and treated with 400–700 cGy of conventionally fractionated radiation to both ovaries.[88] On the other hand, amenorrhea develops in only 68% of prepubescent females treated with higher doses of radiation (1200–1500 cGy).[89] Spinal irradiation for the treatment of ALL and brain tumors appears to result in clinically significant ovarian damage in some young women, although the majority of these women go on to experience normal puberty and menarche (albeit at a slightly older age). Girls treated with whole-abdomen or pelvic irradiation for Hodgkin's disease or Wilms' tumor or other solid tumors are at a high risk of ovarian failure. Patients who receive a BMT with TBI, both single-dose and fractionated, are at a high risk of developing permanent ovarian failure. The extent of gonadal injury depends on age and pubertal status at the time of the irradiation. Almost all patients who undergo BMT after the age of 10 years will develop premature ovarian failure, whereas only 50% of girls given transplants before the age of 10 years will.[90]

Ovarian failure has also been observed after chemotherapy, with alkylating agents showing the best association. Toxicity is dose- and age-dependent. Women older than 40 years may develop amenorrhea with only 1–4 cycles of mechlorethamine, vincristine, prednisone, and procarbazine, compared with 3–12 cycles in the 30% of women who are younger than 35 years and become amenorrheic.[91] Many of these young women demonstrate normalization of FSH levels over time, and only a minority appear to experience irreversible ovarian failure requiring long-term hormone replacement therapy.[92] Females who receive high-dose, myeloablative therapy with alkylating agents in the context of allogeneic or autologous BMT are at high risk of developing ovarian failure.[92]

The diagnostic evaluation of ovarian function in females treated for childhood cancer includes menstrual history, Tanner staging, and determination of serum LH, FSH, and estradiol levels. Because of the increased risk of premature menopause in these patients, follow up should be life-long.

Breast

Radiation in doses of 1000 cGy or higher to the prepubertal breast bud will result in subsequent hypoplasia of the affected breast, and doses of 2000 cGy or higher to any prepubertal breast tissue may prevent breast development in the irradiated area.[93,94] Failure of lactation may also occur as a result of low-dose radiation to breast tissue.[95] Radiation to the pubertal or postpubertal breast may result in decreased elasticity of the skin and fibrosis of breast structures.[96] There is also an increased risk of breast cancer in the irradiated breast tissue.[97] Surveillance includes breast examination and Tanner staging during physical examinations. Anticipatory guidance should be offered to those at risk for breast hypoplasia. As adolescents experiencing an altered body image are particularly vulnerable to low self-esteem, affected patients may need referral for psychological counseling. Breast augmentation may be an option; however, this may be technically difficult owing to fibrosis and delayed healing of irradiated skin. In addition, early detection of secondary malignancy in the area may be hampered by the breast augmentation procedure.[96]

INTEGUMENTARY SYSTEM

Late effects to the skin of childhood cancer survivors include fibrosis, telangiectasia, permanent alopecia, acceleration of aging, increased melanogenesis, and the development of secondary skin cancer, particularly basal cell carcinoma.[96] Most of these late effects can be attributed to radiation; however, increased melanogenesis has also been associated with bleomycin and doxorubicin, and permanent alopecia has been induced by the high-dose busulfan and cyclophosphamide conditioning regimen used for some BMTs.[96]

Surveillance includes thorough physical examination of the skin, with particular attention paid to areas within or near radiation ports. In addition, any suspicious lesions or suspicious changes within melanocytic nevi should be noted, and dermatology consultation should be obtained for excision and definitive biopsy. Patients should be counseled regarding the importance of performing monthly skin self-examination and should be instructed to report any suspicious lesions immediately. Patients should also be educated regarding the importance of avoiding sun exposure whenever possible, particularly of radiation-treated areas. Sunscreens and protective clothing, including hats, should be used for any prolonged sun exposure.

GASTROINTESTINAL FUNCTION

The most common late gastrointestinal (GI) toxicities occurring as a consequence of childhood cancer treatment include adhesions, stricture formations, fibrosis, and malabsorption, most often related to surgery and radiotherapy.[98] Patients who have undergone abdominal surgery for tumor resection or have had radiation with fields involving the GI tract are most likely to be affected. Diagnoses most commonly associated with late GI toxicities include Wilms' tumor, NHL, rhabdomyosarcoma, and neuroblastoma. Long-term survivors of BMT may also be affected, owing to the effects of chronic graft-versus-host disease on the GI tract. Manifestations of toxicity can occur in any area of the GI tract involved in the treatment field, from the esophagus to the rectum. Clinical manifestations may include vomiting, abdominal pain, dysphagia, diarrhea, hematochezia, and fatigue.[98]

Appropriate surveillance includes yearly follow-up evaluations, including complete blood count to detect microcytic anemia associated with GI bleeding or macrocytic anemia associated with malabsorption. Serum albumin and protein levels should be monitored every 3–5 years in those patients at high risk for enteritis (e.g., those who had irradiation or surgery involving the bowel and those with chronic graft-versus-host disease). As these children move into adulthood, routine cancer screening (including sigmoidoscopy and stool for occult blood) should be recommended on the basis of the patients' age and treatment history.[98]

HEPATOBILIARY FUNCTION

Late effects on the hepatobiliary system are most often related to irradiation, hepatotoxic chemotherapy (Table 10.1), and the infectious consequences of blood transfusions (e.g., hepatitis and cytomegalovirus).[99] Fibrosis is the most common long-term hepatic toxicity of childhood cancer therapy. Detection of fibrosis or cirrhosis of the liver may be difficult, as patients may be asymptomatic for years. However, routine liver biopsies or scans are not recommended.[98,99]

Surveillance in at-risk patients includes physical examination, with attention paid to icterus, hepatomegaly, and signs of malabsorption, and measurement of serum transaminases, alkaline phosphatase, and bilirubin every 2–5 years. In addition, patients who have a history of blood transfusion and are found to have elevated serum transaminases should be tested for hepatitis A, B, and C.[98] Patients should be counseled to avoid potentially hepatotoxic agents (e.g., alcohol). Those who do not have adequate immunity to hepatitis should receive the hepatitis A and B vaccines. In addition, patients who received blood products before the initiation of routine screening for hepatitis C (initiated in May 1990) should be tested.

URINARY TRACT FUNCTION

Kidneys

Long-term renal damage in children treated for cancer is most often associated with such drugs as cisplatin or ifosfamide and with radiotherapy. Cisplatin can

TABLE 10.1 Common Late Toxicities by Therapeutic Agent

Agent	Common Late Toxicity
Alkylating agents	
Cyclophosphamide	Bladder fibrosis, hemorrhagic cystitis, cardiac failure (high-dose), gonadal failure, infertility, SMN (leukemia), pulmonary fibrosis, hyperpigmentation of skin
Mechlorethamine	SMN (leukemia), infertility
Ifosfamide	Fanconi's renal syndrome, rickets, hemorrhagic cystitis, bladder fibrosis, gonadal failure, infertility
Melphalan	Infertility
Lomustine, Carmustine	Chronic marrow hypoplasia, pulmonary fibrosis, renal atrophy, hepatic fibrosis, gonadal failure, infertility, hyperpigmentation of skin
Busulfan	Pulmonary fibrosis, gonadal failure, infertility, hyperpigmentation of skin and nails
Cisplatin	Renal tubular dysfunction, hypomagnesemia, hearing loss, peripheral neuropathies, infertility
Carboplatin	Nephrotoxicity, hearing loss, infertility
Dacarbazine	Infertility, hyperpigmentation of skin and nails
Procarbazine	Gonadal failure, infertility, SMN
Antimetabolites	
Methotrexate	Osteoporosis, neurocognitive deficits–leukoencephalopathy (high-dose, IT), hepatic fibrosis, hyperpigmentation of skin, pulmonary fibrosis
Mercaptopurine, thioguanine	Hepatic fibrosis
Cytarabine	Neurocognitive deficits, ataxia, leukoencephalopathy (high-dose, IT)
Fluorouracil	Dry eyes, lacrimal duct fibrosis
Antibiotics	
Doxorubicin, daunorubicin, idarubicin	Cardiomyopathy, CHF (possible cardiac decompensation during pregnancy or at onset of physical fitness programs; reported sudden cardiac deaths associated with anaerobic activities, such as weightlifting)
Bleomycin	Pulmonary fibrosis, hyperpigmentation of skin and nails
Dactinomycin	Hepatic fibrosis, skin and tendon contractures, hyperpigmentation of skin

Plant alkaloids	
Vincristine	Foot drop, peripheral neuropathies
Vinblastine	Peripheral vascular disease (Raynaud's phenomenon)
Etoposide	SMN (leukemia), Leydig's cell damage, peripheral neuropathies
Teniposide	SMN (leukemia)
Corticosteroids	Osteoporosis, AVN, cataracts, slipped capital femoral epiphysis
Enzymes	
L-Asparaginase	Sequelae of CVA
Radiation	
All fields	Increased melanocytic nevi, basal cell carcinoma, skin fibrosis, malignant melanoma
Cranial	Neurocognitive deficits, endocrinopathies (HPA axis), abnormal tooth and root development, dental caries, cataracts, SMN (brain tumor), infertility, leukoencephalopathy, CVA, precocious puberty
Spinal	Dental caries, abnormal tooth and root development, thyroid dysfunction, scoliosis, kyphosis, lordosis, decreased sitting height, myelitis
Brain, head, neck	Neurocognitive deficits, hearing loss, chronic otitis, cataracts, endocrinopathies (HPA axis), thyroid dysfunction, radionecrosis of brain tissue, chronic sinusitis, abnormal tooth and root development, dental caries, salivary gland atrophy, xerostomia, mandibular or maxillary hypoplasia, vocal cord hypoplasia, alopecia
Orbit	Cataracts, dry eyes, conjunctival damage, retinitis, iritis, glaucoma, blepharitis, corneal ulceration, optic nerve damage, orbital hypoplasia
Mediastinum, pulmonary	Thyroid dysfunction, cardiomyopathy, pericarditis, coronary artery disease, pulmonary fibrosis, SMN (breast), hypoplasia of breast tissue, esophageal stricture
Mantle	Thyroid dysfunction, cardiomyopathy, pericarditis, coronary artery disease, pulmonary fibrosis, hypoplasia of breast tissue, SMN (breast)
Abdominal	Hepatic fibrosis, esophageal varices, renal damage, renal artery stenosis, hypertension, scoliosis, intestinal fibrosis, gastritis, enteritis, malabsorption

TABLE 10.1 Continued

Agent	Common Late Toxicity
Testicular	Leydig's cell failure, infertility
Pelvic	Gonadal failure, marrow hypoplasia, bladder and ureteral fibrosis, urethral strictures, uterine and vaginal fibrosis, prostate hypoplasia or atrophy, hemorrhagic cystitis
Bladder	Hemorrhagic cystitis, bladder fibrosis
Extremity	Growth discrepancy of limb (e.g., leg length), SMN (bone, soft tissue), pathological fractures, contractures, muscular hypoplasia, osteonecrosis
Total-body irradiation	Growth failure, hypothyroidism, gonadal failure, cataracts
Surgery	
Limb salvage	Pathological fractures, limited range of motion, graft infection
Laparotomy	Luminal narrowing, fistulas, bowel obstruction (strictures)
Nephrectomy	Hypertension, renal dysfunction
Amputation	Prosthesis and stump complications
Orchiectomy, oophorectomy	Gonadal failure if bilateral (requiring hormone replacement)
Splenectomy	Overwhelming sepsis (usually pneumococcal)
Adrenalectomy	Need for glucocorticoid and mineral corticoid replacement if bilateral
Thyroidectomy	Hypothyroidism
Enucleation	Prosthesis complications, blindness

AVN, avascular necrosis; CHF, congestive heart failure; CVA, cerebrovascular accident; HPA, hypothalamic-pituitary axis; IT, intrathecal; SMN, secondary malignant neoplasm.

damage the glomerulus and distal renal tubules, potentially causing diminished glomerular filtration rate and electrolyte wasting, most commonly involving magnesium, calcium, potassium, and sodium.[100,101] Ifosfamide damages the proximal renal tubule, potentially resulting in Fanconi's renal syndrome (hypokalemia, hypophosphatemia glucosuria, proteinuria, renal tubular acidosis, and rickets).[102] Children at particular risk include those who received treatment with more than one nephrotoxic agent and those with concomitant renal damage related to surgery or irradiation. Although the glomerular filtration rate may improve over time, electrolyte wasting associated with ifosfamide therapy and hypomagnesemia associated with cisplatin therapy appear to persist in some children.[15,101] Yearly surveillance should include monitoring of serum creatinine, blood urea nitrogen, and serum chemistries; urinalysis; and measurement of blood pressure. Ongoing management includes electrolyte replacement, treatment of hypertension, and avoidance of further nephrotoxic agents. In children who have a history of radiation to the renal artery and subsequently develop hypertension, radiologic studies for stenosis of the renal artery should be conducted; if stenosis is present, surgical correction should be undertaken.[103] Patients with a history of nephrectomy should be counseled regarding the importance of protecting the remaining single kidney. These patients should be cautioned to reduce sodium intake, avoid contact sports, avoid potentially nephrotoxic agents (e.g., ibuprofen, aminoglycosides), maintain normal weight, and obtain early intervention for urinary tract infections.

Bladder

Cyclophosphamide and ifosfamide are both capable of inducing hemorrhagic cystitis as a result of accumulation of acrolein in the bladder.[100] Urgency, frequency, and dysuria are symptoms commonly associated with hemorrhagic cystitis, which can be a long-term complication of cancer therapy in some children.[103] Radiation to the pelvis or bladder can result in fibrosis and scarring, with resultant decreased bladder capacity and predisposition to urinary tract infections.[104] Bladder cancer has developed in some patients who received bladder-toxic agents during treatment for childhood cancer, although the risk is not clearly defined.[100] Yearly urinalysis should be performed in these patients to determine the presence of microscopic hematuria.

MUSCULOSKELETAL FUNCTION

Childhood cancer and its treatment can affect bone accretion, resulting in reduced bone mineral density (BMD). Risk factors for decreased BMD and osteoporosis include therapy with corticosteroids, high-dose methotrexate, and cranial irradiation.[15] A recent study reported gonadal dysfunction to be associated with decreased BMD.[105] Because age at study (median age, 25 years) coincided with the normal age of attainment of peak bone mass and because peak bone mass is a major determinant of BMD later in life, the authors concluded that childhood cancer survivors were at increased risk for osteoporosis and fractures. Preventive measures and interventions for osteopenia or asymptomatic osteoporosis include smoking cessation, avoidance of carbonated beverages, supplementation of calcium and vitamin D, bisphosphonates, weight-bearing exercise, and hormonal replacement when indicated.[106] For those with more advanced bone demineralization, orthopedic or endocrine consultation and management should be obtained.

Avascular necrosis is often related to corticosteroid therapy but may be associated with radiotherapy as well.[101,107] Avascular necrosis occurs most frequently in the femoral heads but can occur in other locations and may be multifocal.[99] Treatment should be undertaken in consultation with an orthopedist and includes analgesics, avoidance of weight bearing on the affected extremity, and joint replacement surgery in severe cases.

Other musculoskeletal sequelae related to childhood cancer treatment may include scoliosis, kyphosis, gait disturbances, and growth deficits secondary to radiation effects on bones, soft tissues, and blood vessels. Arm and leg length discrepancies and spinal abnormalities may result from radiation-induced physeal growth injury to the bones in growing children, particularly during phases of rapid growth, such as infancy, early childhood, and adolescence. Higher radiation doses, asymmetric treatment fields, and large tissue treatment volumes also increase the likelihood of musculoskeletal complications.[96,108]

Dental Complications

Irradiation involving the head and neck regions (including cranial radiation and TBI) often results in deleterious effects on oral health. Developing teeth are particularly vulnerable and often sustain delayed or arrested root and enamel formation. Maxillofacial abnormalities may occur in the radiation field, resulting in malocclusion and facial asymmetry. Diminished salivary gland function related to radiation results in xerostomia, predisposing affected children to dental caries and gingivitis and to disturbances in taste that may result in poor nutrition.[104,109] Chemotherapy has also been implicated in dental complications of cancer treatment, usually resulting in qualitative effects on enamel and tooth development.[110] Children younger than 6 years at the time of treatment are most vulnerable to dental complications.[109] Interventions include regular dental visits, panorex radiographs to evaluate root formation, prophylactic fluoride applications, aggressive management of dental caries and periodontal disease, and artificial saliva if indicated.

HEMATOLOGIC AND IMMUNOLOGIC FUNCTION

Long-term sequelae of cancer treatment may involve diminished bone marrow reserve and impairment of immune function. Cell-mediated immunity, as measured by T-cell activity, is most likely to be affected and may persist for up to 10 years after treatment.[111] Patients who have undergone splenectomy experience impaired humoral immunity, placing them at risk for fulminant infections, particularly with encapsulated organisms.[99] Deficits in cell-mediated immunity are of particular concern because of the T-lymphocyte's role in cancer surveillance (i.e., ability to detect and destroy cancer cells that may herald disease recurrence or second malignant neoplasms) and in regulating the function of humoral immunity and the inflammatory response. Risk factors associated with persistent immunologic impairment include higher total radiation dose, large radiation fields, upper-body radiation, total nodal radiation, combined modality treatment, and high-dose chemotherapy regimens given over prolonged periods, especially those involving alkylating agents.[111] Interventions include evaluation for adequate levels of immunity for vaccine-preventable diseases 6 months to 1 year after cancer treatment with reimmunization as indicated. In addition, splenectomized patients require pneumococcal and *Haemophilus influenzae* vaccines and ongoing penicillin prophylaxis. Patients and their families should be counseled regarding the need for medical evaluation and treatment of fevers in the splenectomized patient.

SECOND MALIGNANT NEOPLASMS

Several studies following up large cohorts of childhood cancer survivors have reported a three- to sixfold increased risk of a second cancer as compared with the general population, and this risk continues to increase as the cohort ages.[112,113] The incidence and the type of second malignancy differ with the primary diagnosis, type of therapy received, and presence of genetic conditions. The following are at particularly high risk: patients with Hodgkin's disease, hereditary retinoblastoma, and a genetic form of Wilms' tumor; patients receiving high doses of radiotherapy or alkylating agents; and patients with von Recklinghausen's neurofibromatosis, xeroderma pigmentosum, Klinefelter's disease, or immunodeficiency.

Younger age at diagnosis has been reported to be associated with an increased risk of second cancers,[112] with the exception of secondary myelodysplasia and acute myeloid leukemia, in which the risk increases with older age at diagnosis and treatment of the primary cancer.[114,115] Female gender is associated with an increased risk of second primary cancers. This gender effect is due primarily to the excess number of secondary breast cancers and, to some extent, to the increased occurrence of thyroid cancer in female survivors.[112] Ionizing radiation can cause most types of cancer, but different organs vary in their susceptibility. The risk is highest when the exposure occurs at a younger age.[97,112] It increases with the total dose of radiation[116–120] and with increasing follow up after irradiation.[121] Examples of radiation-associated tumors include breast and lung cancer (following Hodgkin's disease), thyroid cancer (following Hodgkin's disease or ALL), brain tumors (following ALL), and osteosarcoma (following retinoblastoma). The large majority of radiation-associated second cancers develop within the radiation field.

Secondary myelodysplasia and acute myeloid leukemia have been associated with certain chemotherapeutic agents, such as alkylating agents[97,122] and topoisomerase II inhibitors.[123] A dose-dependent relationship is noted with alkylating agents. Cytogenetic abnormalities in the alkylating agent–associated secondary leukemias characteristically involve chromosomes 5 or 7. Topoisomerase II inhibitor–associated secondary leukemias classically have a shorter latency, no preceding dysplastic phase, and cytogenetic abnormalities involving chromosome 11q23. Exposure to alkylating agents has also been shown to increase the risk of bone[124] and bladder cancers.[125]

Patients with a family history of early-onset cancers have been shown to be at an increased risk for developing a second cancer. Members of families with Li-Fraumeni syndrome have been reported to be at increased risk of multiple subsequent cancers.[126] The highest risk was observed among survivors of childhood cancer. Moreover, the excess risk was mainly for cancers characteristic of Li-Fraumeni syndrome. It therefore appears that germline mutations in tumor suppressor genes, as occur in Li-Fraumeni syndrome, might interact with therapeutic exposures and result in an increased risk of second cancers. Genetic predisposition also has a substantial impact on risk of secondary sarcomas among patients with hereditary retinoblastoma. This risk is further increased by radiotherapy and increases with the total dose of radiation delivered.[116]

Another example of underlying genetic characteristics interacting with treatment and resulting in an increased risk of certain second cancers is the presence of a polymorphism in a drug-metabolizing enzyme, such as thiopurine S-methyltransferase (TPMT). TPMT catalyses the S-methylation of thiopurines, including 6-mercaptopurine and 6-thioguanine. TPMT activity exhibits genetic polymorphism, with approximately 1 in 300 inheriting TPMT deficiency as an autosomal recessive trait. There is emerging evidence that the TPMT genotype might influence the risk of secondary cancers, including brain tumors and acute myeloid leukemia.[127]

Several other genetic polymorphisms of enzymes capable of metabolic activation or detoxification of anticancer drugs, such as NAD(P)H:quinone oxidoreductase, glutathione S-transferase-M1 and -T1, and CYP3A4, have been examined for their role in the development of therapy-related leukemia or myelodysplasia. These studies indicate that NQO1 polymorphism is significantly associated with the genetic risk of therapy-related acute leukemia and myelodysplasia. In addition, individuals with CYP3A4-W genotype may be at increased risk of treatment-related leukemia by increasing the production of reactive intermediates that might damage DNA.[128–134]

The incidence of nonhematopoietic second cancers appears to be increasing and, if it is coupled with a long latency period, we anticipate that the incidence and types of second cancers observed and reported is going to change over the next decade. In addition, with newer therapeutic modalities, such as BMT and monoclonal antibody–directed irradiation, insufficient time has elapsed to determine their carcinogenic potential. We therefore recommend lifelong surveillance for second malignancies.

LATE MORTALITY AMONG CHILDHOOD CANCER SURVIVORS

More than 12,000 children and adolescents younger than 20 years receive diagnoses of cancer each year in the United States. With the use of risk-based therapies, the overall 5-year survival rate is approaching 80%.[135] Several investigators have shown a tenfold excess in overall mortality among 5-year survivors, compared to the general population.[136,137] The excess mortality was due to death from primary cancer, second cancer, and noncancer death.

SURVEILLANCE AND HEALTH PROMOTION STRATEGIES

Surveillance

Care of patients who have received treatment for childhood cancer is complex and should be carried out by professionals familiar with current and past treatment of childhood cancer patients. The follow up should involve a multidisciplinary team approach, including medicine, psychology, nursing, education, social work, rehabilitation, and medical subspecialties as indicated (e.g., endocrinology, cardiology, etc.).

Initial follow up should occur every month, then at intervals of every 3 months, then every 6 months, and finally every year. Exact scheduling depends on the disease, intensity of treatment, and treatment sequelae. An annual detailed patient history and physical examination should include evaluation of height, weight, and blood pressure measurements; vision and hearing screening; sexual maturation assessment; complete blood count; and urinalysis. Psychosocial assessment should include evaluation of cognitive (e.g., school performance) and social functioning. Additional studies and interventions should be undertaken as indicated on the basis of patients' diagnosis and treatment history and results of the annual comprehensive evaluation (Table 10.2; see also Table 10.1).

As they enter young adulthood, survivors of childhood cancer should be provided with a summary of their diagnosis and treatment and informed of the importance of sharing this information with health care personnel who may be unfamiliar with their medical history. The written summary given to patients should include diagnosis, name of physician, dates and place of treatment, primary site, metastasis, surgery (including organs removed), irradiation (including sites, dosages, and shielding), chemotherapeutic agents and dosages (especially cumulative anthracycline dose), relapse and treatment (if any), and major treatment complications.[108]

TABLE 10.2 Surveillance Guidelines

Diagnostic Test	Frequency	Toxicity	Anticipatory Guidance
History, physical	Yearly	Special attention to growth, blood pressure, skin, gonadal function, thyroid	Review cancer diagnosis and treatment, review symptoms to report to healthcare providers
CBC, platelet, differential	Yearly	Secondary leukemia, marrow hypoplasia, anemia r/t renal or GI toxicity	Report fatigue, pallor, or petechiae promptly
Urinalysis	Yearly	Renal, bladder	Report dysuria or gross hematuria promptly
Serum chemistries (BUN, creatinine, phosphorus, magnesium, transaminases, bilirubin, alkaline phosphatase)	Every 2–5 yr	Renal, hepatic	Avoid hepatotoxic agents (e.g., alcohol) or nephrotoxic agents (e.g., ibuprofen, aminoglycosides)
Echocardiogram, ECG	Every 2–3 yr for those with hx of anthracyclines or chest irradiation	Cardiac	Consult with physician prior to beginning exercise program or becoming pregnant, notify obstetrician of medical history
CXR	Every 2–5 yr for hx of chest irradiation or bleomycin	Pulmonary fibrosis	Use pneumococcal and influenza vaccines, avoid or stop smoking
LH, FSH, estradiol (females)	Yearly beginning at age 8 years until puberty for patients with hx of cranial or gonadal irradiation or gonadotoxic chemotherapy	Gonadal failure	Learn breast self-examination. Women with regular menses should not delay childbearing (risk of early menopause)

LH, FSH, testosterone (Male)	Yearly beginning at age 8 years until puberty for patients with hx cranial or gonadal irradiation or gonadotoxic chemotherapy; sperm count for postpubertal males	Gonadal failure	Learn testicular self-examination.
T3, T4, TSH	Yearly for minimum of 6 yr for patients with hx of cranial irradiation or irradiation to the neck	Thyroid	Report excessively dry skin, brittle hair, decreased energy level
Bone density study	As clinically indicated, particularly in those with hx of chronic steroid therapy or hypogonadism	Osteoporosis	Use preventive measures (increased calcium intake, weight-bearing exercise, and hormone replacement if indicated)
Neurocognitive testing	As clinically indicated, particularly in those with history of treatment with cranial irradiation or intrathecal or high-dose methotrexate	Learning difficulties, developmental delay	Report school or work difficulties
Nutritional assessment	Yearly height and weight, hemoglobin, serum protein, and albumin every 3–5 yr in patients at high risk for enteritis; additional assessments as clinically indicated	Malabsorption, obesity	Maintain normal weight, regular exercise program, diet rich in fruits, vegetables, and fiber

TABLE 10.2 Continued

Diagnostic Test	Frequency	Toxicity	Anticipatory Guidance
Mammogram	Baseline at age 25 for hx of chest irradiation, every year thereafter	SMN (breast cancer)	Perform monthly breast self-examination, clinical breast examination every 6 mo
Audiogram	Periodically for those who received ototoxic agents	Hearing loss	Avoid loud noises, use ear protection in noisy environments, avoid ototoxic agents (e.g., aminoglycosides, loop diuretics)
Pulmonary function tests	As clinically indicated, based on symptoms and treatment history and before general anesthesia in patients with hx of chest irradiation or bleomycin	Pulmonary fibrosis	Report shortness of breath, decreased exercise tolerance
Vision assessment	Yearly screening, yearly ophthalmology examination for those who received radiation involving the eye	Cataracts, glaucoma, Sjögren's syndrome	Report visual changes promptly
Dental examination	Every 6 mo	Increased risk for dental caries, tooth malformation, xerostomia	Use good dental hygiene habits and routine fluoride prophylaxis

BUN, blood urea nitrogen; CBC, complete blood count; CXR, chest X-ray; ECG, electrocardiogram; FSH, follicle-stimulating hormone; GI, gastrointestinal; hx, history; LH, luteinizing hormone; SMN, secondary malignant neoplasm; TSH, thyroid-stimulating hormone

Health Promotion

All patients treated for malignancy in childhood should be counseled regarding the importance of avoiding potential environmental carcinogens. Information regarding health-promoting strategies aimed at cancer risk reduction should also be provided. Routine cancer screening examinations, including stool testing for occult blood, Papanicolaou smears, and mammograms, should be conducted as indicated on the basis of age, gender, and risk related to patients' specific diagnosis and treatment. Cancer detection methods, including self-examination of breasts or testicular and skin self-examinations, should be part of health education beginning in early adolescence. In addition, patients should be counseled regarding proper nutrition and exercise, risks of sun exposure, and the importance of smoking cessation or avoidance.[138]

ISSUES IN SURVIVORSHIP

Psychosocial Issues

As a group, childhood cancer survivors appear to be within the normally expected range in terms of psychosocial adjustment.[139] Most have been found to have normal self-concept and social relationships and a lifestyle similar to that of controls in regard to education, employment, marriage, and family.[140] However, certain subgroups of children, including survivors of childhood ALL and brain tumors, have a high incidence of neurocognitive treatment sequelae. These neurocognitive deficits have an impact on affected children's functioning in many domains, including poor school achievement, diminished employment potential, and problems in marriage and interpersonal relationships. Children with a history of brain tumors are most severely affected.[139,140] Additionally, a subset of young adult survivors of childhood cancer have recently been identified as suffering from symptoms of posttraumatic stress disorder and from other psychological difficulties,[141] underscoring the importance of continued psychosocial assessment and support in the ongoing management of these patients.[142]

School Issues

Children with neurocognitive deficits may require specific interventions to succeed in school. For some children, allotting additional time to complete examinations may be sufficient. Many children experience difficulties with information processing and may require additional assistance with specific subjects, typically mathematics and spelling. These children may benefit from compensatory strategies that emphasize their strengths so as to circumvent weaknesses. Allowing these children to use electronic devices, such as spell-checkers and calculators, may also increase their academic success.[5]

Some childhood cancer survivors may have developed school avoidance as a consequence of frequent absences during their treatment and may fear educational and social failure on their return to school. Altered body image may be an issue for some children, particularly for those who have experienced excessive weight loss or gain or obvious loss of a body part. Parental overprotectiveness often plays a role in school avoidance problems. School attendance and success allow a return to the world of normal childhood and should be strongly encouraged. Assistance from psychologists experienced with school reintegration issues can prove most helpful to these children.

Employment and Workplace Issues

In general, survivors of childhood cancer have been found to be superior to members of the general public in regard to performance in the workplace. They have fewer absences and superior job performance and job stability.[143] Some require modifications in the physical environment to perform job duties, including wheelchair access or assistive hearing devices. Survivors with neurocognitive deficits, particularly childhood brain tumor survivors, have not fared as well in the workplace[143] and often require remedial job training and placement in a sheltered work environment.

CONCLUSION

Although most long-term survivors of childhood cancer are thought to be cured of their primary malignancy, the possibility of late recurrence must be kept in mind. The greatest cause of death beyond 5 years from diagnosis remains recurrent tumor.[144] Recommendations for laboratory tests should be tailored according to primary disease and therapy received, using a multidisciplinary approach for the surveillance and management of long-term complications after childhood cancer. These recommendations are summarized in Table 10.2.

Most children who receive a diagnosis of cancer today are expected to become long-term survivors. Many of these survivors will experience significant physical, cognitive, and psychosocial sequelae. Care for childhood cancer survivors should involve a multidisciplinary team capable of providing ongoing surveillance, intervention, and support to minimize the consequences of complications and maximize quality of life for these patients.

ACKNOWLEDGMENTS

Supported in part by Grant No. 5 U10 CA13539-26S2 from the National Cancer Institute.

REFERENCES

1. Robison LL. Issues in the consideration of intervention strategies in long-term survivors of childhood cancer. Cancer 1993;71[suppl]:3406–3410.

2. Brown RT, Sawyer MB, Antoniou G et al. A 3-year follow-up of the intellectual and academic functioning of children receiving central nervous system prophylactic chemotherapy for leukemia. J Dev Behav Pediatr 1996;17(6):392–398.

3. Kramer J, Moore IM. Late effects of cancer therapy on the central nervous system. Semin Oncol Nurs 1989;5: 22–28.

4. Packer RJ, Meadows AT, Rorke LB et al. Long-term sequelae of cancer treatment on the central nervous system in childhood. Med Pediatr Oncol 1987;15:241–253.

5. Moore IM, Packer RJ, Karl D, Bleyer WA. Adverse effects of cancer treatment on the central nervous system. In: Schwartz CL, Hobbie WL, Constine LS, Ruccione KS, eds. Survivors of Childhood Cancer: Assessment and Management. St. Louis: Mosby, 1994:81–95.

6. Fochtman D. Follow-up care for survivors of childhood cancer. Nurse Pract Forum 1995;6: 194–200.

7. Packer RJ, Sutton LN, Atkins TE et al. A prospective study of cognitive function in children receiving whole-brain radiotherapy and chemotherapy: 2-year results. J Neurosurg 1989;70: 707–713.

8. Mulhern RK, Reddick WE, Palmer SL et al. Neurocognitive deficits in medulloblastoma survivors and white matter loss. Ann Neurol 1999;46:834–841.

9. Schell MJ, McHaney VA, Green AA et al. Hearing loss in children and young adults receiving cisplatin with or without prior cranial irradiation. J Clin Oncol 1989;7:754–760.

10. Iveskoski I, Saarinen UM, Wiklund T et al. Ototoxicity in children with malignant brain tumors treated with the "8 in 1" chemotherapy protocol. Med Pediatr Oncol 1996;27:26–31.

11. Landier W. Hearing loss related to ototoxicity in children with cancer. J Pediatr Oncol Nurs 1998;15:195–206.

12. Soysal T, Bavunoglu I, Baslar Z, Aktuglu G. Cataract after prolonged busulfan therapy. Acta Haematol 1993;90:213.

13. Schimmer BP, Parker KL. Adrenocorticotropic hormone; adrenocortical steroids and their analogs; inhibitors of the synthesis and actions of adrenocortical hormones. In: Hardman JG, Limbird LE, eds. Goodman and Gilman's The Pharmacological Basis of Therapeutics, 9th ed. New York: McGraw Hill, 1996:1475.

14. Abramson DH, Servodidio CA. Ocular complications due to cancer treatment. In: Schwartz CL, Hobbie WL, Constine LS, Ruccione KS, eds. Survivors of Childhood Cancer: Assessment and Management. St. Louis: Mosby, 1994:111–131.

15. Neglia JP, Nesbit ME. Care and treatment of long-term survivors of childhood cancer. Cancer 1993;71[suppl]:3386–3391.

16. Shan K, Lincoff AM, Young AB. Anthracycline-induced cardiotoxicity. Ann Intern Med 1996; 125:47–58.

17. Grenier MA, Lipshultz SE. Epidemiology of anthracycline cardiotoxicity in children and adults. Semin Oncol 1998;25:72–85.

18. Pai VB, Nahata MC. Cardiotoxicity of chemotherapeutic agents: incidence, treatment and prevention. Drug Saf 2000;22:263–302.

19. Prout MN, Richards MJS, Chung KJ et al. Adriamycin cardiotoxicity in children. Cancer 1977; 39:62.

20. Minow RA, Benjamin RS, Gottlieb JA. Adriamycin (NSC-123127) cardiotoxicity: a clinicopathologic correlation. Cancer Chemother Rep 1975;6:195.

21. Cortes EP, Lutman G, Wanka J et al. Adriamycin (NSC-123127) cardiotoxicity: A clinicopathologic correlation. Cancer Chemother Rep 1975;6:215.

22. Bossi G, Lanzarini L, Laudisa ML et al. M. Echocardiographic evaluation of patients cured of childhood cancer: a single center study of 117 subjects who received anthracyclines. Med Pediatr Oncol 2001;36:593–600.

23. Kremer LC, van delen EC, Offringa et al. Anthracycline-induced clinical heart failure in a cohort of 607 children: long-term follow-up study. J Clin Oncol 2001;19:191–196.

24. Steinherz LJ, Steinherz PG, Tan CT, Murphy ML. Cardiac toxicity 4–20 years after completing anthracycline therapy. JAMA 1991;266:1672.

25. Lipshultz SE, Colan SD, Gelber RD et al. Late cardiac effect of doxorubicin therapy for acute lymphoblastic leukemia in childhood. N Engl J Med 1991;324:808.

26. Fajardo L, Stewart J, Cohn K. Morphology of radiation-induced heart disease. Arch Pathol 1968; 86:512–519.

27. Von Hoff DD, Layard MW, Basa P et al. Risk factors for Adriamycin-induced congestive heart failure. Ann Intern Med 1979;91:710.

28. Kushner JR, Hansen VL, Hammar SP. Cardiomyopathy after widely separated courses of Adriamycin exacerbated by actinomycin D and mithramycin. Cancer 1975;36:1577.

29. Smith PJ, Eckert H, Waters KD, Matthews RN. High incidence of cardiomyopathy in children treated with Adriamycin and DTIC in combination chemotherapy. Cancer Treat Rep 1977;61: 1736.

30. Von Hoff DD, Rozencweig M, Piccart M. The cardiotoxicity of anticancer agents. Semin Oncol 1982;9:23.

31. Lipshultz SE, Lipsitz SR, Mone SM et al. Female sex and higher drug dose at risk for late cardiotoxic effects of doxorubicin therapy for childhood cancer. N Engl J Med 1995;332:1738.

32. Pratt CB, Ransom JL, Evans WE. Age-related Adriamycin cardiotoxicity in children. Cancer Treat Rep 1978;62: 1381.

33. Von Hoff DD, Rozencweig M, Layard M et al. Daunomycin induced cardiotoxicity in children and adults. Am J Med 1977;62:200.

34. Weiss AJ, Manthel RW. Experience with the use of Adriamycin in combination with other anticancer agents using a weekly schedule with particular reference to lack of cardiac toxicity. Cancer 1977;40:2046.

35. Legha SS, Benjamin RS, Mackay B et al. Reduction of doxorubicin cardiotoxicity by prolonged continuous infusion. Ann Intern Med 1982;96:133.

36. Martin RG, Rukdeschel JC, Chang P et al. Radiation-related pericarditis. Am J Cardiol 1975;35: 216.

37. Marks RD Jr, Agarwal SK, Constable WC. Radiation induced pericarditis in Hodgkin's disease. Acta Radiol Ther Phys Biol 1973;12:305.

38. Ruckdeschel JC, Chang P, Martin RG et al. Radiation related pericardial effusions in patients with Hodgkin's disease. Medicine 1975;54:245.

39. Mill WB, Baglan RJ, Kurichetz P et al. Symptomatic radiation induced pericarditis in Hodgkin's disease. Int J Radiat Oncol Biol Phys 1984;10:2061.

40. Kadota RP, Burgert EO, Driscoll DJ et al. Cardiopulmonary function in long-term survivors of childhood Hodgkin's lymphoma: a pilot study. Mayo Clin Proc 1988;63:362.

41. Perraut DJ, Levy M, Herman JD et al. Echocardiac abnormalities following cardiac radiation. J Clin Oncol 1985; 3:546.

42. Scott DL, Thomas RD. Late onset constrictive pericarditis after thoracic radiotherapy. Br Med J 1978;1:341.

43. Haas JM. Symptomatic constrictive pericarditis developing 45 years after radiation therapy to the mediastinum: a review of radiation pericarditis. Am Heart J 1969;77:89.

44. Boivin JF, Hutchison GB. Coronary heart disease mortality after irradiation for Hodgkin's disease. Cancer 1982; 49:2470.

45. Hancock SL, Donaldson SS, Hoppe RT. Cardiac disease following treatment of Hodgkin's disease in children and adolescents. J Clin Oncol 1993;11:1199–1203.

46. Bu'Lock FA, Gabriel HM, Oakhill A et al. Cardioprotection by ICRF187 against high dose anthracycline toxicity in children with malignant disease. Br Heart J 1993;70:185–188.

47. Wexler LH. Ameliorating anthracycline cardiotoxicity in children with cancer: clinical trials with dexrazoxane. Semin Oncol 1998;25:86–92.

48. Iarussi D, Indolfi P, Coppolino P et al. Recent advances in the prevention of anthracycline cardiotoxocity in childhood. Curr Med Chem 2001;8:1667–1678.

49. Steinherz LJ. Guidelines for cardiac monitoring of children during and after anthracycline therapy: report of the Cardiology Committee of the Children's Cancer Study Group. Pediatrics 1992;89: 942.

50. Littman P, Meadows AT, Polgar G et al. Pulmonary function in survivors of Wilms' tumor: patterns of impairment. Cancer 1976;37:2773.

51. Benoit MR, Lemerle J, Jean R et al. Effects on pulmonary function of whole lung irradiation for Wilms' tumor in children. Thorax 1982;37:175.

52. Miller RW, Fusner JE, Fink RJ et al. Pulmonary function abnormalities in long-term survivors of childhood cancer. Med Pediatr Oncol 1986;14:202.

53. Springmeyer SC, Flourney N, Sullivan KM et al. Pulmonary function changes in long-term survivors of allogeneic marrow transplantation. In: Gale RP, ed. Recent Advances in Bone Marrow Transplantation. New York: Alan R. Liss, 1983:343.

54. Gisberg SJ, Comis RL. The pulmonary toxicity of antineoplastic agents. Semin Oncol 1982;9: 34.

55. Bauer KA, Sskarin AT, Balikian JP et al. Pulmonary complications associated with combination chemotherapy programs containing bleomycin. Am J Med 1983;74:557.

56. Goldiner PL, Schweizer O. Hazards of anesthesia and surgery in bleomycin-treated patients. Semin Oncol 1979; 6:121.

57. Samuels ML, Johnson DE, Holoye PY, Lanzotti VJ. Large doses of bleomycin therapy and pulmonary toxicity: a possible role of prior radiotherapy. JAMA 1976;235:1117.

58. Aronin PA, Mahaley MS Jr, Rudnick SA et al. Prediction of BCNU pulmonary toxicity in patients with malignant gliomas: an assessment of risk factors. N Engl J Med 1980;303:183.

59. Nysom K, Holm K, Olsen JH et al. Pulmonary function after treatment for acute lymphoblastic leukaemia in childhood. Br J Cancer 1998;78:21–27.

60. Shaw NJ, Eden OB, Jenney ME et al. Pulmonary function in survivors of Wilms' tumor. Pediatr Hematol Oncol 1991;8:131–137.

61. Nysom K, Holm K, Hertz H, Hesse B. Risk factors for reduced pulmonary function after malignant lymphoma in childhood. Med Pediatr Oncol 1998;30:240–248.

62. Hancock S, Cox R, McDougall I. Thyroid diseases after treatment of Hodgkin's disease. N Engl J Med 1991;325:599.

63. Glatstein E, McHardy-Young S, Brast N et al. Alterations in serum thyrotropin (TSH) and thyroid function following radiotherapy in patients with malignant lymphoma. J Clin Endocrinol Metab 1971;32:833.

64. Rosenthal MB, Goldfine ID. Primary and secondary hypothyroidism in nasophanryngeal carcinoma. JAMA 1976; 236:1591.

65. Denvey RB, Sklar CA, Nesbit ME et al. Serial thyroid function measurements in children with Hodgkin' disease. J Pediatr 1984;105:599.

66. Sklar C, Whitton J, Mertens A et al. Abnormalities of the thyroid in survivors of Hodgkin's disease: data from the Childhood Cancer Survivor Study. J Clin Endocrine Metab 2000;85: 3227–3232.

67. Chin D, Sklar C, Donahue B et al. Thyroid dysfunction as a late effect in survivors of pediatric medulloblastoma/primitive neuroectodermal tumors: a comparison of hyperfractionated versus conventional radiotherapy. Cancer 1997;80:798–804.

68. Sklar CA. Growth and neuroendocrine dysfunction following therapy for childhood cancer. Pediatr Clin North Am 1997;44:489–503.

69. Danoff BF, Cowchock FS, Marquette C et al. Assessment of the long-term effects of primary radiation therapy for brain tumors in children. Cancer 1982;49:1580.

70. Onoyama Y, Mitsuyuki A, Takahashi M et al. Radiation therapy of brain tumors in children. Radiology 1977;115:687.

71. Oberfield SE, Allen JC, Pollack J et al. Long-term endocrine sequelae after treatment of medulloblastoma: prospective study of growth and thyroid function. J Pediatr 1986;108:219.

72. Oliff A, Bode U, Bercu BB et al. Hypothalamic-pituitary dysfunction following CNS prophylaxis in acute lymphocytic leukemia: correlation with CT scan abnormalities. Med Pediatr Oncol 1979;7:141.

73. Robison LL, Nesbit ME, Sather HN et al. Height of children successfully treated for acute lymphoblastic leukemia: a report from the late effects study committee of Children's Cancer Study Group. Med Pediatr Oncol 1985;13:14.

74. Berry DH, Elders MJ, Crsit W et al. Growth in children with acute lymphocytic leukemia: a Pediatric Oncology Group study. Med Pediatr Oncol 1983;11:39.

75. Papadakis V, Tan C, Heller G, Sklar C. Growth and final height after treatment for childhood Hodgkin's disease. J Pediatr Hematol Oncol 1996;18:272–276.

76. Sklar C, Mertens A, Walter A et al. Final height after treatment for childhood acute lymphoblastic leukemia: comparison of no cranial irradiation with 1800 and 2400 centigrays of cranial irradiation. J Pediatr 1993;123:59–64.

77. Verzosa MS, Aur RJA, Simone JV et al. Five years after central nervous system irradiation of children with leukemia. Int J Radiat Oncol Biol Phys 1976;1:209.

78. Hakimi N, Mohammad A, Mayer JW. Growth and growth hormone of children with acute lymphocytic leukemia following central nervous prophylaxis with and without cranial radiation. Am J Pediatr Hematol Oncol 1980;2:311.

79. Blatt J, Bercu BB, Gillin JC et al. Reduced pulsatile growth hormone secretion in children after therapy for acute lymphocytic leukemia. J Pediatr 1984;104:182.

80. Sklar CA, Mertens AC, Walter A et al. Changes in body mass index and prevalence of overweight in survivors of childhood acute lymphoblastic leukemia: role of cranial irradiation. Med Pediatr Oncol 2000;35:91–95.

81. Cifton DK, Bremmer WJ. The effect of testicular x-irradiation on spermatogenesis in man. J Androl 1983;4:387.

82. Rowley MM, Leach DR, Warner GA, Heller CG. Effect of graded doses of ionizing radiation on the human testes. Radiat Res 1974;59:665.

83. Blatt J, Sherins RJ, Niebrugge D et al. Leydig cell function in boys following treatment for testicular relapse of acute lymphoblastic leukemia. J Clin Oncol 1985;3:1227.

84. Brauner R, Czernichow P, Cramer P et al. Leydig-cell function in children after direct testicular irradiation for acute lymphoblastic leukemia. N Engl J Med 1983;309:25.

85. Sherins RJ, DeVita VT. Effects of drug treatment for lymphoma on male reproductive capacity. Ann Intern Med 1973;79:216.

86. da Cunha MF, Meisrich ML, Fuller LM et al. Recovery of spermatogenesis after treatment for Hodgkin's disease with limiting dose of MOPP chemotherapy. J Clin Oncol 1984;2:571.

87. Santaro A, Bonadonna G, Valagussa P et al. Long-term results of combined chemotherapy-radiotherapy approach in Hodgkin's disease: superiority of ABVD plus radiotherapy versus MOPP plus radiotherapy. J Clin Oncol 1987;5:27.

88. Lushbaugh CC, Casarett GW. The effects of gonadal irradiation in clinical radiation therapy: a review. Cancer 1976;37:1111.

89. Stillman RJ, Schilfeld JS, Schiff I et al. Ovarian failure in long-term survivors of childhood malignancy. Am J Obstet Gynecol 1981;139:62.

90. Sarafoglou K, Boulad F, Gillio A, Sklar C. Gonadal function after bone marrow transplantation for acute leukemia during childhood. J Pediatr 1997;130:210–216.

91. Chapman RM, Sutcliffe SB, Malpas JS. Cytotoxic-induced ovarian failure in women with Hodgkin's disease. JAMA 1979;242:1877.

92. Sklar C. Reproductive physiology and treatment-related loss of sex hormone production. Med Pediatr Oncol 1999;33:2–8.

93. Fürst CJ, Lundell M, Ahlbäck SO, Holm L-E. Breast hypoplasia following irradiation of the female breast in infancy and early childhood. Acta Oncol 1989;28:519–523.

94. Rosenfield NS, Haller JO, Berdon WE. Failure of development of the growing breast after radiation therapy. Pediatr Radiol 1989;19:124–127.

95. Rostom AY, O'Cathail S. Failure of lactation following radiotherapy for breast cancer [letter]. Lancet 1986;1(8372):163–164.

96. Marcus RB, McGrath B, O'Conner K, Scarborough M. Long-term effects on the musculoskeletal and integumentary systems and the breast. In: Schwartz CL, Hobbie WL, Constine LS, Ruccione KS, eds. Survivors of Childhood Cancer: Assessment and Management. St. Louis: Mosby, 1994: 263–292.

97. Bhatia S, Robison LL, Oberlin O et al. Breast cancer and other second neoplasms after childhood Hodgkin's disease. N Engl J Med 1996;334:745–751.

98. Blatt J, Neigut D, Robertson JM, Lawrence TS. Late gastrointestinal and hepatic effects. In: Schwartz CL, Hobbie WL, Constine LS, Ruccione KS, eds. Survivors of Childhood Cancer: Assessment and Management. St. Louis: Mosby, 1994:197–211.

99. Blatt J, Copeland DR, Bleyer WA. Late effects of childhood cancer and its treatment. In: Pizzo PA, Poplack DG, eds. Principles and Practice of Pediatric Oncology. Philadelphia: Lippincott, 1997:1303–1329.

100. Raney B, Heyn R, Cassady R, Marks LB. Late effects of cancer therapy on the genitourinary tract in children. In: Schwartz CL, Hobbie WL, Constine LS, Ruccione KS. Survivors of Childhood Cancer: Assessment and Management. St. Louis: Mosby, 1994:245–262.

101. Grossi M. Management of long-term complications of pediatric cancer. Pediatr Clin North Am 1998;45:1637–1658.

102. Pratt CB, Meyer WH, Jenkins JJ et al. Ifosfamide, Fanconi's syndrome and rickets. J Clin Oncol 1991;9:1495–1499.

103. Green DM. Effects of treatment for childhood cancer on vital organ systems. Cancer 1993; 71[suppl]:3299–3305.

104. Marina N. Long-term survivors of childhood cancer: The medical consequences of cure. Pediatr Clin North Am 1997;44:1021–1042.

105. Aisenberg J, Hseigh K, Kalaitzoglou G et al. Bone mineral density in young adult survivors of childhood cancer. J Pediatr Hematol Oncol 1998;20:241–245.

106. Haddy TB, Mosher RB, Reaman GH. Osteoporosis in survivors of acute lymphoblastic leukemia. Oncologist 2001;6(3):278–285.

107. Mattano LA, Sather HN, Trigg ME, Nachman JB. Osteonecrosis as a complication of treating acute lymphoblastic leukemia in children: a report from the Children's Cancer Group. J Clin Oncol 2000;18(18):3262–3272.

108. Ruccione K, Weinberg K. Late effects in multiple body systems. Semin Oncol Nurs 1989;5: 22–28.

109. Donahue B, Meyerowitz C, Handler S, Cooper J. Head and neck. In: Schwartz CL, Hobbie WL, Constine LS, Ruccione KS, eds. Survivors of Childhood Cancer: Assessment and Management. St. Louis: Mosby, 1994:142–146.

110. Maguire A, Craft AW, Evans RGB et al. The long-term effects of treatment on the dental condition of children surviving malignant disease. Cancer 1987;60:2570–2575.

111. Workman ML. Immunologic late effects in children and adults. Semin Oncol Nurs 1989;5: 36–42.

112. Neglia JP, Friedman DL, Yutaka Y et al. Second malignant neoplasms in five-year survivors of childhood cancer: childhood cancer survivor study. J Natl Cancer Inst 2001;93:618–629.

113. Olsen JH, Garwicz S, Hertz H et al. Second malignant neoplasms after cancer in childhood or adolescence. Nordic Society of Paediatric Haematology and Oncology Association of the Nordic Cancer Registries. Br Med J 1993;307:1030–1036.

114. Bhatia S, Ramsay NKC, Steinbuch M et al. Malignant neoplasms following bone marrow transplantation. Blood 1996;87:3633.

115. Darrington DL, Vose JM, Anderson JR et al. Incidence and characterization of secondary myelodysplastic syndrome and acute myelogenous leukemia following high-dose chemoradiotherapy and autologous stem cell transplantation for lymphoid malignancies. J Clin Oncol 1994;12:2527.

116. Wong FL, Boice JD Jr, Abramson DH et al. Cancer incidence after retinoblastoma. Radiation dose and sarcoma risk. JAMA 1997;278:1262–1267.

117. Zang EA, Wynder EL. Differences in lung cancer risk between men and women: examination of the evidence. J Natl Cancer Inst 1996;88:183–192.

118. Hawkins MM, Wilson LM, Burton HS et al. Radiotherapy, alkylating agents, and risk of bone cancer after childhood cancer. J Natl Cancer Inst 1996;88:270–278.

119. Breslow NE, Takashima JR, Whitton JA et al. Second malignant neoplasms following treatment of Wilms' tumor: a report from the National Wilms' Tumor Study Group. J Clin Oncol 1995; 13:1851–1859.

120. Garwicz S, Anderson H, Olsen JH et al. Second malignant neoplasms after cancer in childhood and adolescence: a population-based case-control study in the 5 Nordic countries. The Nordic Society for Pediatric Hematology and Oncology. The Association of the Nordic Cancer Registries. Int J Cancer 2000; 88:672–678.

121. de Vathaire F, Hawkins M, Campbell S et al. Second malignant neoplasms after a first cancer in childhood: temporal pattern of risk according to type of treatment. Br J Cancer 1999;1884–1893.

122. Meadows AT. Risk factors for second malignant neoplasms: report from the Late Effects Study Group. Bull Cancer 1988;75:125–130.

123. Smith MA, Rubinstein L, Anderson JR et al. Secondary leukemia or myelodysplastic syndrome after treatment with epipodophyllotoxins. J Clin Oncol 1999;17:569–577.

124. Tucker MA, D'Angio GJ, Boice JD Jr et al. Bone sarcomas linked to radiotherapy and chemotherapy in children. N Engl J Med 1987;317:588–593.

125. Pedersen-Bjergaardd J, Erbsoll J, Hansen VL et al. Carcinoma of the urinary bladder after treatment with cyclophosphamide for non-Hodgkin's lymphoma. N Engl J Med 1988:1028–1032.

126. Hisada M, Garber JE, Fung CY et al. Multiple primary cancers in families with Li-Fraumeni syndrome. J Natl Cancer Inst 1998;90:606–611.

127. Relling MV, Rubnitz JE, Rivera GK et al. High incidence of secondary brain tumors after radiotherapy and antimetabolites. Lancet 1999;354:34–39.

128. Naoe T, Takeyama K, Yokozawa T et al. Analysis of genetic polymorphism in NQO1, GST-M1, GST-T1, and CYP3A4 in 469 Japanese patients with therapy-related leukemia/myelodysplastci syndrome and de novo acute myeloid leukemia. Clin Cancer Res 2000;6:4091–4095.

129. Felix CA, Walker AH, Lange BJ et al. Association of CYP3A4 genotype with treatment-related leukemia. Proc Natl Acad Sci USA 1998;95:13176–13181.

130. Hayes JD, Pulford DJ. The glutathione S-transferase supergene family: regulation of GST and the contribution of the isoenzymes to cancer chemoprotection and drug resistance. Crit Rev Biochem Mol Biol 1995;30:445–600.

131. Smith G, Stanley LA, Sim E et al. Metabolic polymorphisms and cancer susceptibility. Cancer Surv 1995;25:27–65.

132. Raunio H, Husgafvel-Pursianen K, Anttila S et al. Diagnosis of polymorphisms in carcinogen-activating and -inactivating enzymes and cancer susceptibility. Gene 1995;159:113–121.

133. Wrighton S, Stevens J. The human hepatic cytochromes P450 involved in drug metabolism. Crit Rev Toxicol 1992;22:1–21.

134. Rebbeck TR, Walker AH, Lange BJ et al. Association of CYP3A4 genotype with treatment-related leukemia. Proc Natl Acad Sci USA 1998;95:13176–13181.

135. Ries LAG, Smith MA, Gurney JG et al, eds. Cancer Incidence and Survival Among Children and Adolescents: U.S. SEER Program 1975–1995. Bethesda, MD: National Cancer Institute, National Institutes of Health Publication No. 99–4649, 1999.

136. Mertens AC, Yasui Y, Neglia JP et al. Late mortality experience in five-year survivors of childhood and adolescent cancer: the childhood cancer survivors study. J Clin Oncol 2001;19:3163–3172.

137. Moller TR, Garwicz S, Barlow L et al. Decreasing late mortality among five-year survivors of cancer in childhood and adolescence: a population-based study in the Nordic countries. J Clin Oncol 2001;19:3173–3181.

138. Hudson MM, Tyc VL, Jayawardene DA et al. Feasibility of implementing health promotion interventions to improve health-related quality of life. Int J Cancer 1999;12[suppl]:138–142.

139. Hymovich DP, Roehnert JE. Psychosocial consequences of childhood cancer. Semin Oncol Nurs 1989;5:56–62.

140. Lansky SB, List MA, Ritter-Sterr C. Psychosocial consequences of cure. Cancer 1986;58[suppl]: 529–533.

141. Hobbie WL, Stuber M, Meeske K et al. Symptoms of posttraumatic stress in young adult survivors of childhood cancer. J Clin Oncol 2000;18(24):4060–4066.

142. Van Dongen-Melman JEWM. Developing psychosocial aftercare for children surviving cancer and their families. Acta Oncologica 2000;39(1):23–31.

143. Hays DM. Adult survivors of childhood cancer: employment and insurance issues in different age groups. Cancer 1993;71[suppl]:3306–3309.

144. Nicholson HS, Fears TR, Byrne J. Death during adulthood in survivors of childhood and adolescent cancer. Cancer 1994;73:3094.

Chapter 11

The Use of Spiral Computed Tomography in Lung Cancer Screening

Claudia I. Henschke

David F. Yankelevitz

James P. Smith

Olli S. Miettinen

Lung cancer, more than any other cancer, calls for consideration of screening. Not only is the disease highly fatal—essentially incurable—when diagnosed on the prompting of symptoms or clinical signs (or both), but its occurrence also is highly concentrated in identifiably high-risk persons. Even before computed tomography (CT), radiographic screening provided for earlier diagnosis, and when non-small-cell cancer was diagnosed in Stage I, resection was curative in most cases.[1] With CT screening, the prospects are much brighter, as most of the diagnoses are achieved not only in Stage I but when the tumor still is less than 10 mm in diameter.[2,3] Thus, there cannot be any reasonable question about the usefulness of CT-based screening for lung cancer, or about whether its associated early treatment can be curative in instances in which postsymptomatic treatment would fail. The question is merely quantitative: To what extent does CT-based screening for lung cancer enhance the curability of the disease by earlier intervention that is provided for by the earlier diagnosis?

The degree of usefulness of CT-based screening for lung cancer must be thought of in reference to a particular, presumably optimal regimen of pursuing early, latent-stage diagnosis: an algorithm that begins with the initial test ("screening CT") and ends either in discontinuation of the diagnostic pursuit or in diagnosis (rule-in) of the disease.[4] Integral to the regimen's definition is the interval between its successive repeat applications. In CT-based screening for lung cancer, the regimen's components are principally radiologic, CT-based assessments of growth rate and CT-guided fine-needle aspirations included, with the final element in the process leading to early diagnosis being a matter of pathology.

The diagnosis that the regimen is designed to achieve (insofar as latent cancer indeed is present) is the presurgical one, typically involving a cytologic rather than histologic specimen, even though the postsurgical diagnosis may be better informed on account of intraoperative observations and the availability of histologic specimens. For it is the presurgical and not the postsurgical diagnosis that determines the intervention. Although the most immediate purpose of the pursuit of early diagnosis is to provide for early intervention, that intervention is not part of the concept of screening and, thus, of the screening regimen.[4]

No radiologic facility should accede to, much less actively market, CT screening for lung cancer without a set of prerequisites being satisfied. The natural beginning is the adoption of a presumably optimal regimen and the protocol defining it. The associated added need is to have the requisite competence in its application, both radiologic and pathologic. Moreover, competent surgery for screen-diagnosed cases must be available and accessible. With such readiness to screen and to act on its resultant diagnoses, the team also needs to be able to counsel potential subjects on the implications of the screening, first and foremost on the degree to which it can be presumed to provide for enhanced curability of lung cancer through earlier intervention. Finally, screening for lung cancer should not be offered without also offering, when indicated, suitable information to promote cessation of smoking.[5]

What follows first presents a carefully developed, extensively pilot-tested and critically reviewed, updated protocol for CT-based screening for lung cancer. Then, its implementation is addressed together with quality assurance. Finally, its associated curability rate for lung cancer is addressed in the light of what is knowable or can be surmised on the basis of evidence already available. All this is supplemented by delineation of what else must be known.

SCREENING REGIMEN

The development of a protocol for CT-based screening for lung cancer has been a concern of the Early Lung Cancer Action Project (ELCAP) group for a decade,[2,6] and modifications have been made in the framework of the international conferences[7] organized by this group and in their resultant International Consortium on screening for lung cancer.[8] The latter, I-ELCAP, has adopted a common protocol[6] and has subsequently updated it. This updated protocol is presented in what follows, with the understanding that the pathology aspect of the screening in the I-ELCAP is guided by a separate protocol specific to it.

In this regimen, the initial, low-dose test (involving screening CT) is identical between baseline and repeat screenings. A multislice helical CT scanner (Lightspeed, General Electric, Milwaukee, WI; Volume Zoom, Siemens, Erlangen, Germany; or equivalent) is preferably used at a low-dose setting (GE: 120 kVp, 40 mA with 6 : 1 pitch, 1.25 mm slice thickness, and 0.5s rotation; Siemens: 120 kVp, 20 mAs with a 7:1 pitch at 1 mm slice thickness and 0.5 s rotation). In a single breath hold, contiguous slices from the thoracic inlet to the adrenal glands are obtained. The use of contrast material is not involved.

Although multislice scanners are preferable because they provide higher-resolution images in the initial low-dose test and thus simplify the subsequent workup, single-slice helical (spiral) CT scanners may be used. Again, they are used at a low-dose setting and the images are obtained at the thinnest possible collimation and lowest pitch, even if the attainment of this collimation requires obtaining the images in two breath holds.

The resulting images are read by a radiologist at the site. The reader is aware that the images derive from the initial, low-dose test for early diagnosis of lung cancer and of whether they are from baseline or repeat screening. The reader views the images as they are displayed in a high-resolution monitor at their typical window and level settings with maximal magnification, scrolling through the images one at a time. For purposes of assessing size, however, the following settings are used: lung window width of 1500 and lung window level of –650 for nodules; mediastinal window width of 350 and mediastinal window level of 25 for mediastinal abnormalities.

For a predetermined number of screenings, a second, "central" reading is performed, without knowledge of the results of the first site reading. The site radiologist receives the central reading report with discrepancies, if any, highlighted. In case of discrepancies, the site radiologist may find it necessary to change the site report. In that event, the updated report is also submitted to the central facility, where a record is kept. The site radiologist sends the final report to the subject and to the referring physician.

In both baseline and repeat screening, the reader's first concern with the images from the first, low-dose test is to identify all noncalcified nodules visible in them. A nodule is manifest as a focal nonlinear opacity, whether the nodule be solid or subsolid (the latter corresponding to "ground-glass opacity").[9] A nodule is classified as noncalcified if it fails to meet the usual criteria for benign, noncalcified nodules.[10] Thus, a nodule < 5 mm in diameter is noncalcified if it appears uniformly less dense than the ribs (on bone and lung windows); a nodule 5–20 mm in diameter is noncalcified if less than 50% of it is "calcified;" calcification does not correspond to a classic benign pattern (complete, central, lamellated, popcorn) or the edge is spiculated (to some extent at least); and a nodule larger than 20 mm in diameter is noncalcified unless it is completely calcified. Diameter is the average of length and width.

At baseline, the result of the initial, low-dose test is negative if there are no noncalcified nodules or more than six, with the largest < 5 mm in diameter; otherwise it is positive. Thus, the result is positive if there are one to six noncalcified nodules or more than six, with the largest 5 mm in diameter or larger.

When a single-slice scanner is used with a collimation of > 5 mm, a "positive" result, as just defined, of the initial, low-dose test is only tentative. The tentatively positive result immediately leads to high-resolution CT (HRCT) imaging of the one to six largest nodules that rendered the initial result tentatively positive, except (1) when all nodules are 3 mm or less in diameter, in which case the definitive result is taken to be negative; (2) when the largest nodules are > 3 mm but < 5 mm in diameter, in which case the HRCT images are obtained either immediately or 6 months after the initial, low-dose test; and (3) when recommending antibiotics, in which case the HRCT images are obtained 1 month after the initial, low-dose test. The foregoing criteria for noncalcified nodules are applied to these HRCT images and, on the basis of this classification, the result of the initial test is definitively negative or positive (as defined).

HRCT images, whether obtained on a single-slice scanner (as just described) to verify the tentative result of the initial test or on a multislice scanner for further workup (detailed later), are consistently obtained at the same dose setting (kVp, mA) and 1-mm collimation through the entire nodule, at the lowest possible pitch in a single breath hold. The initial images are taken well above the nodule, and the final images are taken well below it, to ensure that the entire nodule is covered by this set of images (which is critical for accurate assessment of growth). The images are obtained at maximum resolution (GE: targeted field of view of 9.6 cm; Siemens: 10 cm) and they are reconstructed using a high-resolution algorithm. The localization of the nodule prior to obtaining the HRCT images is accomplished using low-dose CT imaging. The use of contrast material is not involved.

The reader documents whether the result of the initial, low-dose test is negative or positive, and if it is positive, the reader also documents each of the one to six noncalcified nodules or the six largest such nodules in case there are more than six in total (and the largest one ≥ 5 mm in diameter). Specifically, as for each of these nodules of record at baseline, the reader documents the location; size; whether solid, part-solid, or nonsolid; presence of calcifications; and edge type. A nodule is classified as part-solid if it has patches within it that completely obscure the lung parenchyma and is considered nonsolid if none of the lung parenchyma in it was totally obscured.[9] In making the distinction between part-solid and nonsolid nodule, blood vessels within the nodule, despite their appearance as solid components, are not regarded as solid components.

On repeat screenings, again the reader's first concern with the initial, low-dose test is to identify all noncalcified nodules, but now the focus, among these, is on those that have grown in size—overall size if solid or the size of the solid component if subsolid—since the previous screen. To determine whether growth has occurred, the reader compares the current images with the corresponding previous ones, displayed side by side with the current images.

On repeat screening, the result of the low-dose test is negative or positive by criteria fully analogous to those at baseline, except that tallied are noncalcified nodules with interim growth. With this same proviso, the documentation of repeat-screen nodules of record is analogous, except that this documentation has to be supplemented by the corresponding characterization of the nodule in the previous screen.

When the result of the initial test is negative, whether at baseline (by baseline criteria) or on repeat screening (by repeat-screening criteria), the pursuit of early diagnosis stops, and the next screening test is scheduled for a time 12 months after the current test (even if the current test is a repeat screen not 12 months after the previous screen). When the result is positive, further workup immediately ensues. At baseline, that workup varies according to the size of the largest nodule of record (defined above).

If this nodule is < 5 mm in diameter, an HRCT limited to the nodules of record is performed 6 months after the initial, low-dose test, and given no growth in any of these nodules, the workup stops. If growth is manifest, fine-needle aspiration is immediately carried out.

If this nodule is 5–9 mm in diameter, HRCT limited to the nodules of record is performed 3 months after the initial, low-dose test, and given no growth in any of these nodules but some of them remaining, the HRCT is repeated 6 months after the initial test. If no nodule remains at 3 months or no growth is manifest in any of the remaining nodules at 6 months, the workup stops. If growth of any of the nodules is manifest at either 3 or 6 months, fine-needle aspiration is immediately carried out.

If this nodule is ≥ 10 mm in diameter, immediate action on the nodules of record in this size range ensues, whereas smaller nodules, if any, are worked up according to one of the guidelines in the paragraphs above, whichever applies. For the large nodules, two options are available.

One option (particularly useful for relatively small nodules having a benign appearance, such as that of hamartoma or focal pneumonia) is to perform HRCT limited to these nodules 1 month after the initial, low-dose test. In the interim, a 2-week course of broad-spectrum antibiotics may be used. Further workup depends on the HRCT result: (1) For the nodules that show complete resolution, the workup stops; (2) nodules showing growth lead to immediate fine-needle aspiration; (3) nodules showing partial or no resolution (but no growth) may, depending on whether their appearance is suggestive of malignancy, lead to immediate fine-needle aspiration, immediate positron emission tomography scanning, or repeat HRCT at 3 months after the initial, low-dose test. For nodules found to be negative on positron emission tomography scan or showing no growth on repeat HRCT, the workup stops. Nodules found to be positive on the positron emission tomography scan or showing growth on repeat HRCT also call for an immediate fine-needle aspiration. If the result is negative and benign-specific, workup stops or, if the result is negative but nonspecific, repeat HRCT in 6 months after the initial, low-dose test is performed; for nodules showing no growth at 6 months, the workup stops, while nodules showing growth lead to a surgical biopsy.

Another option is immediate fine-needle aspiration, notably if the nodule is relatively large or has an appearance suggestive of malignancy. When the regimen at baseline does not lead to the diagnosis of malignancy, repeat screening is scheduled (as was noted) for a time 12 months subsequent to the initial, low-dose test at baseline. Similarly, when malignancy is not diagnosed in the first repeat screening, the second repeat screening is scheduled to follow 12 months subsequent to the first one, and so on. Also, if Stage I or Stage II malignancy is diagnosed, screening is continued with the original schedule.

At repeat screening, a positive result of the low-dose test routinely leads to an immediate 2-week course of broad-spectrum antibiotics followed by an HRCT of the nodules of record at 1 month after the initial, low-dose test. Further workup depends on the HRCT result in respect to resolution or growth of the nodules of record on repeat screening (as defined). If all these nodules have completely resolved, the workup stops; otherwise, the first concern is to identify the nodules still showing growth since the previous screen (13 months ago), thus updating the nodules of record. Among these, any nodule ≥ 5 mm in diameter immediately undergoes biopsy. For the remaining nodules of record (if any), the HRCT is repeated at 3 months after the initial, low-dose test. Given complete resolution of all nodules, the workup stops. Any nodule showing growth (over the 2 months) immediately undergoes biopsy. If there are any remaining nodules of record, the HRCT is repeated 6 months after the initial, low-dose test. The result is handled as it was at 3 months, including scheduling another HRCT, only in this instance at 12 months; if need be, yet another HRCT is scheduled at 24 months. With any one of these successive HRCTs, the assessment of growth is based on this one in comparison with the HRCT at 1 month.

The short-term assessment of growth based on HRCT images[10,11] includes consideration of whether the rate of growth is consistent with malignancy. In this assessment, the screening site has access to collaboration from the central facility, as electronic image transmission is provided for by ELCAP, the Web-based management system.

At the biopsy procedure, CT-guided percutaneous transthoracic fine-needle aspiration is preferable, as this is a 1-hour outpatient procedure. If this is not feasible, video-assisted thoracoscopic biopsy can be used; however, use of this procedure requires a stronger suspicion of malignancy than for those undergoing fine-needle aspiration. The images of the resulting cytology and histology specimens are also entered into the Web-based management system.

The Web-based management system calls for documentation of the actions and findings, including those that may not accord with the protocol.

PROTOCOL IMPLEMENTATION

The screening coordinator at the site provides information about the available screening to each potential screenee and schedules the initial, low-dose test for baseline screening. The coordinator provides information about the nature and benefits and risks of the screening regimen, with particular attention paid to the radiation dose and its carcinogenic effects. This information may be provided, in part at least, through brochures together with the consent form. The coordinator obtains all contact information when scheduling the initial, low-dose test and the detailed information pertaining to the indication and contraindications in an interview just before the test is administered. She or he performs data entry and scheduling of the follow-up appointments, including repeat screenings. Weekly or biweekly, he or she reports all new enrollments and forthcoming appointments, with particular attention paid to scheduled invasive procedures, to the radiologist to ensure coordinated communication and follow-through.

The technologist at the site prepares and positions the screenee on the CT table and obtains the images in the manner prescribed by the protocol, all the while ensuring the comfort of the screenee. A radiologist at the site reads the images from the initial, low-dose test and those from subsequent tests and supervises the entry of the test results into the management system. The same radiologist is also responsible for communicating the results to both the referring physician and the screenee. A radiologist is in charge of regular weekly or biweekly meetings with the coordinator and other relevant personnel to ensure that communication of the results and recommendations to the referring physician and screenee has occurred.

A negative result of the initial test (at baseline or on repeat screening) is communicated by the radiologist to the referring physician and separately to the screenee, stating the result and recommending return in 1 year for the next screening, specifying the date and enclosing an appointment card. If the test result is positive, the written report again is sent to the referring physician, but a phone call also is made to the physician (as per the American College of Radiology Communications Standards). The management system is used to document the contacts and follow-up.

Each month, the site physicist ensures and documents that the CT number for air and water and for distance accuracy are at acceptable levels (i.e., CT number of water is 0 ± 10 HU, that of air is between –1000 and –985, and the distance accuracy is within 2 mm for actual linear distance of 100 mm). Image quality (low-contrast detection, high-contrast spatial resolution, and distance accuracy) and multiple scan average dose (MSAD) are documented for both low-dose and standard-dose scannings with each scanner used for screening, and the

MSAD measurement is ensured to accord with the American Association of Physicists in Medicine (AAPM) standards.[13,14] These measurements are documented on quality control logs, and they are reviewed at least quarterly by the local quality control coordinator and physicist. Service to correct performance outside of specified parameters is documented and provided to the physicist prior to continuing screening studies. Each month, the physicist ensures and documents the scanner measurement accuracy using an anthropomorphic lung phantom with nodules of known size, using the low-dose and standard-dose techniques.[15]

QUALITY ASSURANCE

Qualifications of the radiologist consist of board certification in radiology together with subspecialization in chest radiology, supplemented by on-site training at a center experienced in applying the I-ELCAP protocol and by that center's recognition of readiness to practice CT screening for lung cancer. The required continuing education consists of review of I-ELCAP teaching files (electronically available through the Web-based management system), participation in the International Conferences on Screening for Lung Cancer,[7] and the comparisons of the site readings with the central reading reports.

For the CT technologist, qualifications consist of certification by the American Registry of Radiologic Technologists or equivalent and training and experience in such CT image acquisition as is involved in the I-ELCAP protocol. The medical physicist is qualified when certified by the American Board of Radiology or equivalent in radiologic physics or its diagnostic subspecialty and pursuing continuing education in diagnostic physics according to American College of Radiology Standards for Continuing Medical Education. A qualified CT screening coordinator is trained to understand the screening protocol and to provide the necessary information to the potential subjects, to schedule the activities, and to use the reports provided by the management system to ensure appropriate follow-up of each screenee.

Even though the collaboration in the I-ELCAP is motivated by concerns for collaborative research in addition to providing presumably useful care, the quality assurance built into it is no more ambitious than what befits good practice.[6] As outlined, quality assurance begins with the qualifications of the key personnel, including their continuing education.[13] In the I-ELCAP, its Web-based management system is an integral part of quality assurance, as it guides adherence to the protocol at every step of the screening regimen as to what to do and what to record, scheduling included. It also provides for image transfer to a central facility, for communication with it through its internal messaging system, and for receiving reports on central readings and identified problems with data entry. Monitoring of quality is accomplished by the central facility using site visits and review of the data and images routinely and instantaneously flowing to the central facility.

EFFECTIVENESS AND UTILITY

The clinician helping people to decide whether to avail themselves of screening for lung cancer needs to be able to answer two closely related questions, first and foremost. The first question naturally is about the regimen's effectiveness in producing its intended result: not a question of whether it is effective but how effective it is. As the intent of the regimen's application is attainment of early diagnosis, the effectiveness question is: How early is lung cancer diagnosed under the screening regimen at issue? The first, baseline screen is different from the subsequent, repeat screens (likely to be many). Thus, the effectiveness question is, in essence, specific to the diagnoses after the baseline screen (i.e., to the repeat screen and interim diagnoses combined). It also is specific to non-small-cell diagnoses as the prospect of enhanced curability by earlier intervention is currently confined to this type of cancer. Of course, this question of effectiveness refers to the span in which the screening regimen is being followed. Conversely, it is reasonable to presume that the effectiveness is essentially invariant over the successive "cycles" of repeat screening.

In these terms, then, what can be said about the effectiveness of the I-ELCAP regimen? It typically provides for diagnosis at tumor diameter < 10 mm, the majority of all cases—some 80%—being of Stage IA at diagnosis.[3,16,17] As the screening regimen thus can be taken to be quite effective in attaining early diagnosis, its effectiveness may have considerable utility in providing for cure through early (in lieu of late) intervention, but to what extent, to be specific? Of stage I cases of non-small-cell cancer detected under such experimental screening as was most promising a quarter-century ago, with these tumors typically approximately 20 mm in diameter at diagnosis, some 60% were curable by resection.[1,18] For the distinctly smaller Stage I cases diagnosed under the I-ELCAP regimen, a 70% curability rate thus would be a reasonable surmise.[19] If curability is taken to be confined to stage I cases of non-small-cell cancer, on this somewhat conservative premise, that 70% curability rate would apply to the majority of the lung cancer cases diagnosed under the I-ELCAP regimen (after the baseline screen, while the screening continues). This compares very favorably with the approximate 5%–15% curability that recently has been prevailing in near-total absence of screening.

FURTHER CONSIDERATIONS

Recommendation for or against screening requires knowledge inputs beyond the central one: the gain in curability of non-small-cell lung cancer previously considered, or its corresponding reduction in case-fatality rate (from 85%–95% to perhaps 40%–50%). Principal among these further considerations are two that have critical bearing on the definition of the indication for the screening: person's risk for lung cancer (in the near future) and their life expectancy (when spared from death from lung cancer). These two inputs bear on when, if ever, to begin the screening on a given person and, insofar as it has been initiated, when to discontinue screening.[20] Related to the life-expectancy consideration is that of the time from lung cancer diagnosis to death from the cancer, preventable by early intervention. Finally, cost-effectiveness of the screening program should be considered.[20–22]

The question of whether to recommend for or against lung cancer screening, on a particular person at a particular time, for now should be addressed on a background of institutional, official beliefs. Some authorities and institutions currently hold that the utility of CT screening for lung cancer remains unknown, even qualitatively, and that resolution of even this qualitative issue would require a very large, very expensive long-term study (costing hundreds of millions of dollars). Specifically, a randomized controlled trial (RCT) contrasting CT screening with more traditional radiographic screening, earlier deemed useless,[23] is being contemplated. The object of the trial would be to test (inconclusively perhaps) whether CT screening reduces mortality from lung cancer when used in lieu of its traditional radiographic alternative.

Insofar as this authoritative view indeed does arise, the pursuit of practice decision begins with choosing between the following two outlooks.

The Outlook Here

CT screening obviously provides for earlier diagnosis of lung cancer (usually fairly early in Stage IA), and the earlier interventions rendered possible by the screening clearly have enhanced effectiveness in preventing death from lung cancer. Therefore, CT screening for lung cancer clearly provides for increased curability of lung cancer and, thereby, for reduced case-fatality rate and reduced lung-cancer mortality in any screened population at risk for the disease. As for the second premise in this, no one is so equivocal about the relative merits of early and late intervention as to favor a RCT contrasting the two in whatever subset of cases of screen-diagnosed cancer of the lung, or to otherwise delay intervention in the context of early diagnosis of the disease.

The Alternative Outlook

Individual deductive reasoning by practitioners, even if founded on strong premises and on formally correct deduction from them (as in *The Outlook Here*), must be rejected in favor of public policy based on evidence from an RCT, even if the context might be something other than intervention research, as in the context of screening research here. With this outlook, one needs to find a way to avoid being discouraged by the previous RCT experiences and their associated controversies, in particular in the context of breast cancer screening.

If the latter outlook is adopted, everything presented here is irrelevant, for now at least, as the time for officially sanctioned CT screening for lung cancer is many years away, if it ever arrives at all. If it does arrive, devotees of this outlook will have to make decisions about the screening without the RCT having produced any quantitative information about the fatality-rate reduction—and thus about the curability gain—provided for by the screening.[24]

REFERENCES

1. Flehinger BJ, Kimmel M, Melamed MR. Survival from early lung cancer: implications for screening. Chest 1992;101:1013–1018.
2. Henschke CI, McCauley DI, Yankelevitz DF et al. Early Lung Cancer Action Project: overall design and findings from baseline screening. Lancet 1999;354:99–105.
3. Henschke CI, Naidich DP, Yankelevitz DF et al. Early Lung Cancer Action Project: initial findings on repeat screening. Cancer 2001;92:153–159.
4. Miettinen OS. The modern scientific physician: 6. The useful property of a screening regimen. Can Med Assoc J 2001;165:1219–1220.
5. Ostroff J, Buckshee N, Mancuso CA et al. Smoking cessation following CT screening for early detection of lung cancer. Prev Med 2001;33:613–621.
6. Henschke CI, Yankelevitz DF, Smith JP, Miettinen OS. International Early Lung Cancer Action Program: origins, principles and protocol. Lung Cancer 2002;55:143–148.
7. International Collaboration to Screen for Lung Cancer. Proceedings of the First, Second, Third, and Fourth International Conference on Screening for Lung Cancer. New York: (Web site: http://ICScreen.med.cornell.edu).
8. International Early Lung Cancer Action Program (Web site: http://www.IELCAP.org)
9. Henschke CI, Yankelevitz DF, Mirtcheva R et al. CT screening for lung cancer: frequency and significance of part-solid and non-solid nodules. Am J Roentgenol AJR 2002; in press.
10. Zerhouni EA, Stitik FP, Siegelman SS et al. CT of the pulmonary nodule: a cooperative study. Radiology 1986;160:319–327.
11. Yankelevitz DF, Gupta R, Zhao B, Henschke CI. Repeat CT scanning for evaluation of small pulmonary nodules. Radiology 1999;212:561–566.
12. Yankelevitz DF, Reeves AP, Kostis WJ et al. Determination of malignancy in small pulmonary nodules based on volumetrically determined growth rates. Radiology 2000;217:251–256.
13. American College of Medical Physics. Radiation Control and Quality Assurance Surveys, Report No 1. Reston VA. American College of Medical Physics, 1986.
14. AAPM Report No. 39: Specification and Acceptance Testing of Computed Tomography Scanners. Diagnostic X-ray Imaging Committee Task Group No. 2; ISBN:1-56396-230-6, 1993.
15. Workshop III Summary: Quality Assurance in Screening for Lung Cancer. Third International Conference on Prevention and Early Detection of Lung Cancer. Lung Cancer 2002; in press.
16. Sone S, Takashima S, Li F et al. Mass screening for lung cancer with mobile spiral computed tomography scanner. Lancet 1998;351(9111):1242–1245.
17. Sone S, Li F, Yank Z-G et al. Characteristics of small lung cancers invisible on conventional chest radiography and detected by population based screening using spiral CT. Br J Radiol 2000;73: 137–145.
18. Yankelevitz DF, Kostis W, Braz-Parente D, Henschke CI. Evidence against overdiagnosis of lung cancer in the context of chest radiographic screening for lung cancer [abstract]. Radiol Soc North Am 2001;11:

19. Henschke CI, Wisnivesky JP, Yankelevitz DF, Miettinen OS. Screen-diagnosed small Stage I cancers of the lung: genuineness and curability. Submitted.

20. Miettinen OS. Screening for lung cancer: Can it be cost-effective? Can Med Assoc J 2000;162: 1431–1436.

21. Wisnivesky JP, Mushlin AI, Sicherman N, Henschke CI. The cost-effectiveness of low-dose computed tomography screening for lung cancer: Preliminary results of baseline screening. Chest 2002; in press.

22. Marshall D, Simpson KN, Earle CC, Chu CW. Economic decision analysis model of screening for lung cancer. Eur J Cancer 2001;37:1759–1767.

23. Eddy DM. Screening for lung cancer. Ann Intern Med 1989;111:232–237.

24. Miettinen OS, Henschke CI. CT Screening for lung cancer: coping with nihilistic recommendations. Radiology 2001;221:592–596.

Chapter 12

Prognostic Factors and Staging of Melanoma

Charles M. Balch

Seng-Jaw Soong

John F. Thompson

Antonio Buzaid

Clinical and pathological factors predicting outcome of melanoma patients have been studied for more than 30 years. The first multivariate analyses of prognostic factors from a single institution were published in 1978,[1,2] and the first multivariate analysis from a multi-institutional experience was published in 1981.[3] Although a multitude of well-designed single-institution analyses have subsequently added to our understanding of prognostic factors in melanoma, few attempts have been made to unify these results into a melanoma staging system to be used in clinical research and clinical practice. However, the design and analysis of melanoma clinical trials depends on the use of relevant predictive or prognostic factors that must be taken into account. Otherwise, treatment differences, or lack thereof, may be influenced more by the mix of the patient's prognostic factors than by the treatment effect being studied. For example, some melanoma adjuvant therapy trials use such different stratification and patient eligibility criteria that it is difficult, if not impossible, to compare across-clinical trials conducted by cooperative groups or institutions or even to compare reliably results of sequential trials conducted by the same investigators.

Over the last few years, a series of multidisciplinary conferences attended by melanoma investigators from major melanoma centers throughout the world provided a forum for revising the melanoma staging system.[4–6] A newly constituted melanoma staging committee of the American Joint Commission on Cancer (AJCC), formed in 1999, proposed a new staging system that was approved by the AJCC in 2001.[5]

THE AJCC MELANOMA STAGING PROJECT

The AJCC Melanoma Staging Committee used the following criteria to select independent prognostic features of melanoma to be used in the revised melanoma TNM classification and the stage groupings.[4,5] First, the staging system must be practical, reproducible, and applicable to the diverse needs of all medical disciplines. Second, the criteria must accurately reflect the biology of melanoma on the basis of consistent outcome results for patients treated at multiple institutions from multiple countries. Third, the criteria used must be evidence-based and reflect the dominant prognostic factors consistently identified in Cox multivariate regression analyses. Fourth, the criteria must be relevant to current clinical practice and regularly incorporated in clinical trials. Fifth, the required data had to be sufficiently easy for tumor registrars to identify in medical records to code staging information.

Independent prognostic factors were considered by the AJCC Melanoma Committee for defining the TNM categories and stage grouping, based on the results published in the literature. In addition, members of the Melanoma Staging Committee and additional consultants agreed to an unprecedented collaboration to share prospectively accumulated melanoma outcome data and established the AJCC Melanoma Staging Database.[7] This is a single, large database involving melanoma patients from 13 cancer centers and is a cooperative group created for the purpose of validating the proposed revisions to the melanoma staging system. The data were merged from prospective databases of patients who did not receive any adjuvant systemic therapy and for all of whom quality control measures were in place regarding data entry, pathology, and surgery. Details about the data collection, statistical methodologies, and results have been published.[7] The resultant collaborative research project is the largest prognostic factors analysis of melanoma ever conducted.

The AJCC Melanoma Database consisted of a total of 30,450 melanoma patients, of whom 17,600 (58%) had information available for all the 15 clinical and pathological factors required for the proposed TNM classification and stage grouping.[7] Of the 17,600 patients included in this analysis, 12,837 (73 %) had at least 5 years of follow up information, 8633 (49%) had at least 10 years follow up, and 2485 (14%) had at least 20 years of follow up. Melanoma-specific survival curves were generated according to the Kaplan-Meier product-limit method and were compared using the log-rank test. Multivariate analyses of prognostic factors were based on the Cox proportional hazards model.

The revised version of the melanoma TNM categories are listed in Table 12.1, and the stage groupings are found in Table 12.2. Fifteen-year survival curves for patients with Stages I–IV melanoma are shown in Figure 12.1. The final version of the melanoma staging system will become official with publication of the sixth edition of the AJCC Cancer Staging Manual in the year 2002. In addition, these melanoma staging criteria have been approved and adopted by the International Union Against Cancer TNM Committee, by the World Health Organization Melanoma Program, and by the European Organization for Research and Treatment of Cancer Melanoma Group.

The major changes in the new version as compared to the previous (1997) version of the melanoma staging system are summarized in Table 12.3. For example, this version retains the anatomic compartmentalization, consistent with staging for other cancers, that categorizes patients with localized melanoma (i.e., without any evidence of metastases) to Stages I and II, those with regional metastases to Stage III, and those with distant metastases to Stage IV. Major changes in the staging include the following:

- Melanoma thickness and ulceration, but not level of invasion, are used in the T category (except for T1 melanomas).
- The number of metastatic lymph nodes, rather than their gross dimensions, and the delineation of clinically occult (i.e., "microscopic") versus clinically apparent (i.e., "macroscopic") nodal metastases are to be used in the N category.
- The site of distant metastases (nonvisceral vs lung vs all other visceral metastatic sites) and the presence of elevated serum lactic dehydrogenase (LDH) are to be used in the M category.
- All patients with Stage I, II, and III disease will be upstaged on determination by histopathologic criteria that a primary melanoma is ulcerated.
- T4 melanomas are relocated into Stage II from Stage III in the previous version so that Stage III is confined to regional metastases.
- Satellite metastases around a primary melanoma and in-transit metastases are merged into a single staging entity that is grouped into Stage III disease.
- A new convention is provided for defining clinical and pathological staging so as to incorporate pathological information gained from lymphatic mapping and sentinel node biopsy.

PROGNOSIS AND STAGING FOR LOCALIZED MELANOMA (STAGES I AND II)

Independent Prognostic Factors

Although much has been published about prognosis of Stage I and Stage II melanoma, this staging revision was largely determined by the results of the prognostic factors analysis of data from the AJCC Melanoma Staging Database.[7] In a multivariate analysis of 13,581 patients with localized melanoma (either

TABLE 12.1 Melanoma TNM Classification

T Classification	Thickness	Ulceration Status
T1	≤ 1.0 mm	
T1a		Without ulceration and level II/III
T1b		With ulceration or level IV/V
T2	1.01–2.0 mm	
T2a		Without ulceration
T2b		With ulceration
T3	2.01–4.0 mm	
T3a		Without ulceration
T3b		With ulceration
T4	> 4.0 mm	
T4a		Without ulceration
T4b		With ulceration
N classification	**Number of Metastatic Nodes**	**Nodal Metastatic Mass**
N1	1 node	
N1a		Micrometastasis[a]
N1b		Macrometastasis[b]
N2	2–3 nodes	Micrometastasis[a]
N2a		Macrometastasis[b]
N2b		In-transit metastasis(es)/ satellite(s) without metastatic nodes
N2c		
N3	4 or more metastatic nodes, or matted nodes, or in-transit metastasis(es)/ satellite(s) with metastatic node(s)	
M Classification	**Site**	**Serum Lactate Dehydrogenase**
M1a	Distant skin, subcutaneous, or nodal metastases	Normal
M1b	Lung metastases	Normal
M1c	All other visceral metastases	Normal
	Any distant metastasis	Elevated

[a]Micrometastases are diagnosed after sentinel or elective lymphadenectomy.
[b]Macrometastases are defined as clinically detectable nodal metastases confirmed by therapeutic lymphadenectomy or when nodal metastasis exhibits gross extracapsular extension.

TABLE 12.2 Revised Stage Groupings for Cutaneous Melanoma

Clinical Staging[a]				Pathological Staging[b]			
0	Tis	N0	M0	0	Tis	N0	M0
IA	T1a	N0	M0	IA	T1a	N0	M0
IB	T1b	N0	M0	IB	T1b	N0	M0
	T2a	N0	M0		T2a	N0	M0
IIA	T2b	N0	M0	IIA	T2b	N0	M0
	T3a	N0	M0		T3a	N0	M0
IIB	T3b	N0	M0	IIB	T3b	N0	M0
	T4a	N0	M0		T4a	N0	M0
IIC	T4b	N0	M0	IIC	T4b	N0	M0
III	Any T	Any N	M0	IIIA	T1–4a	N1a	M0
					T1–4a	N2a	M0
				IIIB	T1–4b	N1a	M0
					T1–4b	N2a	M0
					T1–4a	N1b	M0
					T1–4a	N2b	M0
					T1–4a/b	N2c	M0
				IIIC	T1–4b	N1b	M0
					T1–4b	N2b	M0
					Any T	N3	M0
IV	Any T	Any N	Any M	IV	Any T	Any N	Any M

[a]Clinical staging includes microstaging of the primary melanoma and clinical-radiologic evaluation for metastases. By convention, it should be used after complete excision of the primary melanoma with clinical assessment for regional and distant metastases.
[b]Pathological staging includes microstaging of the primary melanoma and pathological information about the regional lymph nodes after partial or complete lymphadenectomy. Pathological Stage 0 or Stage IA patients are the exception; they do not require pathological evaluation of their lymph nodes.

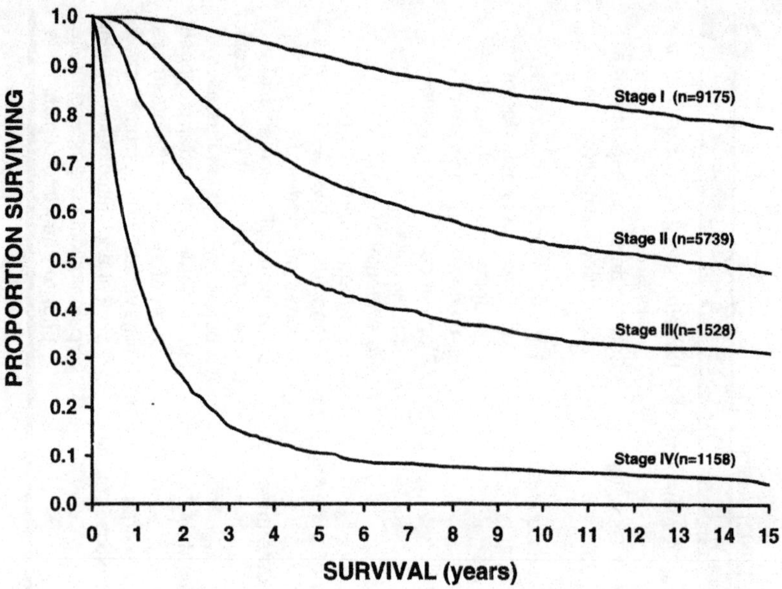

FIGURE 12.1 Fifteen-year survival curves for the melanoma staging system comparing localized melanoma (Stages II and I), regional metastases (Stage III), and distant metastases (Stage IV). The numbers in parentheses are the numbers of patients from the American Joint Commission on Cancer Melanoma Staging Database used to calculate the survival rates. The differences between the curves are significant ($P < 0.0001$). (From Balch C et al, J Clin Oncol 2001;19:3635–3648. Reprinted with permission.)

clinically or pathologically) from the AJCC Melanoma Staging database, the two most powerful independent characteristics of the primary melanoma were tumor thickness and ulceration, among all the prognostic variables analyzed (Table 12.4). Other statistically significant prognostic factors were patient age, site of the primary melanoma, level of invasion, and gender (see Table 12.4). A more detailed description of each independent factor is described below.

Melanoma Thickness The use of melanoma thickness was first described by Breslow,[8–12] who quantitatively measured the maximum vertical dimension of a melanoma on cross-section using an ocular micrometer. In virtually all published studies analyzing the prognosis of patients with Stage I and Stage II melanoma, tumor thickness was the most quantitative and strongest predictor of outcome. Thus, there is uniform agreement in the literature that melanoma thickness is the strongest predictor of survival outcome as evidenced by multivariate analyses reported from single institutions, from multiinstitutional studies, and from population-based studies that spanned countries in North America, Europe, and Australia.[1,3,13–41]

TABLE 12.3 Changes in Melanoma Staging Comparing Previous (1997) and New (2002) Versions

Factor	Old System	New System	Comments
Level of invasion	Primary determinant of T staging	Used only for defining T1 melanomas	Correlation significant only for thin lesions
Thickness	Second prognostic factor of T staging; thresholds of 0.75, 1.50, 4.00 mm	Primary determinant of T staging; thresholds of 1.0, 2.0, 4.0 mm	Correlation of metastatic risk a continuous variable
Ulceration	Not included	Included as a second determinant of T and N staging category	Signifies a locally advanced lesion; dominant prognostic factor for grouping Stage I, II, and III
Satellite metastases	In T category	In N category	Merged with in-transit lesions
Thick melanomas (> 4.0 mm)	In Stage IIIA	In Stage IIC	Stage III defined as regional metastasis
Dimensions of nodal metastases	Primary determinant of N staging	Not used	No evidence of significant prognostic correlation
Number of nodal metastases	Not included	Primary determinant of N staging	Thresholds of 1 vs. 2–3 vs. ≥ 4 metastatic nodes
Metastatic tumor burden	Not included	Included as second determinant of N staging	Clinically occult (microscopic) vs. clinically apparent (macroscopic) burden of nodal metastases
Lung metastases	Merged with all other visceral metastases	Separate category as M1b	Has a somewhat better prognosis than other visceral metastases
Clinical vs. pathological staging	Did not account for sentinel node technology	Sentinel node results incorporated into definition of pathological staging	Large variability in outcome between clinical and pathological staging; pathological staging encouraged prior to entry into clinical trials

From Balch C et al, J Clin Oncol 2001;19:3635–3648. Reprinted with permission.

TABLE 12.4 Cox Regression Analysis for 13,581 Melanoma Patients Without Evidence of Nodal or Distant Metastases

Variable	DF	Chi-Square Value (Wald)	*P* Value	Risk Ratio	95% CI
Variable	DF	Chi-Square Value (Wald)	*P* Value	Risk Ratio	95% CI
Thickness	1	244.3	< 0.00001	1.558	1.473–1.647
Ulceration	1	189.5	< 0.00001	1.901	1.735–2.083
Age	1	45.6	< 0.00001	1.101	1.071–1.132
Site	1	41.0	< 0.00001	1.338	1.224–1.463
Level	1	32.7	< 0.00001	1.214	1.136–1.297
Gender	1	15.1	0.001	0.836	0.764–0.915

DF, degrees of freedom; CI, confidence interval.
From Balch C et al, J Clin Oncol 2001;19:3622–3634. Reprinted with permission.

Through use of the AJCC Melanoma Staging Database, a nonlinear model was fitted to the data to describe the relationship between tumor thickness and mortality. Increasing melanoma thickness was highly correlated with 10-year melanoma-specific mortality ($P < 0.00001$; Fig. 12.2). This model demonstrated

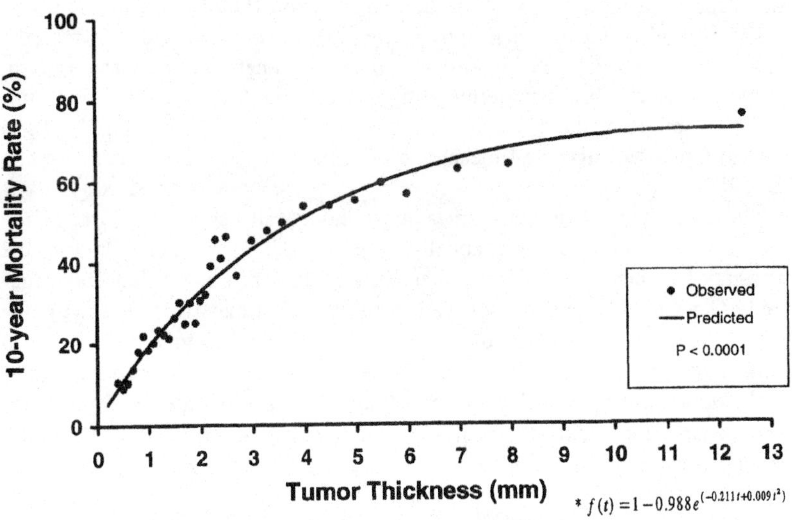

FIGURE 12.2 Observed and predicted 10-year mortality rate of 15,320 patients with clinically localized melanoma based on a mathematical model derived from the American Joint Commission on Cancer Melanoma database. The correlation is highly significant ($P < 0.0001$). There are no naturally occurring breakpoints or thresholds of tumor thickness and mortality. (Reproduced from Balch C et al, J Clin Oncol 2001;19:3622–3634. Used with permission.)

no naturally occurring breakpoints that delineated different biologic risks for melanoma-specific mortality. Increasing melanoma thickness correlated with increasing risk for local recurrences, regional metastases, distant metastases, and melanoma-specific survival.

This finding of melanoma thickness as a continuous variable without any natural breakpoints has also been a consistent conclusion in the literature.[1,3,6,13,21,22,29,42–44] In the previous (1997) version of the melanoma staging system, the threshold of a T1-T2 melanoma was defined as 0.75 mm, which had been empirically recommended by Breslow in 1970.[8] Subsequently, many melanoma investigators have used a threshold of ≤ 1.0 mm to define a "thin" or a "good-risk" melanoma. In the new staging version, the T category thresholds of melanoma thickness are defined in even integers (i.e., at 1.0, 2.0, and 4.0 mm) because they represent both a statistical "best fit" and are most compatible with current thresholds in clinical decision making and the classification of prognostic groups of "node negative" (N0) patients.[1,11,13,21,30,35,45]

Melanoma Ulceration A highly significant and underreported feature of melanoma is the presence or absence of ulceration overlying the primary melanoma. Melanoma ulceration is defined as the absence of an intact epidermis overlying a major portion of the primary melanoma based on microscopical examination of the histologic sections.[1,13,19,46] The interpretation of melanoma ulceration is one of the most reproducible of all the major histopathologic features.[47–50]

The term *ulceration* is a descriptive term for this biologic event, in which the melanoma invades through the overlying epidermis rather than pushing it upward, manifesting as an absent epidermis overlying the tumor. It can easily be distinguished from artifactual or traumatic disruption of the epidermis (Fig. 12.3). In most instances, an ulcerated melanoma does not have an ulcer crater (see Fig. 12.3).[19]

Ulcerated melanomas represent a more biologically aggressive form of the disease, associated with a substantially increased risk of metastases. Indeed, the metastatic capacity of an ulcerated melanoma is similar to that of cancers categorized as "poorly differentiated" or "locally advanced" primary tumors. In virtually every Cox regression analysis of prognostic factors that has included ulceration in the model,[1,6,13-20,23,25,26,29-31,33,39,41,46,51-59] melanoma ulceration portends a significantly worse prognosis and a higher risk for metastatic disease as compared to nonulcerative melanomas of equivalent thickness. This observation was valid even for thin melanomas (≤ 1.0 mm), even although the incidence of ulceration was low overall (6%).

In the AJCC Melanoma Staging Database, the presence or absence of primary tumor ulceration (as documented on histologic sections of each melanoma) was the second most powerful predictor of survival from among those independent prognostic factors analyzed. Although this was clearly a predictive feature independent of tumor thickness, the incidence of melanoma ulceration increased with

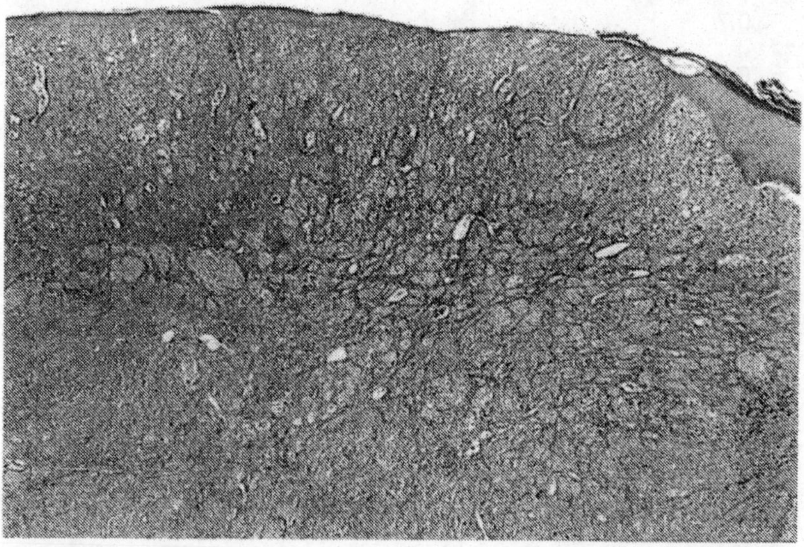

FIGURE 12.3 Typical "ulcerated" melanoma. The epidermis above the primary melanoma is absent, with a tapering of the epidermis at the periphery of the lesion. (From Balch C et al, J Clin Oncol 2001;19:3635–3648. Reprinted with permission.)

increasing tumor thickness, ranging from 6% for thin (≤ 1.0 mm) melanomas to 63% for thick (> 4.0 mm) lesions (Fig. 12.4). Thus, the presence of melanoma ulceration had to be taken into accounted in the stage groupings because ulceration had a negative impact on survival rates in stage I, II, and III disease as compared to nonulcerated melanomas.[6,7,18,60] This was true for every combination of prognostic factors used to assemble various substages.

The presence of melanoma ulceration heralds such a high risk for metastases that it "upstages" the prognosis of all such patients as compared to patients with melanomas of equivalent thickness but without ulceration. Indeed, the survival rates for thick, ulcerated melanomas (i.e., T4b) without nodal metastases are actually worse than for some substages of nodal metastases.[5] Melanoma ulceration correlates with increased mitotic rate within a primary melanoma, further evidence that this factor is associated with increased metastatic behavior.[29]

Melanoma Level of Invasion The level of invasion has been a gold standard of melanoma prognostic features since it was first defined in the 1960s by Clark.[61] It has been a primary factor in the melanoma TNM staging system and has been widely used as a prognostic factor for decades. However, the substantial limitations to using the level of invasion have gradually caused it to be replaced. It requires an interpretation of its maximum depth (especially for levels III and IV), it does not take into account the varying skin thickness of different anatomic parts (e.g.,

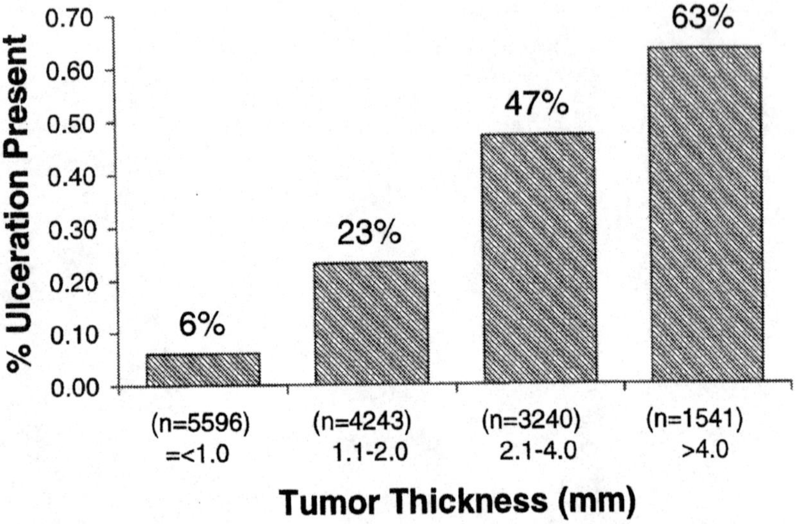

FIGURE 12.4 Incidence of melanoma ulceration (determined histopathologically) correlated with tumor thickness for 14,620 patients with localized melanoma. Number of patients is shown in parentheses. The correlation is highly significant ($P < 0.0001$) by chi-square analysis. (Reproduced from Balch C et al, J Clin Oncol 2001;19:3622–3634. Used with permission.)

skin of the back and the face), and each level is associated with a wide range of melanoma thicknesses. Four studies comparing accuracy of histopathologic prognostic factors used by pathologists showed that ulceration and thickness were much more reproducible as compared to level of invasion.[47–50,62] Moreover, when there is a discrepancy in the prognosis between measured tumor thickness and level of invasion (e.g., "thin" level IV or "thick" level III), the former is more accurate in predicting survival outcome.[6,7,13,14,21,30,45,51]

One of the controversies that could be addressed with the AJCC Melanoma Staging Database was the prognostic interaction between melanoma thickness, level of invasion, and ulceration. This was particularly important for thin melanomas (i.e., ≤ 1.0 mm thickness), for which published data had suggested that deeper levels were associated with a poor outcome.[21,57,63–67] To determine the relative predictive strength of these prognostic features within cohorts of tumor thickness, the Cox regression analysis was performed within each of the major thickness subgroups used in the melanoma T categories (Table 12.5). In comparing level of invasion and ulceration within thickness subgroups, there was a hierarchy of relative predictive strength for thin melanomas (i.e., ≤1.0 mm) that was different from all other thickness groups. Thus, level of invasion does provide additional prognostic discrimination in the specific subgroup of thin (i.e., T1) melanomas.[64,68] The opposite was true for all melanomas thicker than 1.0 mm,

TABLE 12.5 Cox Regression Analysis by Tumor Thickness Category for Stages I and II Primary Melanoma

Variable	DF	Chi-Square Value (Wald)	*P* Value	Risk Ratio	95% CI
Thickness ≤ 1.00 (n = 5299)					
Level	1	24.778	< 0.00001	1.451	1.253–1.680
Ulceration	1	17.239	< 0.00001	2.073	1.469–2.924
Age	1	12.563	0.0004	1.156	1.067–1.253
Site	1	6.940	0.0084	1.394	1.089–1.784
Gender	1	5.506	0.0189	0.744	0.581–0.952
Thickness 1.01–2.00 mm (n = 3943)					
Ulceration	1	57.215	< 0.00001	1.965	1.650–2.341
Site	1	24.085	< 0.00001	1.567	1.310–1.876
Age	1	11.613	0.0007	1.101	1.042–1.164
Level	1	6.656	0.0099	1.211	1.047–1.400
Gender	1	2.668	0.1024	0.861	0.719–1.030
Thickness 2.01–4.00 mm (n = 2959)					
Ulceration	1	62.291	< 0.00001	1.766	1.634–2.034
Age	1	12.529	0.0004	1.087	1.038–1.138
Site	1	12.342	0.0004	1.306	1.125–1.516
Level	1	4.451	0.0349	1.143	1.010–1.294
Gender	1	3.165	0.0752	0.872	0.750–1.014
Thickness > 4.00 mm (n = 1380)					
Ulceration	1	47.246	< 0.00001	1.932	1.601–2.331
Age	1	8.745	0.0031	1.087	1.028–1.148
Level	1	4.065	0.0438	1.139	1.004–1.293
Gender	1	2.875	0.0951	0.858	0.716–1.027
Site	1	2.547	0.1106	1.154	0.968–1.376

DF, degrees of freedom; CI, confidence interval.
From Balch C et al, J Clin Oncol 2001;19:3622–3634. Reprinted with permission.

where ulceration was clearly the most predictive, and level of invasion ranked below that of patient age and anatomic site of the primary melanoma (see Table 12.5).

The multivariate analysis demonstrated that a deep level of invasion (i.e., IV or V) is not a surrogate for ulceration but an independent factor that eclipses the predictive value for ulceration in this specific subgroup of patients. The incidence of ulceration was only 6% for patients with thin melanomas ($\geq$1.0 mm), whereas 16% of thin melanomas had level IV invasion (and < 0.01% with level V).[7] Overall, 10-year survival was significantly lower for thin melanomas with ulceration than for those without ulceration (76% vs 86%; $P < 0.0001$; see Fig. 12.5). Only 8% of these level IV thin melanomas were ulcerated, and these patients had a lower survival as compared to level IV thin melanomas without ulceration (70% vs 82% 10-year survival; $P < 0.001$).[7] These relationships were not true for melanomas > 1.0 mm because the level of invasion was no longer as significant a predictor of survival outcome, relative to ulceration (presence or absence), increasing age, or the anatomic site of the primary melanoma (trunk or head and neck vs extremity).

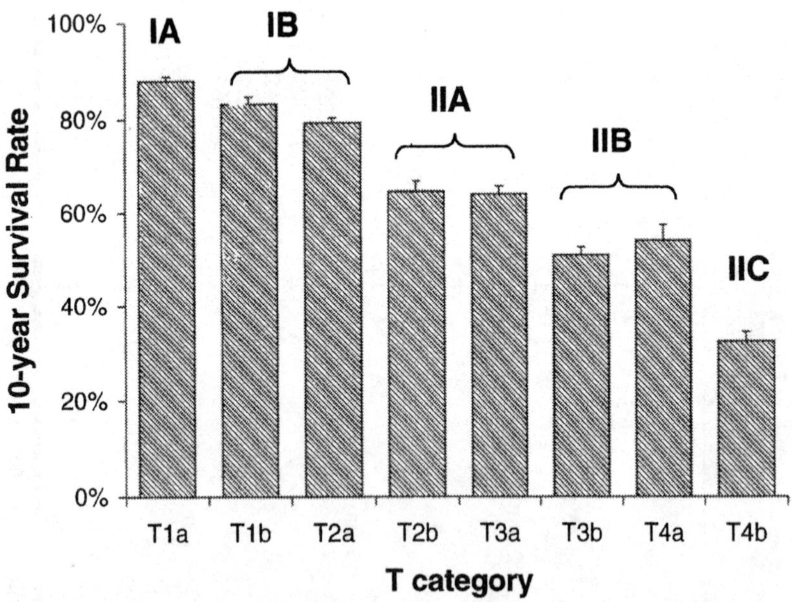

FIGURE 12.5 Ten-year survival rates from the American Joint Commission on Cancer Melanoma Staging Database comparing the different T categories and the stage groupings for Stages I and II melanoma. Note that the stage groupings involve upstaging to account for melanoma ulceration, where thinner melanomas with ulceration are grouped with the next greatest T substage for nonulcerated melanomas. (From Balch C et al, J Clin Oncol 2001;19: 3635–3648. Reprinted with permission.)

Patient Age Even although older patients have thicker melanomas and a higher incidence of ulcerated melanomas, their age is an independent adverse prognostic factor after adjusting for these other factors in a multivariate analysis.[23,32,41,52,69,70] In the AJCC Melanoma Staging Database, there was a consistent and incremental decline in both 5- and 10-year survival rates with each decade increase of age.[7] Increasing patient age was also an independent prognostic factor with respect to survival overall (see Table 12.1) and within each of the thickness subgroups (see Table 12.5). In addition to the patient's age, their gender (males worse than females) and the anatomic site of their primary melanoma (trunk and head and neck sites worse than extremities) correlated significantly with survival, although their chi-square test values were much lower than those for melanoma thickness and ulceration. Numerous other studies have demonstrated that older-age melanoma patients have a lower survival rate, especially those older than 60 years.[23,31,32,41,52,70–73] This has included a number of multiinstitutional clinical trials involving various stages of melanoma, age groups and treatment effects.[41,52,74–76] Indeed, national cancer statistics demonstrate that melanoma has the second highest mortality rate increases among Americans 65 years of age or older (1973–1997), especially for men.[77]

TNM Staging Criteria and Stage Grouping

TNM Criteria The primary criteria for the T classification are tumor thickness (measured in millimeters) and the presence or absence of ulceration (determined histopathologically). Ten-year survival rates for each of the T categories in clinically staged patients are shown in Figure 12.5.

In the new staging version, the T category thresholds of melanoma thickness are defined in even integers (i.e., at 1.0, 2.0, and 4.0 mm) because they represent both a statistical "best fit" and are most compatible with current thresholds in clinical decision making. The presence of melanoma ulceration heralds such a high risk for metastases that its presence upstages the prognosis of all such patients as compared to patients with melanomas of equivalent thickness without ulceration (Table 12.6). Thus, survival rates for patients with an ulcerated melanoma are remarkably similar to those of patients with a nonulcerated melanoma of equivalent T category but are remarkably similar to those of patients with a nonulcerated melanoma of the next highest T category (see Fig. 12.5 and Table 12.6). The level of invasion was incorporated into the staging definitions of T1N0M0 melanomas because it was demonstrated to be an independent prognostic factor for this cohort of patients.

For T1 melanomas, the assignment of T1a is restricted to patients with three criteria: (1) ≤ 1.0 mm thick, (2) absence of ulceration, and (3) depth of invasion limited to level II or level III. Those melanomas with a thickness ≤ 1.0 mm and with the more aggressive features of level IV or V or with ulceration (regardless of level) are defined as T1b melanomas. Approximately 75% of patients with T1

TABLE 12.6 Five-Year Survival Rates of Pathologically Staged Patients

Pathological Stage	1A	IB	IIA	IIB	IIC	IIIA	IIIB	IIIC
Ta: nonulcerated	T1: 95%	T2: 89%	T3: 79%	T4: 67%		N1a, N2a: 67%	N1b, N2b: 54%	N3: 28%
Tb: ulcerated		T1: 91%	T2: 77%	T3: 63%	T4: 45%		N1a, N2a: 52%	N1b: N2b, N3: 24%

From Balch C et al, J Clin Oncol 2001;19:3635–3648. Reprinted with permission.

melanomas are T1a and have a 95% 5-year survival, whereas the remaining T1 patients have T1b lesions and experience a somewhat lower 91% 5-year survival (see Table 12.6).

The data used to derive the TNM categories were largely based on melanomas with superficial spreading and nodular growth patterns. At present, the same staging criteria should be used for melanomas with other growth patterns (i.e., acral lentiginous, lentigo maligna, and desmosplastic melanomas) even though their prognosis may differ somewhat from the more commonly occurring superficial spreading and nodular growth patterns.

Special Features Patients with melanoma in situ are categorized as Ti. Those patients with melanoma presentations that are indeterminate or cannot be microstaged should be categorized as Tx. Two examples of indeterminate staging of melanoma would be a diagnosis with a shave or a curettage biopsy that transected the base of the melanoma or an unknown primary melanoma presenting with regional or distant metastases. When patients present with multiple primary melanomas, the T category staging is based on the melanoma with the worst prognostic features.

The data used in the AJCC melanoma prognostic factors analysis and in other studies reported in the literature are largely based on melanomas with superficial spreading and nodular growth patterns. These two growth patterns, reflecting differences in vertical and radial growth phases, constitute approximately 90% of melanomas seen in most practices; they are not independent prognostic factors because their survival rates are almost the same when their thickness is taken into account.[1,13,30] There is some evidence that other growth patterns—lentigo maligna melanoma, acral lentiginous melanoma, and desmoplastic melanoma—may have different etiologies and prognosis.[15,30,78–84]

Stage Groupings Stage grouping for localized melanomas that are either clinically or pathologically staged are defined in Table 12.2. The sole difference in the definitions of clinical versus pathological stage grouping is whether the regional lymph nodes are staged by clinical-radiologic examination or by pathological examination (after partial or complete lymphadenectomy). Because level of invasion is an independent predictive feature for thin (T1) melanomas (but not for thicker lesions), it is incorporated into the stage grouping definitions for T1 melanomas.[7] Patients with primary melanomas with no evidence of regional or distant metastases (either clinically or pathologically) are divided into two stages: Stage I for early-stage patients with "low risk" for metastases and melanoma-specific mortality or Stage II for those with "intermediate risk" for metastases and melanoma-specific mortality. Furthermore, Stage I patients constitute two subgroups: Stage IA are T1 melanomas without ulceration or level IV or V depth of invasion (T1aN0M0 melanomas), and Stage IB are either T1 melanomas with histopathologic evidence of level IV-V depth of invasion or ulceration of their surface (T1bN0M0) or those T2 melanomas without ulceration (T2aN0M0). Stage II patients constitute three subgroups: Stage IIA are T2 melanomas with ulceration (T2bN0M0) or T3 melanomas without ulceration (T3aN0M0); Stage IIB are either T3 melanomas with ulceration (T3bN0M0) or T4 melanomas without ulceration (T4aN0M0); and Stage IIC are T4 melanomas with ulceration (T4bN0M0). Survival rates for these stage groupings are shown in Figure 12.5 and are listed in Table 12.6.

The determination of stage grouping for patients with T4bN0M0 melanomas was a dilemma because the patients are at particularly high risk for harboring both regional and distant metastases. These thick, ulcerated melanomas are biologically aggressive and are associated with mortality rates that are the same as or even higher than those in some groups of patients with nodal metastases (see Table 12.6). Such patients were grouped as Stage III in the 1997 version of the melanoma staging system because of commensurate risk for melanoma-specific mortality. The Melanoma Staging Committee concluded that such a categorization would add significant complexity to the new stage groupings. To stay within the conventional anatomic definitions, T4 melanomas were, therefore, assigned to Stage II in the final version. This includes T4b melanomas that would still be grouped with other localized melanomas but are designated separately as Stage IIC because these patients are at especially high risk for clinically occult nodal and systemic metastases.

Data-Recording Criteria In entering melanoma TNM data into tumor registries for the purposes of stage grouping, the electronic data fields must record the measured tumor thickness (in millimeters), the presence or absence of ulceration (based on histopathologic examination), and the level of invasion to derive stage groupings for localized melanomas. In those circumstances in which there has been an incisional (or punch) biopsy, generally the maximum tumor thickness in *either* the biopsy or definitive excision should be recorded (i.e., the measurements should not be added). Other prognostic features of localized melanomas were not incorporated into the new TNM categories. Nevertheless, these are potentially important for other types of data analysis and for stratification of patients in clinical trials and should be recorded in medical records and tumor registries. These include the patient's age and gender, the anatomic site of the primary melanoma (i.e., trunk, extremities, or head and neck), mitotic rate, regression (if present), and the growth pattern (superficial spreading, nodular, lentigo maligna melanoma, acral lentiginous melanoma, or desmoplastic melanoma).

PROGNOSIS AND STAGING FOR REGIONAL METASTASES (STAGE III)

Independent Prognostic Factors

Stage III melanoma patients include those with regional metastases either in the regional lymph nodes or with intralymphatic metastases manifesting as either satellite or in-transit metastases. In the AJCC Melanoma Staging Database, complete clinical and histopathologic data were available for 1201 patients with lymph node metastases. A Cox multivariate analysis demonstrated that three factors were most significant (with $P < 0.0001$): the number of metastatic nodes, the tumor burden at the time of staging (i.e., microscopic vs macroscopic), and the presence or absence of ulceration of the primary melanoma (Table 12.7).[7]

These three predictive factors discriminated significant survival differences, even within each of the Stage III subgroups examined, including a three-way comparison that integrated subgroups according to all three of the most important prognostic factors: ulceration of the primary melanoma, nodal tumor burden (microscopic vs macroscopic), and the number of metastatic nodes (Table 12.8). Overall, only 49% of all patients with nodal metastases survived 5 years (37%

TABLE 12.7 Cox Regression Analysis for 1151 Stage III (Nodal Metastases) Patients

Variable	DF	Chi-Square Value (Wald)	*P* Value	Risk Ratio	95% CI
No. of metastatic nodes	1	57.616	< 0.00001	1.257	1.185–1.334
Tumor burden	1	40.301	< 0.00001	1.792	1.497–2.146
Ulceration	1	23.282	< 0.00001	1.582	1.313–1.906
Site	1	17.843	0.0001	1.461	1.225–1.746
Age	1	13.369	0.0003	1.118	1.053–1.187
Thickness	1	1.964	0.1611	1.091	0.966–1.233
Level	1	0.219	0.6396	1.033	0.901–1.186
Gender	1	0.006	0.9407	1.007	0.836–1.213

DF, degrees of freedom; CI, confidence interval.
From Balch C et al, J Clin Oncol 2001;19:3622–3634. Reprinted with permission.

TABLE 12.8 Five-Year Survival Rates for Stage III (Nodal Metastases) Patients Stratified by Number of Metastatic Nodes, Ulceration, and Tumor Burden

	Microscopic (% ± SEM)			Macroscopic (% ± SEM)		
Melanoma Ulceration	1+ nodes	2–3 nodes	> 3+ nodes	1+ nodes	2–3 nodes	> 3+ nodes
Absent	69 ± 3.7 (n = 252)	63 ± 5.6 (n = 130)	27 ± 9.3 (n = 57)	59 ± 4.7 (n = 122)	46 ± 5.5 (n = 93)	27 ± 4.6 (n = 109)
Present	52 ± 4.1 (n = 217)	50 ± 5.7 (n = 111)	37 ± 8.8 (n = 46)	29 ± 5.0 (n = 98)	25 ± 4.4 (n = 109)	13 ± 3.5 (n = 104)

SEM, standard error of the mean.

From Balch C et al, J Clin Oncol 2001;19:3622–3634. Reprinted with permission.

at 10 years), but the range of melanoma-specific survival was large, ranging from 13% at 5 years for patients with the highest risk combination of factors to 69% at 5 years for the lowest-risk combination of predictive factors (see Table 12.8). The site of the primary melanoma and the patient's age had a somewhat lower—but still statistically significant—correlation with survival (see Table 12.7).

Features of Primary Melanomas Based on the AJCC analysis and results in the literature, the presence or absence of ulceration is the only prognostic feature of a primary melanoma that independently predicts outcome in Stage III melanoma (Table 12.7).[6,7,18,60] Thus, all other predictive features for Stage I and Stage II melanoma were not independent factors for Stage III melanomas, including melanoma thickness and level of invasion.

Number of Metastatic Lymph Nodes In almost all published studies analyzing prognosis using Cox regression analysis, either the number or the percentage of metastatic lymph nodes was the strongest predictor of survival outcome.[6,30,60,85–96] In all studies that have examined prognosis based on the number of metastatic nodes, patients with one metastatic node did better than did those with any combination of two or more metastatic nodes.[6,30,85,87,89–91,94] This was true regardless of whether the patient presentation involved macroscopic or microscopic nodal metastases. Thus, survival correlated best with the number of metastatic lymph nodes even for patients with microscopic (or clinically occult) metastases.

In the AJCC Melanoma Staging Database, the actual number of nodal metastases was the most significant predictor of outcome in these patients (see Table 12.7). Melanoma-specific survival (calculated from the onset of primary melanoma diagnosis) decreased significantly with increasing nodal involvement ($P < 0.0001$; Fig. 12.6). The best grouping for the number of metastatic nodes that correlated with 5-year survival was one versus two to three versus ≥ four metastatic nodes.[7]

Micrometastases Versus Macrometastases of Lymph Nodes A second significant prognostic feature for patients with nodal metastases is the tumor burden of nodal metastases, so designated operationally but not by actual measurements. Tumor burden was defined as whether the nodal metastases were clinically occult (i.e., not palpable) and detected by sentinel or elective node dissection (designated operationally as "micrometastases") or clinically apparent (i.e., palpable) metastases and confirmed by therapeutic lymphadenectomy (designated operationally as "macrometastases"). Published results from two randomized surgical trials also confirmed that the survival rates for these two patient groups are significantly different.[7,41,97]

In the AJCC Melanoma Staging database, there was a significantly lower survival for those patients who presented with clinically apparent or macroscopic (i.e., palpable) nodal metastases than for those with clinically occult or microscopic (i.e., nonpalpable) nodal metastases, even after accounting for lead-time bias ($P < 0.0001$; Fig. 12.7). Diminishing 5-year survival with increasing number of

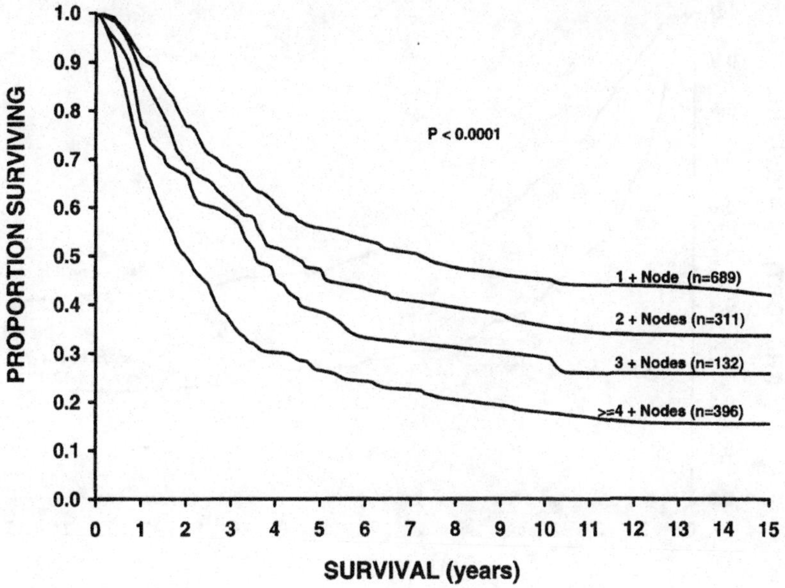

FIGURE 12.6 Survival curves of 1528 melanoma patients with lymph node metastases subgrouped by the actual number of metastatic nodes. The correlation is highly significant ($P < 0.0001$). (Reproduced from Balch C et al, J Clin Oncol 2001;19:3622–3634. Used with permission.)

metastatic nodes present was observed for all subgroups ($P < 0.0001$; see Table 12.8).

Intralymphatic Metastases The fourth criterion for defining pathological stage III melanoma is the presence or absence of intralymphatic metastases (i.e., satellites or in-transit metastases). The presence of clinical or microscopic satellite metastases around a primary melanoma and in-transit metastases between the primary melanoma and the regional lymph nodes represents intralymphatic metastases and portends a poor prognosis.[6,98–101] The available data show no substantial difference in survival outcome for these two anatomically defined entities (Fig. 12.8).[6] Furthermore, the available data demonstrate that patients with a combination of satellites and in-transit metastases *plus* nodal metastases have a worse outcome than do patients who experience either event alone.[6,87]

Special Features By convention, regional nodal metastases refer to disease confined to one nodal basin or two contiguous nodal basins, such as seen in patients with nodal disease in combinations of femoral-iliac, axillary-supraclavicular, cervical-supraclavicular, axillary-femoral, or bilateral axillary or femoral metastases. All such patients would be categorized as having Stage III melanoma.

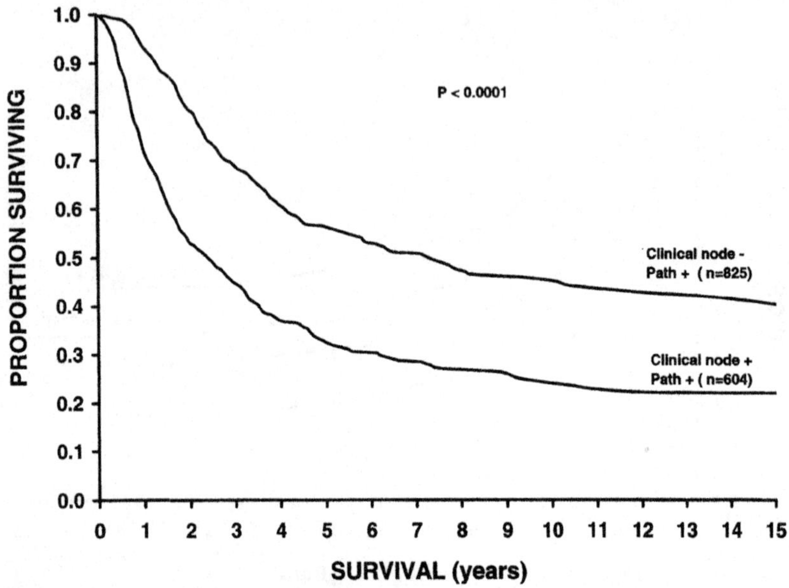

FIGURE 12.7 Survival curves of 1429 patients with lymph node metastases subgrouped by their presenting clinical stage. There were 825 patients with clinically occult nodal metastases diagnosed pathologically after either sentinel or elective lymphadenectomy and 604 patients who presented with clinically evident nodal metastases confirmed pathologically after a therapeutic lymphadenectomy. Survival rates were calculated from the onset of the primary melanoma diagnosis. The difference in survival rates is highly significant ($P < 0.0001$). (Reproduced from Balch C et al, J Clin Oncol 2001;19:3622–3634. Used with permission.)

TNM Staging Criteria and Stage Grouping

Stage III melanoma patients include those with regional metastases either in the regional lymph nodes or as intralymphatic metastases manifesting as either satellite or in-transit metastases. The marked diversity in the natural history of Stage III melanoma is demonstrated by fivefold differences in 5-year survival rates for defined substages. These substages range from 69% for patients who had a nonulcerated melanoma (regardless of thickness) and had a single clinically occult nodal metastasis (detected by sentinel or elective lymphadenectomy) to a low of 13% for patients with an ulcerated melanoma (regardless of thickness) with four or more clinically apparent nodal metastases (detected by therapeutic lymphadenectomy; see Table 12.8).[7]

The ability to stage patients more accurately with sentinel node technology has markedly changed our understanding of the natural history of melanoma.[17,85] This has had a profound impact on the staging, treatment planning, and conduct

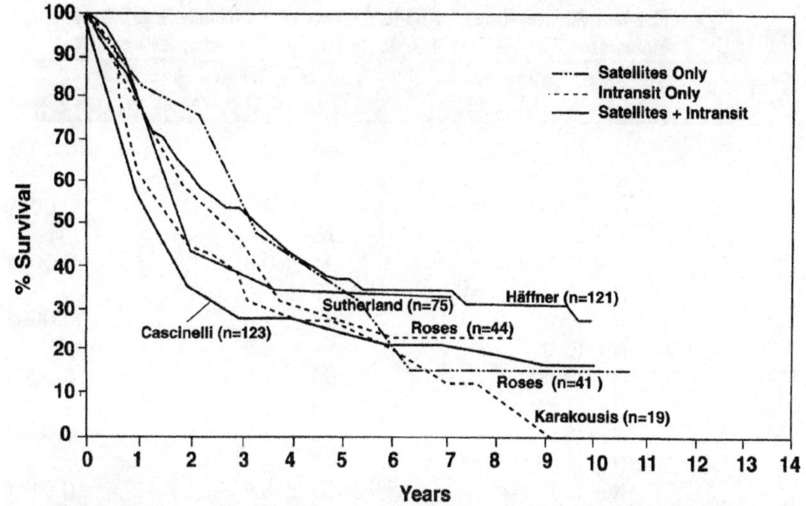

FIGURE 12.8 Survival curves of patients presenting with either satellite or in-transit metastases. Note that there is little difference between these two manifestations of intralymphatic metastases. (Reproduced from Buzaid AC et al, J Clin Oncol 1997;15:1039–1051. Used with permission.)

of clinical trials involving melanoma patients.[18,39,56,96,102–108] This powerful new staging technology has caused a significant stage migration that is now accounted for in this version of melanoma staging. In response to more precise nodal staging of melanoma patients using the technology of sentinel node biopsy, separate designations must be applied for patients who have clinical-radiologic staging of the regional lymph nodes as compared to the more accurate method of pathological staging using lymphatic mapping and sentinel lymphadenectomy.

Historically, the distinction between clinical staging and pathological staging of melanoma has not been emphasized because the definitions did not delineate any specific prognostic groups. With the widespread use of sentinel lymphadenectomy, the range of survival rates among various subgroups of pathological Stage III patients is enormous because of upstaging based on a direct examination of the sentinel lymph nodes by histopathologic exam.[7,85] Thus, significant differences were identified when survival rates for melanoma patients who were first clinically staged as having no evidence of nodal metastases were subsequently staged pathologically after either sentinel or elective node dissection (Table 12.9).[7,18,96,109] These survival differences were statistically significant among all T substages except for T4b (see Table 12.9). The differences were most striking in patients with clinical T2bN0M0, T3aN0M0, T3bN0M0, and T4aN0M0 disease. In this instance, 5-year survival rates for the clinically node-negative patients when staged

TABLE 12.9 Five-Year Survival Rates for 5346 Patients with Clinically Negative Nodal Metastases Who Were Pathologically Staged After Either RND or SLN

T Stage	Pathological Nodes (N)	5-Year Survival (% ± SEM)	P Value[a]
T1a	N− (379)	94 ± 2.0	0.0035
	N+ (15)	64 ± 17.7	
T1b	N− (319)	90 ± 2.5	0.0039
	N+ (18)	76 ± 14.9	
T2a	N− (1480)	94 ± 0.8	< 0.0001
	N+ (150)	73 ± 5.6	
T2b	N− (408)	83 ± 2.3	< 0.0001
	N+ (62)	56 ± 8.8	
T3a	N− (808)	86 ± 1.6	< 0.0001
	N+ (177)	59 ± 6.0	
T3b	N− (639)	72 ± 2.1	< 0.0001
	N+ (176)	49 ± 4.5	
T4a	N− (203)	75 ± 3.9	0.0116
	N+ (66)	61 ± 7.4	
T4b	N− (330)	53 ± 3.1	0.2403
	N+ (116)	44 ± 5.5	

RND, regional lymph node dissection; SEM, standard error of the mean; SLN, sentinel lymphadenectomy.

[a] *P* value based on the comparison of survival curves using the log rank test.

From Balch C et al, J Clin Oncol 2001;19:3635–3648. Reprinted with permission.

on the basis of their pathological nodal status varied significantly with diminished survival ranging from 14% to 30% among clinically versus pathologically staged patients of equivalent T categories (see Table 12.9). These results highlight the compelling prognostic value of knowing the nodal status as identified by lymphatic mapping and sentinel lymphadenectomy in those situations in which accurate staging is important.

Clinical Stage III groupings rely on clinical or radiologic assessment of the regional lymph nodes. Clinical staging of nodal metastases is inherently difficult, especially with respect to assessing the number of metastatic nodes present. As a result, there are no subgroups of clinically staged patients with nodal or intralymphatic regional metastases. All are categorized as having clinical Stage III disease (see Table 12.2)

In contrast to clinical staging of regional metastases, there is greater accuracy (both qualitatively and quantitatively) in delineating distinctive prognostic subgroups within pathological Stage III using information from pathological examination of the regional lymph nodes after lymphadenectomy. The numerical classification for pathological staging requires that pathologists perform a careful examination of the surgically resected nodal basin and report on the actual number of nodal metastases identified.

TNM Criteria Patients with one metastatic node are categorized as N1, those with two to three metastatic nodes as N2, and those with ≥ four metastatic nodes as N3. Survival rates for these N subgroupings, including the impact of melanoma ulceration on survival and stage grouping, are shown in Figure 12.9. The staging process should also delineate the tumor burden of nodal metastases (microscopic or clinically occult nodal metastases vs macroscopic or clinically evident and pathologically confirmed metastatic deposits). The third most significant prognos-

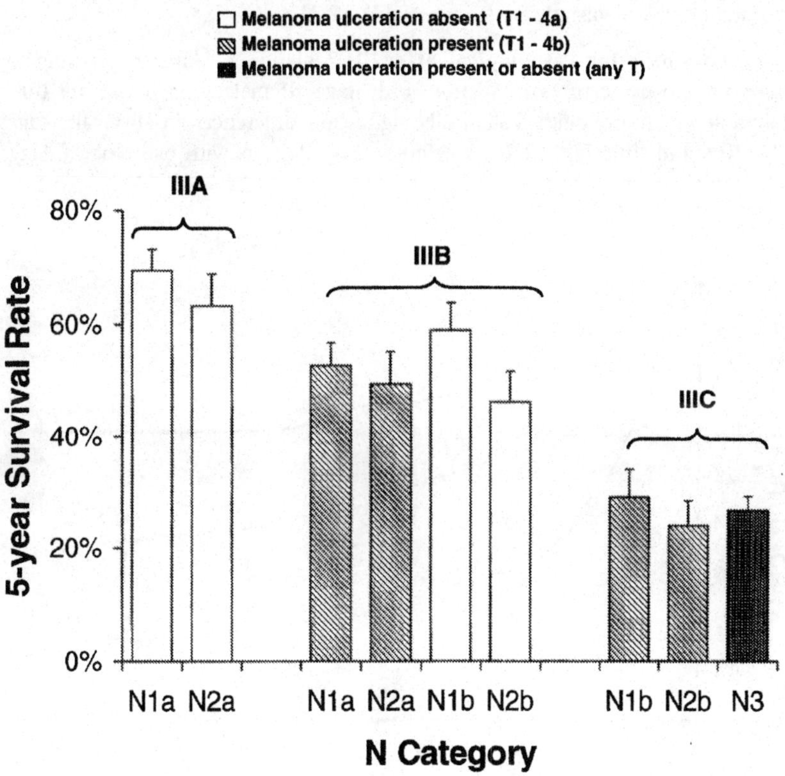

FIGURE 12.9 Five-year survival rates from the American Joint Commission on Cancer Melanoma Staging Database comparing the different N categories and the stage groupings for stage III melanoma. The survival results are significantly different when the primary melanoma is ulcerated as compared to equivalent N category of patients without ulceration. See Tables 12.1 and 12.2 for definitions. (From Balch C et al, J Clin Oncol 2001;19:3635–3648. Reprinted with permission.)

tic factor in defining pathological Stage III melanoma is the presence or absence of melanoma ulceration.[7] The AJCC Melanoma Staging Committee accounted for this by upstaging all Stage III patients by one substage when the primary melanoma was ulcerated. The survival correlation was remarkable when the stage subgroupings were analyzed using these definitions (Fig. 12.9; see Table 12.6). Intralymphatic metastases portend a poor prognosis (see Fig. 12.8). Therefore, both are assigned to a separate N2c classification in the absence of synchronous nodal metastases because both have a prognosis equivalent to multiple nodal metastases (see Tables 12.1 and 12.2). Furthermore, the available data demonstrate that patients with a combination of satellite-in-transit metastases *plus* nodal metastases have a worse outcome than do patients who experience either event alone. Thus, these patients were assigned to an N3 classification regardless of the number of synchronous metastatic nodes (see Table 12.2).[6]

Stage Grouping for Pathological Stage III Melanoma After accounting for these prognostic features in pathological Stage III melanoma, there are three definable subgroups with statistically significant differences in survival: Stages IIIA, IIIB, and IIIC (Fig. 12.10; see Table 12.6). Patients with pathological Stage

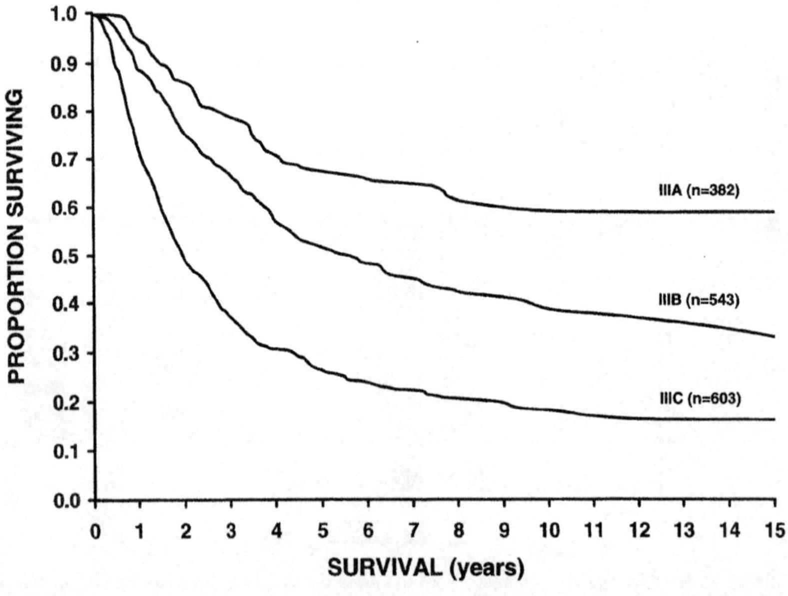

FIGURE 12.10 Fifteen-year survival curves for the stage groupings of patients with regional metastatic melanoma (Stage III). See Table 12.2 for the stage grouping definitions. Numbers of patients from the American Joint Commission on Cancer Melanoma Staging Database are shown in parentheses. The differences between the survival curves are significant ($P < 0.0001$). (From Balch C et al, J Clin Oncol 2001;19:3635–3648. Reprinted with permission.)

IIIA are only those who have one to three microscopic lymph node metastases (detected by sentinel or elective lymphadenectomy) and whose primary melanoma is not ulcerated (T1-4aN1aM0 or T1-4aN2aM0). The 5-year survival rate for such patients is 67% (see Figs. 12.9 and 12.10; see Table 12.6).

With respect to pathological Stages IIIB and IIIC, the final version of the melanoma staging criteria varies slightly from that originally proposed.[4] In the prior proposal for stage grouping, all patients with pathological evidence of lymph node metastases and an ulcerated melanoma would have been upstaged to N3 regardless of the number of metastatic nodes or the tumor burden, based on the published literature at that time.[4] However, the actual data analysis demonstrated that patients with one to three macroscopic lymph node metastases and a nonulcerated primary melanoma (i.e., T1-4aN1bM0 or T1-4aN2bM0) had approximately the same prognosis as those with one to three microscopic lymph node metastases and an ulcerated primary melanoma (T1-4bN1bM0 or T1-4bN2aM0; see Fig. 12.9 and Table 12.8).[7] In the final version, such patients are now grouped as pathological Stage IIIB melanoma, along with N2c patients (intralymphatic metastases without nodal metastases). The estimated 5-year survival for Stage IIIB patients is 53% (see Figs. 12.9 and 12.10 and Table 12.6). Patients grouped as Stage IIIC melanoma are defined as those with a one to three macroscopic lymph node metastases and an ulcerated primary melanoma (T1-4bN1bM0 or T1-4bN2bM0) or any patient with N3 disease regardless of T status or whether the nodal metastases are microscopic or macroscopic (see Table 12.2). The estimated 5-year survival rate for pathological Stage IIIC patients is significantly lower at 26% (see Table 12.6 and Figs. 12.9 and 12.10).

Data Recording Criteria Electronic data fields for melanoma should incorporate all the foregoing information for the primary melanoma. In addition, they should include the number of metastatic lymph nodes identified by the pathologist (of a total number of lymph nodes examined), the presence or absence of intralymphatic metastases (satellites or in-transits), and the intent of the surgical procedure that led to the detection of the nodal metastases (i.e., a therapeutic lymphadenectomy for clinically detectable metastatic lymph nodes or either a sentinel or elective lymphadenectomy that detected clinically occult metastases). The former defines macroscopic nodal disease, and the latter would define microscopic nodal disease. It is acknowledged that these terms are operational definitions simply used for communicating a level of tumor burden and are not intended to be used as a more strict definition of microscopic disease (i.e., that cannot be observed without a microscope). It is not necessary to measure the dimensions of the nodal metastases for the purposes of staging. Nevertheless, the extent of tumor involvement in a sentinel lymph node should be noted (and measured where possible) to examine whether future subgroups should account for this, as has been suggested by some investigators.[110]

With the availability of immunohistochemical staining, it is now possible to detect nodal metastases in tumors at a level of < 0.1 mm or even aggregates of a few cells.[108] The reverse transcriptase polymerase chain reaction technique may even be able to detect metastases not identified by the light microscope.[111–113] Such sophisticated detection procedures may be incorporated into future staging criteria but are not sufficiently available or standardized to warrant their inclusion at this time. Immunohistochemical staining does help to direct pathologists to suspicious areas and does help to distinguish melanoma cells from other cell types in a lymph node. Nevertheless, for the purposes of staging for nodal metastases, there must be histopathologic confirmation using standard hematoxylin and eosin staining.

PROGNOSIS AND STAGING OF DISTANT METASTASES (Stage IV)

Independent Prognostic Features

In all studies using a Cox regression analysis to assess prognosis in patients with distant metastases, the site of metastases, the number of metastatic sites, and elevated serum LDH levels were most predictive of poor survival.[114–118] In the AJCC Melanoma Staging Database, using various combinations of sites of metastases, the prognostic influence of different distant metastatic sites was analyzed in 1158 stage IV patients. The most significant differences were noted when visceral versus nonvisceral sites (i.e., skin, subcutaneous, distant lymph nodes) were compared. Although significant 1-year survival differences were observed when patients with lung metastases were compared to those patients with metastases in other visceral sites ($P < 0.0001$), no differences were noted when 2-year survival data were compared (Fig. 12.11).

Site of Distant Metastases Patients with distant metastasis in the skin, subcutaneous tissue, or distant lymph nodes have a relatively better prognosis than those patients with metastases located in any other anatomic site (see Fig. 12.11).[7,30,60,115,118,119] In several studies, patients with metastasis to lung had an "intermediate" prognosis as compared to skin and subcutaneous ("better prognosis") and all other visceral sites ("worse prognosis").[76,114,115]

Number of Distant Metastases The number of metastases at distant sites has previously been documented as an important prognostic factor.[30,60,115,118] However, this feature was not incorporated into the staging system, owing to the significant variability in the deployment of diagnostic tests to search comprehensively for distant metastases. These may range from a chest x-ray film in some centers to positron emission tomography scanning in others. Until the indications and types of tests used are better standardized, the number of metastases cannot reliably be used for staging purposes.

Elevated Serum LDH Elevated serum LDH was among the most predictive independent factors of diminished survival in all published studies when it was

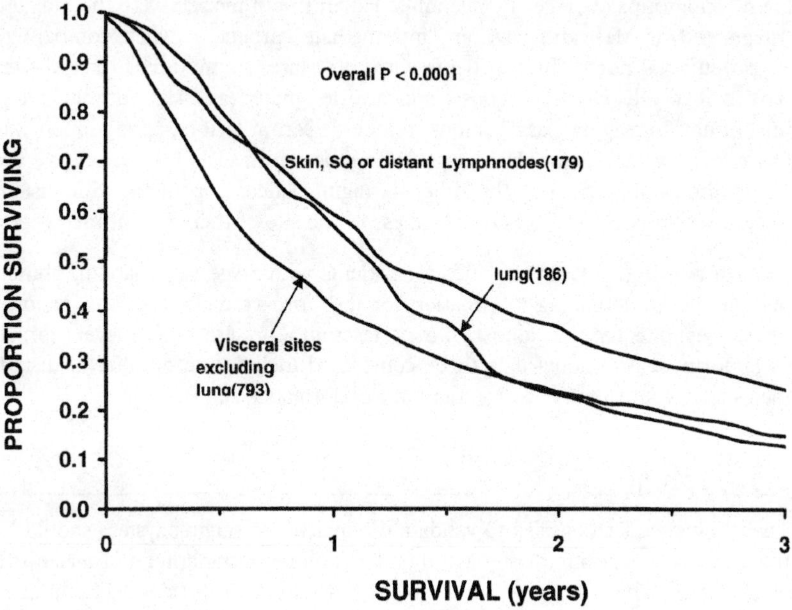

FIGURE 12.11 Survival curves of 1158 patients with metastatic melanomas at distant sites subgrouped into three categories or sites: skin, subcutaneous, or distant lymph nodes vs lung vs all other visceral sites. The number of patients is shown in parentheses. Note that the survival rate for patients with lung metastases is similar to that for nonvisceral sites for 1 year and then approaches that of other visceral sites after 2 years. Survival differences are significantly greater for skin, subcutaneous, or distant lymph node metastases than for lung metastases ($P = 0.003$) or other visceral sites of metastases ($P < 0.0001$). (Reproduced from Balch C et al, J Clin Oncol 2001;19:3622–3634. Used with permission.)

analyzed in a multivariate analysis, even after accounting for site and number of metastases.[116,117,120–123] Therefore, when the serum LDH is elevated past the upper limits of normal at the time of staging, affected patients with distant metastases are assigned to M1c regardless of the site of their distant metastases. The use of an elevated serum LDH should be used only when there are two or more determinations obtained more than 24 hours apart because an elevated serum LDH on a single determination can be falsely positive due to hemolysis or other factors unrelated to melanoma metastases.

TNM Staging

TNM Criteria In patients with distant metastases, the site of metastases and elevated serum LDH levels are used to delineate the M categories into three groups: M1a, M1b, and M1c, with 1-year survival rates ranging from 40% to 60%.[7] Because the survival differences between the M categories are small, there are no subgroups of Stage IV melanoma. Patients with metastasis to the lung are categorized as M1b and have an "intermediate" prognosis when comparing 1-year survival rates. Those patients with metastases to any other visceral sites have a relatively worse prognosis and are designated as M1c. Although it is uncommon in staging classifications to include serum factors, an exception was made for elevated serum LDH levels. When the serum LDH is elevated past the upper limits of normal at the time of staging, affected patients with distant metastases are assigned to M1c regardless of the site of their distant metastases.

Data Recording Electronic fields for patients with Stage IV melanoma should include all the foregoing information for the primary melanoma and regional metastases, plus the sites of distant metastases and the serum LDH level (normal vs abnormal). Additional data to be considered include the number of distant metastases, the patient's age, gender, and performance status.

DISCUSSION

The prognostic factors used to validate the melanoma staging system should be the primary stratification criteria and end-results reporting criteria of melanoma clinical trials. These differences were so great that the AJCC Melanoma Committee has strongly recommended that all patients with clinical T2N0M0, T3N0M0, and T4N0M0 melanomas have pathological nodal staging with sentinel lymphadenectomy prior to entry into melanoma clinical trials to ensure prognostic homogeneity within assigned treatment groups. In this way, investigators will be better able to discern between the impact of natural history and treatment when interpreting results of melanoma clinical trials. Moreover, the use of a consistent set of criteria will facilitate the comparability of melanoma clinical trials and thereby accelerate the progress of multidisciplinary melanoma treatment approaches. Understanding these differences in clinical outcome will be important not only in the design and analysis of melanoma clinical trials but in calibrating therapeutic intensity to metastatic risk. Indeed, some of the problems in interpreting and comparing past clinical trials involving melanoma has been the inability to account fully for the pathological differences in nodal status in a heterogeneous group of T3 and T4 patients: Some had pathological assessment of their regional nodes, whereas others had only clinical assessment.

This importance of accurate staging is best illustrated in Stage III patients, a group of patients who are presumed to be at particularly high risk for distant metastases and therefore should be entered into clinical trials involving very intensive forms of systemic therapy (e.g., biochemotherapy) with attendant morbidity and cost. However, this analysis clearly demonstrates that Stage III melanoma patients are a very heterogeneous group with respect to their risk for distant metastases and melanoma-specific mortality.[6,14,30,60,64,74,75,86–89,91,95,124] Many Stage III patients actually have a good prognosis (or intermediate risk for distant metastases). Patients with nodal metastases should not be considered as a homogeneous high-risk group, and recommendations to enter patients into intensive clinical trials should take into account the fact that some Stage III patients actually have a good prognosis (or intermediate risk for distant metastases). This was demonstrated by more than fivefold differences in 5-year survival rates for defined subgroups that ranged from 69% for patients who had nonulcerated melanomas (regardless of thickness) and a single clinically occult nodal metastasis (detected by sentinel or elective lymphadenectomy) to a low of 13% for patients with ulcerated melanomas (regardless of thickness) with four or more clinically apparent nodal metastases (detected by therapeutic lymphadenectomy).

Once a patient had progressed to Stage IV disease, survival rates were measured more in months than in years. Indeed, there was no prognostic feature in this analysis that substantially separated survival rates by more than a few months, and only a minority of Stage IV patients survived beyond 1 year.[76,114,115,117,118,122] In general, the only Stage IV patients who live beyond 1 or 2 years are those who have limited disease and have had a complete surgical resection of the distant metastases.[115,125–128] Whether the long-term results reflect a more favorable biology of disease or a therapeutic benefit of surgery (or a combination of the two) is a difficult issue to address in the absence of any randomized trials.

It is evident that the next phase of staging melanoma will evolve as new technology allows clinicians to diagnose metastatic melanoma reliably at a level of tumor burden well short of that achievable with the light microscope or routine x-ray films. These include molecular diagnostic approaches, such as reverse transcriptase polymerase chain reaction, to detect relevant gene expression, positron emission tomography scanning, use of anti–melanoma antibodies, and serum markers of tumor-related DNA and RNA species that will more accurately detect and stage metastatic melanoma.[111–113,120,129–132] Some of these advances will no doubt be incorporated into subsequent revisions of the melanoma staging system.

APPENDIX

The following institutions, organizations, and cancer cooperative groups generously contributed their patient database for the AJCC prognostic factors study described in the chapter. The clinician or biostatistician who contributed the database is listed in parenthesis.

- Sydney Melanoma Unit, Royal Prince Alfred Hospital (John F. Thompson, MD; Marjorie Colman, BSc)
- University of Texas M.D. Anderson Cancer Center (Jeffrey E. Gershenwald, MD; Merrick I. Ross, MD)
- Memorial Sloan Kettering Cancer Center (Daniel G. Coit, MD)
- University of Alabama at Birmingham Cancer Center (Marshall Urist, MD; Seng-Jaw Soong, PhD; Rene Desmond, PhD)

- University of South Florida–Moffitt Cancer Center (Douglas S. Reintgen, MD; Gary Lyman, MD)
- National Tumor Institute, Milan (Natale Cascinelli, MD; Aberto Morabito, PhD)
- University of Washington Cancer Center (David Byrd, MD)
- Eastern Cooperative Oncology Group (John M. Kirkwood MD; Michael B. Atkins, MD)
- Southwest Oncology Group (John A. Thompson, MD; Ping-Yu Liu, PhD)
- Intergroup Melanoma Surgical Trial (Charles M. Balch, MD; Seng-Jaw Soong, PhD; Renee Desmond, PhD)
- World Health Organization Melanoma Program (Natale Cascinelli, MD; Aberto Morabito, PhD)
- Sunbelt Melanoma Group (Kelly M. McMasters, MD; Patricia B. Cerrito, PhD)

REFERENCES

1. Balch CM, Murad TM, Soong SJ et al. A multifactorial analysis of melanoma: prognostic histopathological features comparing Clark's and Breslow's staging methods. Ann Surg 1978;188:732–742.
2. Eldh J BB, Peterson LE. Prognostic factors in cutaneous malignant melanoma in Stage I. A clinical, morphological and multivariate analysis. Scand J Plast Reconstr Surg Hand Surg 1978; 12:243–255.
3. Van Der Esch EP, Cascinelli N, Preda F et al. Stage I melanoma of the skin: evaluation of prognosis according to histologic characteristics. Cancer 1981;48:1668–1673.
4. Balch CM, Buzaid AC, Atkins MB et al. A new American Joint Committee on Cancer staging system for cutaneous melanoma. Cancer 2000;88:1484–1491.
5. Balch C, Buzaid AC, Soong SJ et al. Final version of the American Joint Committee on Cancer staging system for cutaneous melanoma. J Clin Oncol 2001;19:3635–3648.
6. Buzaid AC, Ross MI, Balch CM et al. Critical analysis of the current American Joint Committee on Cancer staging system for cutaneous melanoma and proposal of a new staging system [see comments]. J Clin Oncol 1997;15:1039–1051.
7. Balch C, Soong SJ, Gershenwald JE et al. Prognostic factors analysis of 17,600 melanoma patients. Validation of the American Joint Committee on Cancer melanoma staging system. J Clin Oncol 2001;19:3622–3634.
8. Breslow A. Thickness, cross-sectional areas and depth of invasion in the prognosis of cutaneous melanoma. Ann Surg 1970;172:902–908.
9. Breslow A. Tumor thickness, level of invasion and node dissection in stage I cutaneous melanoma. Ann Surg 1975;182:572–575.
10. Breslow A. Problems in the measurement of tumor thickness and level of invasion in cutaneous melanoma. Hum Pathol 1977;8:1–2.
11. Breslow A, Macht SD. Evaluation of prognosis in Stage I cutaneous melanoma. Plast Reconstr Surg 1978;61:342–346.
12. Breslow A. Tumor thickness in evaluating prognosis of cutaneous melanoma [letter]. Ann Surg 1978;187:440.
13. Balch CM, Soong SJ, Murad TM et al. A multifactorial analysis of melanoma: II. Prognostic factors in patients with stage I (localized) melanoma. Surgery 1979;86:343–351.

14. Balch CM, Soong SJ, Milton GW et al. A comparison of prognostic factors and surgical results in 1,786 patients with localized (stage I) melanoma treated in Alabama, USA, and New South Wales, Australia. Ann Surg 1982;196:677–684.

15. Urist MM, Balch CM, Soong SJ et al. Head and neck melanoma in 534 clinical Stage I patients. A prognostic factors analysis and results of surgical treatment. Ann Surg 1984;200:769–775.

16. Cascinelli N, Marubini E, Morabito A et al. Prognostic factors for stage I melanoma of the skin: a review. Stat Med 1985;4:265–278.

17. Essner R, Conforti A, Kelley MC et al. Efficacy of lymphatic mapping, sentinel lymphadenectomy, and selective complete lymph node dissection as a therapeutic procedure for early-stage melanoma [see comments]. Ann Surg Oncol 1999;6:442–449.

18. Gershenwald JE, Thompson W, Mansfield PF et al. Multi-institutional melanoma lymphatic mapping experience: the prognostic value of sentinel lymph node status in 612 stage I or II melanoma patients. J Clin Oncol 1999;17:976–983.

19. Balch CM, Wilkerson JA, Murad TM et al. The prognostic significance of ulceration of cutaneous melanoma. Cancer 1980;45:3012–3017.

20. Soong SJ, Shaw HM, Balch CM et al. Predicting survival and recurrence in localized melanoma: a multivariate approach. World J Surg 1992;16:191–195.

21. Buttner P, Garbe C, Bertz J et al. Primary cutaneous melanoma. Optimized cutoff points of tumor thickness and importance of Clark's level for prognostic classification. Cancer 1995;75: 2499–2506.

22. Meyskens FL, Berdeaux DH, Parks B et al. Cutaneous malignant melanoma (Arizona Cancer Center experience): I. Natural history and prognostic factors influencing survival in patients with stage I disease. Cancer 1988;62:1207–1214.

23. Averbook BJ, Russo LJ, Mansour EG. A long-term analysis of 620 patients with malignant melanoma at a major referral center. Surgery 1998;124:746–756.

24. Sondergaard K. Depth of invasion and tumor thickness in primary cutaneous malignant melanoma. A study of 2012 cases. Acta Pathol Microbiol Immunol Scand A 1985;93:49–55.

25. Thorn M, Ponten F, Bergstrom R et al. Clinical and histopathologic predictors of survival in patients with malignant melanoma: a population-based study in Sweden. J Natl Cancer Inst 1994;86:761–769.

26. Kuehnl-Petzoldt C, Wiebelt H, Berger H. Prognostic groups of patients with stage I melanoma. Arch Dermatol 1983;119:816–819.

27. Wanebo HJ, Cooper PH, Young DV et al. Prognostic factors in head and neck melanoma. Effect of lesion location. Cancer 1988;62:831–837.

28. Schuchter L, Schultz DJ, Synnestvedt M et al. A prognostic model for predicting 10-year survival in patients with primary melanoma. Ann Intern Med 1996;125:369–375.

29. Ostmeier H, Fuchs B, Otto F et al. Can immunohistochemical markers and mitotic rate improve prognostic precision in patients with primary melanoma? Cancer 1999;85:2391–2399.

30. Balch CM. Cutaneous melanoma: prognosis and treatment results worldwide. Semin Surg Oncol 1992;8:400–414.

31. Masback A, Westerdahl J, Ingvar C et al. Cutaneous malignant melanoma in southern Sweden 1965, 1975, and 1985. Prognostic factors and histologic correlations. Cancer 1997;79:275–283.

32. Sahin S, Rao B, Kopf AW et al. Predicting ten-year survival of patients with primary cutaneous melanoma: corroboration of a prognostic model. Cancer 1997;80:1426–1431.

33. Shaw HM, Balch CM, Soong SJ et al. Prognostic histopathological factors in malignant melanoma. Pathology 1985;17:271–274.

34. Soong SJ, Harrison RA, McCarthy WH et al. Factors affecting survival following local, regional, or distant recurrence from localized melanoma. J Surg Oncol 1998;67:228–233.

35. Haffner AC, Garbe C, Burg G et al. The prognosis of primary and metastasising melanoma. An evaluation of the TNM classification in 2,495 patients. Br J Cancer 1992;66:856–861.

36. Haddad FF, Stall A, Messina J et al. The progression of melanoma nodal metastasis is dependent on tumor thickness of the primary lesion. Ann Surg Oncol 1999;6:144–149.

37. Day CLJ, Mihm MCJ, Lew RA et al. Prognostic factors for patients with clinical stage I melanoma of intermediate thickness (1.51–3.39 mm). A conceptual model for tumor growth and metastasis. Ann Surg 1982;195:35–43.

38. McGovern VJ, Shaw HM, Milton GW et al. Prognostic significance of the histological features of malignant melanoma. Histopathology 1979;3:385–393.

39. Wagner JD, Gordon MS, Chuang TY et al. Predicting sentinel and residual lymph node basin disease after sentinel lymph node biopsy for melanoma. Cancer 2000;89:453–462.

40. Straume O, Akslen LA. Independent prognostic importance of vascular invasion in nodular melanomas. Cancer 1996;78:1211–1219.

41. Balch CM, Soong S-j, Ross MI et al. Long-term results of a multi-institutional randomized trial comparing prognostic factors and surgical results for intermediate thickness melanomas (1.0 to 4.0 mm.). Ann Surg Oncol 2000;7:87–97.

42. Keefe M, Mackie RM. The relationship between risk of death from clinical stage I cutaneous melanoma and thickness of primary tumour: no evidence for steps in risk. Br J Cancer 1991; 64:598–602.

43. Karakousis CP, Emrich LJ, Rao U. Tumor thickness and prognosis in clinical stage I malignant melanoma. Cancer 1989;64:1432–1436.

44. Day CL Jr, Lew RA, Mihm MC Jr et al. The natural break points for primary-tumor thickness in clinical Stage I melanoma. N Engl J Med 1981;305:1155.

45. Balch CM, Murad TM, Soong SJ et al. Tumor thickness as a guide to surgical management of clinical stage I melanoma patients. Cancer 1979;43:883–888.

46. McGovern VJ, Shaw HM, Milton GW et al. Ulceration and prognosis in cutaneous malignant melanoma. Histopathology 1982;6:399–407.

47. Lock-Andersen J, Hou-Jensen K, Hansen JP et al. Observer variation in histological classification of cutaneous malignant melanoma. Scand J Plast Reconstr Surg Hand Surg 1995;29:141–148.

48. Corona R, Mele A, Amini M et al. Interobserver variability on the histopathologic diagnosis of cutaneous melanoma and other pigmented skin lesions. J Clin Oncol 1996;14:1218–1223.

49. Larsen TE, Little JH, Orell SR et al. International pathologists congruence survey on quantitation of malignant melanoma. Pathology 1980;12:245–253.

50. Heenan PJ, Matz LR, Blackwell JB et al. Inter-observer variation between pathologists in the classification of cutaneous malignant melanoma in western Australia. Histopathology 1984;8: 717–729.

51. Vollmer R. Malignant melanoma. A multivariate analysis of prognostic factors. Pathol Annu 1989; 24:383–407.

52. Balch CM, Soong SJ, Bartolucci AA et al. Efficacy of an elective regional lymph node dissection of 1 to 4 mm thick melanomas for patients 60 years of age and younger. Ann Surg 1996;224: 255–263 [discussion 263–266].

53. Balch CM, Urist MM, Karakousis CP et al. Efficacy of 2-cm surgical margins for intermediate-thickness melanomas (1 to 4 mm). Results of a multi-institutional randomized surgical trial [see comments]. Ann Surg 1993;218:262–267 [discussion 267–269].

54. Heaton KM, Sussman JJ, Gershenwald JE et al. Surgical margins and prognostic factors in patients with thick (> 4 mm) primary melanoma. Ann Surg Oncol 1998;5:322–328.

55. Kim SH, Garcia C, Rodriguez J et al. Prognosis of thick cutaneous melanoma. J Am Coll Surg 1999;188:241–247.

56. Mraz-Gernhard S, Sagebiel RW, Kashani-Sabet M et al. Prediction of sentinel lymph node micrometastasis by histological features in primary cutaneous malignant melanoma. Arch Derm 1998; 134:983–987.

57. Marghoob AA, Koenig K, Bittencourt FV et al. Breslow thickness and Clark level in melanoma: support for including level in pathology reports and in American Joint Committee on Cancer Staging [see comments]. Cancer 2000;88:589–595.

58. MacKie RM, Aitchison T, Sirel JM et al. Prognostic models for subgroups of melanoma patients from the Scottish Melanoma Group database 1979–86, and their subsequent validation. Br J Cancer 1995;71:173–176.

59. Day CL Jr, Lew RA, Harrist TJ. Malignant melanoma prognostic factors 4: ulceration width. J Dermatol Surg Oncol 1984;10:23–24.

60. Balch CM, Soong SJ, Murad TM et al. A multifactorial analysis of melanoma: III. Prognostic factors in melanoma patients with lymph node metastases (stage II). Ann Surg 1981;193:377–388.

61. Clark WH Jr, From L, Bernardino EA, Mihm MC. The histogenesis and biological behavior of primary human malignant melanoma of the skin. Cancer Res 1969;29:705–727.

62. Prade M, Sancho-Garnier H, Cesarini JP et al. Difficulties encountered in the application of Clark classification and the Breslow thickness measurement in cutaneous malignant melanoma. Int J Cancer 1980;26:159–163.

63. Mansson-Brahme E, Carstensen J, Erhardt K et al. Prognostic factors in thin cutaneous malignant melanoma. Cancer 1994;73:2324–2332.

64. Morton DL, Davtyan DG, Wanek LA et al. Multivariate analysis of the relationship between survival and the microstage of primary melanoma by Clark level and Breslow thickness. Cancer 1993;71:3737–3743.

65. Finley JW, Gibbs JF, Rodriguez LM et al. Pathologic and clinical features influencing outcome of thin cutaneous melanoma: correlation with newly proposed staging system. Am Surg 2000; 66:527–531 [discussion 531–532].

66. Salman SM, Rogers GS. Prognostic factors in thin cutaneous malignant melanoma [see comments]. J Dermatol Surg Oncol 1990;16:413–418.

67. Kelly JW, Sagebiel RW, Clyman S, Blois MS. Thin level IV malignant melanoma. Ann Surg 1985; 202:98–103.

68. Shaw HM, McCarthy WH, McCarthy SW et al. Thin malignant melanomas and recurrence potential. Arch Surg 1987;122:1147–1150.

69. Austin PF, Cruse CW, Lyman G et al. Age as a prognostic factor in the malignant melanoma population. Ann Surg Oncol 1994;1:487–494.

70. Cohen HJ, Cox E, Manton K et al. Malignant melanoma in the elderly. J Clin Oncol 1987;5: 100–106.

71. Austin PF, Cruse CW, Lyman G et al. Age as a prognostic factor in the malignant melanoma population. Ann Surg Oncol 1994;1:487–494.

72. Loggie B, Ronan SG, Bean J et al. Invasive cutaneous melanoma in elderly patients. Arch Dermatol 1991;127:1188–1193.

73. Shaw HM, McGovern VJ, Milton GW et al. The female superiority in survival in clinical stage II cutaneous malignant melanoma. Cancer 1982;49:1941–1944.

74. Kirkwood JM, Ibrahim JG, Sondak VK et al. High- and low-dose interferon alfa-2b in high-risk melanoma: first analysis of intergroup trial E1690/S9111/C9190. J Clin Oncol 2000;18: 2444–2458.

75. Kirkwood JM, Strawderman MH, Ernstoff MS et al. Interferon alfa-2b adjuvant therapy of high-risk resected cutaneous melanoma: the Eastern Cooperative Oncology Group Trial EST 1684 [see comments]. J Clin Oncol 1996;14:7–17.

76. Manola J, Atkins M, Ibrahim J et al. Prognostic factors in metastatic melanoma: a pooled analysis of Eastern Cooperative Oncology Group trials [in process citation]. J Clin Oncol 2000;18: 3782–3793.

77. NCI Fact Book. Bethesda, MD: National Cancer Institute, 2000.

78. Cascinelli N, Zurrida S, Galimberti V et al. Acral lentiginous melanoma. A histological type without prognostic significance. J Dermatol Surg Oncol 1994;20:817–822.

79. McGovern VJ, Shaw HM, Milton GW et al. Is malignant melanoma arising in a Hutchinson's melanotic freckle a separate disease entity? Histopathology 1980;4:235–242.

80. Kuchelmeister C, Schaumburg-Lever G, Garbe C. Acral cutaneous melanoma in Caucasians: clinical features, histopathology and prognosis in 112 patients. Br J Dermatol 2000;143:275–280.

81. Slingluff CL Jr, Vollmer R, Seigler HF. Acral melanoma: a review of 185 patients with identification of prognostic variables. J Surg Oncol 1990;45:91–98.

82. Garbe CBP, Bertz J et al. Primary cutaneous melanoma: prognostic classification of anatomic location. Cancer 1995;75:2492.

83. Carlson J, Dickersin GR, Sober AJ et al. Desmoplastic neurotropic melanoma. Cancer 1995;75: 478.

84. Quinn MJ, Crotty KA, Thompson JF et al. Desmoplastic and desmoplastic neurotropic melanoma: experience with 280 patients. Cancer 1998;83:1128–1135.

85. Morton DL, Wanek L, Nizze JA et al. Improved long-term survival after lymphadenectomy of melanoma metastatic to regional nodes. Analysis of prognostic factors in 1134 patients from the John Wayne Cancer Clinic. Ann Surg 1991;214:491–499 [discussion 499–501].

86. Buzaid AC, Tinoco LA, Jendiroba D et al. Prognostic value of size of lymph node metastases in patients with cutaneous melanoma. J Clin Oncol 1995;13:2361–2368.

87. Coit DG, Rogatko A, Brennan MF. Prognostic factors in patients with melanoma metastatic to axillary or inguinal lymph nodes. A multivariate analysis. Ann Surg 1991;214:627–636.

88. Koh HK, Sober AJ, Day CL Jr et al. Prognosis of clinical stage I melanoma patients with positive elective regional node dissection. J Clin Oncol 1986;4:1238–1244.

89. Drepper H, Biess B, Hofherr B et al. The prognosis of patients with stage III melanoma. Cancer 1993;71:1239–1246.

90. Cascinelli N, Vaglini M, Nava M et al. Prognosis of skin melanoma with regional node metastases (stage II). Surg Oncol 1984;25:240–247.

91. Slingluff CL Jr, Vollmer R, Seigler HF. Stage II malignant melanoma: presentation of a prognostic model and an assessment of specific active immunotherapy in 1,273 patients. J Surg Oncol 1988;39:139–147.

92. Karakousis CP, Hena MA, Emrich LJ et al. Axillary node dissection in malignant melanoma: results and complications. Surgery 1990;108:10–17.

93. Kissin MW, Simpson DA, Easton D et al. Prognostic factors related to survival and groin recurrence following therapeutic lymph node dissection for lower limb malignant melanoma. Br J Surg 1987;74:1023–1026.

94. Roses DF, Provet JA, Harris MN et al. Prognosis of patients with pathologic stage II cutaneous malignant melanoma. Ann Surg 1985;201:103–107.

95. Calabro A, Singletary SE, Balch CM. Patterns of relapse in 1001 consecutive patients with melanoma nodal metastases. Arch Surg 1989;124:1051–1055.

96. Gershenwald JE, Prieto V, Colome-Grimmer MI et al. The prognostic significance of microscopic tumor burden in 925 melanoma patients undergoing sentinel lymph node biopsy. Proc Am Soc Clin Oncol 2000;19:551a.

97. Cascinelli N, Belli F, Santinami M et al. Sentinel lymph node biopsy in cutaneous melanoma: the WHO Melanoma Program experience [in process citation]. Ann Surg Oncol 2000;7:469–474.

98. Cascinelli N, Bufalino R, Marolda R et al. Regional non-nodal metastases of cutaneous melanoma. Eur J Surg Oncol 1986;12:175–180.

99. Day CJ, Harrist T, Gorstein F et al. Malignant melanoma: prognostic significance of "microscopic satellites" in the reticular dermis and subcutaneous fat. Ann Surg 194:108–112, 1981

100. Leon P, Daly JM, Synnestvedt M et al. The prognostic implications of microscopic satellites in patients with clinical stage I melanoma. Arch Surg 126:1461–1468, 1991

101. Harrist T, Rigel D, Day Jr. C et al. "Microscopic satellites" are more highly associated with regional lymph node metastases than with primary melanoma thickness. Cancer 1984;53:2183–2187.

102. Morton DL, Thompson JF, Essner R et al. Validation of the accuracy of intraoperative lymphatic mapping and sentinel lymphadenectomy for early-stage melanoma: a multicenter trial. Multicenter Selective Lymphadenectomy Trial Group. Ann Surg 1999;230:453–463 [discussion 463–465].

103. Morton DL, Chan AD. Current status of intraoperative lymphatic mapping and sentinel lymphadenectomy for melanoma: Is it standard of care? J Am Coll Surg 1999;189:214–223.

104. Gershenwald JE, Tseng CH, Thompson W et al. Improved sentinel lymph node localization in patients with primary melanoma with the use of radiolabeled colloid. Surgery 1998;124:203–210.

105. Gershenwald JE, Mansfield PF, Lee JE, Ross MI. The role for lymphatic mapping and sentinel lymph node biopsy in patients with thick (> 4 mm) primary melanoma. Ann Surg Oncol 2000; 7:160–165.

106. O'Brien CJ, Uren RF, Thompson JF et al. Prediction of potential metastatic sites in cutaneous head and neck melanoma using lymphoscintigraphy. Am J Surg 1995;170:461–466.

107. Pu LL, Cruse CW, Wells KE et al. Lymphatic mapping and sentinel lymph node biopsy in patients with melanoma of the lower extremity [see comments]. Plast Reconstr Surg 1999;104:964–969.

108. Yu LL, Flotte TJ, Tanabe KK et al. Detection of microscopic melanoma metastases in sentinel lymph nodes. Cancer 1999;86:617–627.

109. Gershenwald JE, Colome MI, Lee JE et al. Patterns of recurrence following a negative sentinel lymph node biopsy in 243 patients with stage I or II melanoma. J Clin Oncol 1998;16:2253–2260.

110. Wagner JD, Davidson D, Coleman JJ 3rd et al. Lymph node tumor volumes in patients undergoing sentinel lymph node biopsy for cutaneous melanoma. Ann Surg Oncol 1999;6:398–404.

111. van der Velde-Zimmermann D, Schipper ME, de Weger RA et al. Sentinel node biopsies in melanoma patients: a protocol for accurate, efficient, and cost-effective analysis by preselection for immunohistochemistry on the basis of Tyr-PCR. Ann Surg Oncol 2000;7:51–54.

112. Van der Velde-Zimmermann D, Roijers JF, Bouwens-Rombouts A et al. Molecular test for the detection of tumor cells in blood and sentinel nodes of melanoma patients. Am J Pathol 1996; 149:759–764.

113. Shivers SC, Wang X, Li W et al. Molecular staging of malignant melanoma: correlation with clinical outcome. JAMA 1998;280:1410–1415.

114. Balch CM, Soong S-J, Murad TM et al. A multifactorial analysis of melanoma: IV. Prognostic factors in 200 melanoma patients with distant metastases (stage III). J Clin Oncol 1983;1: 126–134.

115. Barth A, Wanek LA, Morton DL. Prognostic factors in 1,521 melanoma patients with distant metastases. J Am Coll Surg 1995;181:193–201.

116. Keilholz U, Conradt C, Legha SS et al. Results of interleukin-2-based treatment in advanced melanoma: a case record-based analysis of 631 patients. J Clin Oncol 1998;16:2921–2929.

117. Eton O, Legha SS, Moon TE et al. Prognostic factors for survival of patients treated systemically for disseminated melanoma. J Clin Oncol 1998;16:1103–1111.

118. Brand CU, Ellwanger U, Stroebel W et al. Prolonged survival of 2 years or longer for patients with disseminated melanoma. Cancer 1997;79:2345–2353.

119. Bowen GM, Chang AE, Lowe L et al. Solitary melanoma confined to the dermal and/or subcutaneous tissue: evidence for revisiting the staging classification [in process citation]. Arch Dermatol 2000;136:1397–1399.

120. Deichmann M, Benner A, Bock M et al. S100-Beta, melanoma-inhibiting activity, and lactate dehydrogenase discriminate progressive from nonprogressive American Joint Committee on Cancer stage IV melanoma. J Clin Oncol 1999;17:1891–1896.

121. Franzke A, Probst-Kepper M, Buer J et al. Elevated pretreatment serum levels of soluble vascular cell adhesion molecule 1 and lactate dehydrogenase as predictors of survival in cutaneous metastatic malignant melanoma. Br J Cancer 1998;78:40–45.

122. Sirott MN BD, Wong GYC, Tao YT et al. Prognostic factors in patients with metastatic malignant melanoma. A multivariate analysis. Cancer 1993;72:3091–3098.

123. Agrawal S, Yao T-J, Coit DG. Surgery for melanoma metastatic to the gastrointestinal tract. Annals of Surgical Oncology 1999;6:336–344.

124. Bevilacqua RG, Coit DG, Rogatko A et al. Axillary dissection in melanoma: prognostic variables in node-positive patients. Ann Surg 1990;212:125–131.

125. Balch C. Surgical treatment of advanced melanoma. In: Balch C, Houghton AN, Sober AJ, Soong S-J, eds. Cutaneous Melanoma. St. Louis: Quality Medical Press, 1998:373–388.

126. Ollila DW, Hsueh EC, Stern SL et al. Metastasectomy for recurrent stage IV melanoma. J Surg Oncol 1999;71:209–213.

127. Wong JH, Skinner KA, Kim KA et al. The role of surgery in the treatment of nonregionally recurrent melanoma. Surgery 1993;113:389–394.

128. Eton O, Legha SS, Moon TE et al. Prognostic factors for survival of patients treated systemically for disseminated melanoma. J Clin Oncol 1998;16:1103–1111.

129. Bostick PJ, Morton DL, Turner RR et al. Prognostic significance of occult metastases detected by sentinel lymphadenectomy and reverse transcriptase–polymerase chain reaction in early-stage melanoma patients. J Clin Oncol 1999;17:3238–3244.

130. Curry BJ, Farrelly M, Hersey P. Evaluation of S-100 beta assays for the prediction of recurrence and prognosis in patients with AJCC stage I-III melanoma. Melanoma Res 1999;9:557–567.

131. Kelley MC, Ollila DW, Morton DL. Lymphatic mapping and sentinel lymphadenectomy for melanoma. Semin Surg Oncol 1998;14:283–290.

132. von Schoultz E, Hansson LO, Djureen E et al. Prognostic value of serum analyses of S-100 beta protein in malignant melanoma. Melanoma Res 1996;6:133–137.

Chapter 13.1

Prevention of Cervical Cancer: Chemoprevention

Hakan Akbulut

Albert Deisseroth

Cervical cancer is the third most common cancer in women worldwide and is a major cause of overall mortality among young women in developing countries.[1] By the end of 2001, approximately 12,900 new cases of cervical cancer and 4400 deaths from this cancer are estimated to occur in the United States.[2] Since the introduction of regular gynecologic examinations and screening Papanicolaou (Pap) smear tests, the incidence and mortality of cervical cancer have decreased in developed countries,[3] although for the last decade, the decline in incidence and mortality in those countries has begun to reverse.[3,4] Meanwhile, the prognosis of cervical cancer patients is somewhat better than that for patients with most other solid tumors because of screening programs. Patients with early-stage disease have 5-year survival rates of approximately 80%,[5,6] whereas this rate in patients with advanced disease does not exceed 10%. Currently, no efficient methods exist for treating the cancer in this group of patients.

The screening programs are useful not only for making an early diagnosis of cancer but also for identifying premalignant lesions that carry high potential for cervical cancer. Since the term *carcinoma in situ* (CIS) for premalignant lesions was first introduced almost 100 years ago, the spectrum of cervical mucosal abnormalities leading to invasive cervical cancer has been well defined. The precursor lesions vary from mild to severe dysplasia and CIS. Richart's term,[7] *cervical intraepithelial neoplasia* (CIN), refers to all lesions representing different stages of the same disease process for cervical cancer. The simplicity of the CIN terminology, classified as CIN1–CIN3 and representing the degree of dysplasia (from mild to severe) and CIS, has led to its wide use in clinical trials. The Bethesda System for Reporting Cervical/Vaginal Cytological Diagnoses classifies the lesions as *low-grade squamous intraepithelial lesions*, which are equivalent to CIN1, or *high-grade squamous intraepithelial lesions*, including the CIN2–CIN3 and CIS lesions.[8] Abnormalities that do not fulfill the criteria for squamous intraepithelial lesions are defined as *atypical squamous cells of undetermined significance*. Although this new system has been used widely for the reporting of Pap test results, it is not used widely in clinical prevention trials.

Although previously reported studies on cervical dysplasia demonstrate a degree of selection bias, misclassification of cytopathologic findings, and neglect of some of the known important risk factors, they have shed light on the natural history of the disease. Mild and moderate dysplasias (CIN1 and CIN2) usually regress. The spontaneous regression rates for mild dysplasia within 5 years vary between 30% and 90%, whereas the regression rates for moderately dysplastic lesions vary between 20% and 54%.[9–12] CIN3 and CIS lesions generally tend to progress.

The well-known precursor lesions, the ease with which the organ can be examined, and the known role of these lesions in the development of cancer have made cervical cancer a good candidate for chemoprevention. Nonetheless, since the first trial more than 20 years ago, no important advances have been achieved. The potential for success of chemoprevention is tightly linked to the mechanisms of carcinogenesis. As the carcinogenic mechanisms of cervical cancer become better understood, new, more effective drugs will be available for clinical chemoprevention trials. In this chapter, the current status of chemoprevention in cervical cancer is reviewed.

RISK FACTORS

Various carcinogenic agents, including chemical, physical, and viral, target the genetic material of the cell during carcinogenesis. As a consequence of genetic changes, the proliferative and differentiating control of normal cervical mucosal cells is disrupted. For most cancers, the etiologic agent and exact mechanism of carcinogenesis is not fully understood, although some risk factors are usually known. Many risk factors have also been reported for cervical cancer.

The well-known strong risk factors for cervical cancer include early age at first intercourse ($\leq$ 16 years), a high lifetime number of sexual partners, a history of genital human papillomavirus (HPV) infection or other sexually transmitted diseases, the presence of other genital tract neoplasia, and prior squamous intraepithelial lesions.[13,14] A number of less relevant risk factors for cervical cancer, including smoking, immunodeficiency, poor nutrition, human immunodeficiency virus positivity, HPV antibody positivity, intercourse with a sexual partner having risk factors for sexually transmitted disease, long-term use of oral contraceptives, and grand multiparity, have also been reported.[14–16] Although recent findings suggest that HPV is a causative agent for cervical cancer, a small number of patients without documented HPV positivity exist, and the small incidence of cancer as contrasted to the high incidence of HPV infection raises the possibility that the aforementioned risk factors are cofactors. However, recent epidemiological data show that most of the previously well-known risk factors are important for HPV-induced cervical carcinogenesis.[17]

Genital HPV infection is one of the most common sexually transmitted diseases. Up to 90% of abnormal cell changes in Pap smears are reportedly related to HPV.[18,19] As mentioned earlier, whereas most of the low-grade squamous intraepithelial lesions (CIN1)—the most common cytopathologic manifestations of cervical HPV infection—generally regress spontaneously over time, high-grade squamous intraepithelial lesions (CIN2–3) usually persist and may lead to invasive cancer. However, the reasons for development of high-grade squamous intraepithelial lesions and progression to cancer in HPV-infected women are as yet unclear. Among the more than 100 genotypes of HPV, types 16, 18, 31, 33, 35, 39, 45, 51, 52, 56, 58, 59, and 68 are classified as high-risk viruses, and infections with these types of HPV are most likely to progress to cancer.[20,21] HPV16 is the most prevalent type in CIN2–3 and invasive cancers,[21–23] but it is also the most common type found in women with normal cytologic findings.[21]

CERVICAL CARCINOGENESIS

HPV Infection as the First Step

HPV is now accepted as the primary etiologic agent for cervical cancer. In conjunction with the epidemiological studies that demonstrate the close relationships between HPV infections and cervical cancer, the data on HPV DNA integrated to the cancer cell genome lend strength to the plausibility of HPV's etiologic role.[24,25] The prevalence of HPV DNA, though dependent on the method used, has been as high as 20%–50% among young women between the ages of 20 to 25.[25,26] The cohort studies have shown that cervical HPV DNA detection declines with age.[27] However, the antibodies against HPV particles increase with age, which indirectly indicates the possible role of humoral immunity in the clearance of virus.[27]

Most individuals who are exposed to HPV clear the infection on the basis of the cellular and humoral immune response to the viral antigens expressed on the surface of the infected cells.[28] Only in a small fraction of women does the HPV infection persist and do lesions induced by the virus in these chronically infected individuals progress to CIN2–3 and, eventually, to invasive cancer. Individuals who harbor chronic HPV infection may have a cryptic immune response defect that accounts for their inability to clear the chronic infection.[28] Genetic or acquired immunosuppression (i.e., human immunodeficiency virus infection) is known to be a cofactor for progression of HPV-induced lesions.[28,29]

Papillomaviruses are circular, double-stranded DNA viruses that infect the squamous epithelium. The virus, generally spread through sexual contact, enters through a break in the skin and infects the basal cells of the cervical mucosa. The interval between entry of the virus to development of a lesion varies from several weeks to months. After an initial period in which the copy number of HPV episomal DNA increases to 50 copies per cell,[30] the copy number stabilizes and, thereafter, the HPV DNA replicates as an episome in synchrony with the replication of the host cell, using the host DNA polymerase. This process is called *latent viral DNA replication*. As the cells in the mucosa mature to the point at which they no longer have the capacity to undergo cellular division, the copy number of the HPV episomal DNA increases dramatically in a manner independent of cellular division.[31] After this occurs, the late viral genes are expressed and sufficient levels of envelope proteins are produced to promote the packaging of infectious particles. This process is called *vegetative viral DNA replication*.

Carcinogenic Switch: Transition from Chronic Infection and Dysplasia to Invasive Cancer

The HPV viral genome consists of approximately 8 kb, and the protein-coding genes are located on only one of the DNA strands. Within the HPV genome are three distinct regions. The *early region* encodes the viral proteins for viral DNA replication, transcriptional regulation, and cellular transformation. The second distinct region, the *late region*, encodes the viral capsid proteins. The third region, known as the *long control region* (LCR) or *upstream regulatory region*, contains cis-regulatory elements as the origin of the DNA replication and some important transcriptional enhancers.[32]

The genes located in the early region are important for HPV-induced lesions. The *E1* and *E2* genes usually take part in the regulation of the LCR. The *E1* gene encodes a viral DNA helicase, which is a DNA-specific binding protein necessary for the initiation of viral DNA synthesis.[33] Likewise, the *E2* gene encodes a DNA binding protein that promotes the binding with host cell DNA polymerase and E1. E2 also regulates the transcription of transforming genes, depending on the level of E2 and E2 binding sites within the promoter sequences.[34] Both *E6* and *E7* genes of the HPV early region encode cellular transforming proteins. The E6 oncoprotein binds to several cellular proteins, activating the ubiquitin pathway of proteolysis, which finally targets p53 tumor suppressor protein.[35] The E7 protein of HPV binds pRb and members of the pRB family such as p107 and p130, leading the release of active E2F transcription factor, which finally stimulates cell cycle progression.[36] The high- and low-risk HPV viral types mainly differ in the expression of those transforming genes, the process of genetic integration, and the mechanisms by which the LCR is influenced.[37]

Once a chronically HPV-infected mucosal surface is established, the *E6* and *E7* HPV genes are expressed sufficiently to reduce the intracellular level of p53 and to functionally inactivate the RB protein. As a consequence, the cervical mucosal cell loses its control of cell cycle progression at the G_1/S restriction point, and genomic instability eventually occurs. In addition, the sensitivity of the cell to DNA damage–induced apoptosis is reduced. This produces an environment in which the probability of acquisition of somatic mutations and chromosomal abnormalities is increased. Thus, a chronically HPV-infected dysplastic mucosa often has chromosomal rearrangements.[38] At some point, the HPV DNA episome integrates, often at the site of the HPV *E2* gene, and the integrated HPV DNA, no longer under the restrictive influence of the E1 or E2 protein, produces higher levels of E6 and E7 expression. The consequent increase of the expression of the *E6* and *E7* genes finally leads to invasive cervical cancer.

The continued replication of the HPV episomal DNA is necessary to maintain chronic infection. The first step in the assembly of a replication initiation complex is the binding of the dimeric E2 protein to the origin of replication contained within the LCR of the HPV DNA. This is followed by the binding of E1 (helicase), which then enables the host cell DNA polymerase to bind to the origin of replication. In the absence of E2, the E1 protein cannot bind sufficiently stably to the LCR to initiate the replication initiation complex. The effect of the *E2* gene on gene transcriptional activation at other sites in the HPV DNA may depend in part on the level of E2 in the cells. At low E2 levels, HPV E2 is a transactivator and, at very high levels, HPV E2 is a transcriptional repressor.[39,40] Both E1 and E2 are necessary for papilloma virus formation induced by papillomavirus genes.[34]

CERVICAL CANCER CHEMOPREVENTION TRIALS

Endpoints for Chemoprevention Trials

Chemoprevention, the method of inhibiting carcinogenesis before the invasive cancer is established, has attracted a great deal of attention thus far. Chemoprevention trials in cancer have two major endpoints. The first is, in the clinical setting, to prevent or delay the development of clinical cancer. Although this is the main goal of chemoprevention trials, it is not useful as an endpoint for *clinical* chemoprevention trials. To achieve the primary endpoint of reducing cervical cancer incidence, large, long-term, randomized studies are required. Managing and conducting such studies is extremely difficult, because they involve a large number of patients and require years of follow up. The natural history of cervical cancer has already been outlined. The existence of effective treatment modalities for patients with CIN3, which constitutes the optimal target group for chemoprevention, is likely to lead to problems with recruitment for and compliance with prevention trials.

Instead of using the ultimate goal of reducing cervical cancer incidence as an endpoint, biomarkers may serve as intermediate or surrogate endpoints for chemoprevention trials. Surrogate endpoint biomarkers (SEBs) are useful for randomized phase II trials, which are usually preferred for cervical chemoprevention. Such a marker should be on the pathway to carcinogenesis and ideally should change as the process progress. Aside from their sensitivity and specificity, potential chemopreventive drugs are chosen on the basis of their ability to modulate the surrogate markers of carcinogenesis. Although not yet validated by large clinical chemoprevention trials, numerous SEBs, such as quantitative cytopathologic markers, proliferation markers such as proliferating cell nuclear antigen, Ki67, cell cycle regulation markers, differentiation markers, genomic instability markers, and tissue maintenance markers, have been used in cervical cancer prevention trials. These SEBs have been well outlined in a recent review.[41] Among these SEBs, cytopathologic markers of altered nuclear features and tissue architecture have been widely used in clinical trials.[42,43] These markers have also been used as the inclusion criteria of almost all of trials conducted thus far.

The apparent role of viral carcinogenesis in cervical cancer relates the SEBs to HPV. Among those markers used previously, histopathologic nuclear features, HPV viral load, mitotic frequency (MPM-2 antibody staining), proliferating cell nuclear antigen, epidermal growth factor receptor, and aneuploidy demonstrated by flow cytometry are promising factors for cervical chemoprevention trials.[43–46]

Chemopreventive Agents and Clinical Trials

Study design in chemoprevention trials is somewhat problematic. After the toxicity tests in Phase I trials have been conducted, which sometimes also evaluate the activity of a given drug in high-risk patients, the activity of the drug is tested in a short-term Phase IIa trial, which also evaluates the predictability of endpoint biomarkers. After an effective drug and useful SEBs are available, definitive randomized Phase IIb trials are conducted. In some studies, Phase II and I designs have been overlapped. Phase III trials should include a large number of patients and aim at long-term efficacy in decreasing cancer incidence. An ideal Phase III trial, therefore, requires thousands of patients and usually more than 10 years of follow up. However, the clinical trials conducted to date for cervical cancer chemoprevention have been mostly randomized Phase IIb or small Phase III studies that included a mere few hundred patients (Table 13.1.1). Therefore, from a statistical perspective, the power of such studies is usually low.

Another important problem encountered in cervical chemoprevention trials is patient selection criteria. Cytopathologic markers, the most widely used SEBs at the tissue level, generally are used to select the target population for clinical chemoprevention trials in cervical carcinoma. Most previous studies aimed to reverse the premalignant lesion. All grades of cervical premalignant lesions have been included in chemoprevention trials (see Table 13.1.1). The results of these

TABLE 13.1.1 Randomized (Phase II–III) Clinical Trials of Cervical Cancer Chemoprevention

Study	No. Evaluable Responses/ No. Recruited	Drug, Dose, Time Period	Target Population	Spontaneous Responses: Overall Response (%)	Spontaneous Responses: Complete Response (%)
de Vet et al[68] (1991)	278/369	β-Carotene, 10 mg, vs placebo, PO, 3 mo	CIN1–3	32	11
Butterwoth et al[58] (1992)	47/78	Folic acid, 10 mg, vs placebo, PO, 6 mo	CIN1–2	—	66
Meyskens et al[85] (1994)	232/301	β-*trans*-Retinoic acid vs placebo, topical, 6 mo	CIN2	—	27[a]
			CIN3	—	31
Chiklders et al[60] (1995)	246/331	Folic acid, 5 mg, vs placebo, PO, 6 mo	CIN1–2	—	6
Fairley et al[69] (1996)	111/117	β-Carotene, 30 mg, vs placebo, PO, 12 mo	CIN2	60	—•
Romney et al[70] (1997)	69/98	β-Carotene, 30 mg, vs placebo, PO, 9 mo	CIN1–3	50	47[a]

TABLE 13.1.1 Continued

Study	No. Evaluable Responses/ No. Recruited	Drug, Dose, Time Period	Target Population	Spontaneous Responses Overall Response (%)	Complete Response (%)
Ruidi et al[86] (1997)	74/74	Retinamide II, 10 mg, vs placebo, suppository, 6 mo	CIN1–2	56	48[b]
Mackerras et al[71] (1999)	141/147	β-Carotene, 30 mg, vs placebo Vitamin C, 500 mg, vs placebo β-carotene + vitamin C, PO, 6 mo	CIN1	—	29
Bell et al[100] (2000)	27/30	Indole-3-carbinole, 200 or 400 mg, vs placebo, 3 mo	CIN2–3	—	0
Keefe et al[72] (2001)	103/124	β-Carotene, 30 mg, vs placebo, PO, 24 mo	CIN2–3	—	47

CIN, cervical intraepithelial neoplasia; PO, per os (orally).
[a]$P < .05$ for only complete response.
[b]$P < .05$ for overall response.

trials should be reviewed with regard to the spontaneous regression rates, which are as high as 90% in CIN1 lesions. The higher spontaneous regression rate of CIN1–CIN2 lesions has often caused previous trials to fail to show any beneficial effect. Hence, because of the natural history of the disease, patients with severe dysplasia (CIN3) lesions appear to be reasonable candidates for cervical chemoprevention trials.

Many effective drugs have been tested in vitro as treatment for cervical lesions. However, the toxic effects of some of those drugs prevent their use in a prevention trial, which usually requires long-term administration of the drug. Also, because the majority of women being targeted for the cervical cancer chemoprevention trials are of reproductive age, use of the retinoids, which have been shown to be effective in some other solid tumor prevention trials, is problematic.

In randomized cervical cancer prevention trials, micronutrients such as folic acid, β-carotene, retinoids, and indole compounds have been used thus far (see Table 13.1.1).

Micronutrients Case-control studies investigating the effects of micronutrients on cervical cancer risk have shown that high intake of dietary carotene, vitamins C and E, and folate are associated with reduced risk.[47,48] Likewise, the epidemiological studies suggest an increased risk for CIN and cervical cancer with low vitamin A intake.[49] However, most of these studies investigating the relation between micronutrients and cervical cancer risk were conducted before reliable testing methods for HPV were available. Recent studies of the role of diet in cervical cancer risk have usually taken into account the HPV association. Although an association between HPV persistence and micronutrients has been reported,[50] the more recent studies report conflicting results with regard to a protective role of micronutrients.[51,52] In addition, recent reports do not support an association between folate and HPV infection.[53,54] Among the micronutrients investigated thus far, folic acid and β-carotene have been used in clinical chemoprevention trials.

Although results are conflicting with regard to the association of folate levels and cervical cancer risk, the rationale for folic acid to be used in clinical trials is based mainly on its role in DNA synthesis, repair, and methylation.[55,56] However, the randomized folate trials published to date reported negative results for its efficacy in CIN.

An early study by Butterworth et al[57] reported a significantly increased response rate for folic acid, 10 mg/day for 3 months, as compared to placebo (vitamin C, 10 mg) in patients using oral contraceptives.[57] However, the second largest study of the same group did not show any beneficial treatment effect of the same drug at the same dose in low-income women.[58] In the second study, involving patients with CIN1–CIN2 lesions, the spontaneous regression rate was 66%, which constituted one of the leading causes of failure of the trial. The beneficial effect seen in the first study might be related to the reversal effects of folic acid on megaloblastic changes seen in women using oral contraceptives. The lack of a relationship between folic acid and HPV makes unlikely a reversing effect for this nutrient in HPV-induced lesions of cervical mucosa.[59] In the Phase III trial conducted by the Southwest Oncology Group,[60] folic acid was used at a dose of 5 mg/day for 6 months in patients with CIN1–CIN2 lesions. Again, the regression rates of lesions assessed by Pap smear and colposcopy did not differ between folic acid and placebo groups.

Although the aforementioned trials suffer from several limitations—short duration of the intervention and recruiting of patients with CIN1–CIN2 lesions, which have high spontaneous regression rates—the unfavorable results have prevented the use of folic acid in further trials. Nevertheless, testing of this agent in combination with other drugs for chemoprevention might be warranted on the basis of folic acid's known effects on DNA synthesis and methylation.

β-Carotene is a precursor of vitamin A (retinol). Other than being a provitamin A, it exhibits a broad range of activities, such as modulation of immune response, inhibition of viral gene expression, and antioxidant activity.[61–63] Epidemiological studies have shown an inverse relationship between β-carotene levels and cervical cancer and CIN risk.[48,64,65] Although a similar relationship has been reported with chronic HPV infection,[63] this finding is not supported in other studies.[66,67] Therefore, the exact role of β-carotene in HPV infection and HPV-induced carcinogenesis remains unclear.

As with the folate trials, the randomized β-carotene trials published thus far have failed to show any beneficial effect of this micronutrient. deVet et al,[68] in their randomized trial of β-carotene using 10 mg/day for 3 months, as compared with placebo, have reported similar response rates for both arms. Although this study included CIN1–CIN3 lesions, no significant difference was found with respect to the degree of dysplasia after treatment. In another randomized trial, Fairley et al[69] were unable to show a beneficial effect of 30 mg/day β-carotene for 12 months on the lesions of CIN1–CIN2. On the contrary, Romney et al[70] reported a significantly higher complete remission rate for the placebo arm as compared to the β-carotene arm of a trial involving administration of 30 mg/day for 9 months, although the overall response rates of the placebo and drug groups were similar. Moreover, no significant relationship between plasma β-carotene levels and regression of CIN was found in that trial. In the trial by Mackerras et al,[71] patients were randomized among three arms: β-carotene only, 30 mg/day; β-carotene plus vitamin C, 500 mg/day; and placebo, for 6 months. Although not significant, the combination arm had the worst response rate. In the very recent Phase III study by Keefe et al,[72] even the prolonged use of β-carotene, 30 mg/day for 24 months, did not enhance the regression rates of CIN2–CIN3 lesions, especially in patients positive for human immunodeficiency virus. The outlined results of these randomized studies suggest no beneficial treatment effect of β-carotene in cervical cancer chemoprevention.

Retinoids Retinoids are potent modulators of epithelial cell growth and differentiation. They have been reported to inhibit cell proliferation and to induce cell differentiation.[73] Both the metabolites of vitamin A and its synthetic analogs binding retinoid receptors are the most effective drugs studied thus far in solid tumor chemoprevention trials. Two main types of retinoid receptors in the nucleus have been identified. Whereas the first identified receptor type, retinoic acid receptors α, β, and γ, binds both all-*trans*-retinoic acid and *cis*-retinoic acid, the second group of receptors, retinoid X receptors α, β, and γ, binds only 9-*cis*-retinoic acid.[74,75] The studies on tissues from both premalignant and malignant lesions suggest that the decreased expression of retinoid receptors might be related to tumor promotion.[76] Also, the reduced expression of retinoic acid receptors α, β, and γ has been reported in CIN1–CIN3 lesions.[77] As the molecular aspects of retinoid receptors become clearer, the number of new synthetic analogs of retinol may increase.

The exact mechanisms of the antiproliferative effect of retinoids on HPV-induced cells are not well understood. Although in a clinical report 13-*cis*-retinoic acid has been shown to decrease the titer of high-risk HPVs, its molecular effects on HPV-induced transformation are potentially more important.[78] Earlier studies have reported that the suppressive effects of retinoic acid on HPV16-transformed cells might be related to the inhibition of E6/E7 oncoproteins.[79,80] Recent studies show that besides their E6/E7 inhibitory effects, retinoids may induce the expression of p53 in HPV-infected cells, which might partially reverse the E6-induced degradation of this tumor suppressor protein.[81] Also, the growth inhibitory effects of these compounds on HPV-induced lesions were found to be mediated by transforming growth factor-β, which seems to augment the HPV-induced decrement of both p53- and pRb-dependent functions.[81,82] This finding suggests that the loss of retinoid sensitivity seen in the later phases of HPV-induced carcinogenesis, shown in vitro and in vivo, might be related to transforming growth factor-β–mediated resistance. Further studies demonstrated that the increasing effects of retinoids on insulinlike growth factor binding proteins 3 and 5 levels also contribute to antiproliferative effect.[83,84] These many effects of retinoids underscore the importance of these compounds in cervical cancer chemoprevention trials.

Hundreds of retinoic acid receptor and retinoid X receptor ligands have been synthesized and tested. However, their important side effects, especially the teratogenic effects, limit the use of these compounds in cervical chemoprevention trials. Because most patients in the target population for cervical cancer chemoprevention studies are of reproductive age (unlike the women who compose the populations for other solid tumor prevention studies), no randomized clinical trial using systemic administration of retinoids has been published thus far. In lieu of systemic administration, topical application has been widely used. In the first Phase III cervical cancer prevention trial of retinoids, Meyskens et al[85] reported a significant regression of CIN2 lesions with topical use of b-*trans*-retinoic acid as a 0.375%

cream. However, no significant response was found for CIN3 lesions. In a recent interim analysis of a randomized study from China, retinamide II suppositories were shown to incite a significant therapeutic effect on CIN1–CIN2 lesions.[86] Further randomized trials will determine the exact role of topical retinoids in cervical cancer prevention.

The systemic administration of retinoid compounds in the chemoprevention of other solid tumors has yielded positive results.[87] However, as mentioned earlier, the toxicity of these drugs limits their systemic use in patients with CIN lesions. Trials with new and less toxic retinoid compounds, as in the ongoing trial of fenretidine [N-(4-hidroxyphneyl) retinamide] by Fullen et al,[88] will determine the efficacy of oral administration of these compounds.

Indole Compounds Many vegetables and fruits, which are found on the American Cancer Society's daily recommended diet for cancer prevention, include indole compounds. Indole-3-carbinol, one of these indole compounds, has been approved by the U.S. Food and Drug Administration as a nutritional supplement. No significant toxicity of this compound has been reported.[89] Indole-3-carbinol has been reported to exert various indirect and direct inhibitory effects on carcinogenesis. Its indirect effects include induction of the detoxification action of cytochrome P450,[90] reduction of the activation of carcinogens by binding to the aryl hydrocarbon receptor,[91] and induction of C2 hydroxylation of estrogen, which may play an additive role in HPV-induced carcinogenesis of the cervical mucosa.[92] The direct effects include induction of apoptosis in some tumor cell lines (e.g., MCF-7 breast cancer cells)[93] and of cell cycle arrest at G_1/S restriction points by inhibition of cyclin-dependent kinase 6.[94] In a cottontail rabbit papillomavirus animal model, Wu et al[95] reported that while the wild-type cottontail rabbit papillomavirus genome, intradermally inoculated within a gene gun, induced papilloma formation on inoculation sites, no papillomas were seen with frame shift mutations into the *E1* and *E2* genes of the cottontail rabbit papillomavirus genome. Therefore, drugs that could inhibit the functions of E1 and E2 in promoting both the latent and vegetative replication of HPV could eradicate HPV infections in individuals unable to clear such infections and might be used as chemopreventive agents. Indole compounds have recently been shown to inhibit the binding of proteins to E2.[96] In a mouse model, indole-3-carbinol has been shown to inhibit HPV-induced cervical carcinogenesis.[97]

Indole-3-carbinol also has been tested and proven successful as a treatment of HPV11-associated laryngeal papillomatosis in a few children[98] and in 18 adults with recurrent HPV11-related laryngeal papillomatosis.[99] This experience showed a 30% response rate and 30% stabilization of disease rate in the involved patients. In a recent small randomized trial of indole-3-carbinol by Bell et al,[100] a 50% complete remission rate in patients with CIN2–CIN3 lesions has been reported. Nonetheless, further randomized trials are required to establish the efficacy of indole compounds in cervical cancer prevention. A randomized, double-blind trial of indole-3-carbinol in cervical dysplasia sponsored by a grant from the NIH is about to begin.

Other Chemopreventive Agents

Some other agents also are under investigation for possible chemopreventive effects. A strong correlation between the levels of polyamines and cell proliferation has led to the synthesis of the inhibitors of ornithine decarboxylase enzyme, a key enzyme in polyamine biosynthesis. Difluoromethylornitihine, a specific inhibitor of ornithine decarboxylase, has already been used in chemoprevention trials of some solid tumors. However, its high potential for toxicity, especially ototoxiciy, has limited its use.[101] Nonetheless, in a Phase I trial of this drug in patients with CIN3 lesions, Mitchell et al[102] reported no significant toxicity. This same research group has already completed patient accrual for a Phase II study of eflornithine in patients with CIN2–CIN3 lesions.[103] Further trials are needed to establish the chemopreventive role of polyamine synthesis inhibitors in cervical cancer.

FUTURE CONSIDERATIONS

Although the availability of effective screening programs in some countries has already decreased its incidence and mortality, cervical cancer continues to be the second leading cause of cancer death among women. Chemoprevention trials for cervical cancer have been disappointing so far. With our increased understanding of the mechanisms that lead to cervical cancer, the processing, designing, synthesizing, and testing of new and promising drugs has begun. However, these trials are still in their infancy. The role of HPV in cervical carcinogenesis has also led to vaccine trials, but this research too is in its beginning stages. Along with the chemoprevention and vaccine strategies, risk avoidance and new, efficient early detection technologies may help to decrease the incidence and mortality of cervical cancer.

ACKNOWLEDGMENTS

The authors recognize support from the Bush Leukemia Research Foundation, support from the National Cancer Institute for Dr. Hakan Akbulut's fellowship in the Deisseroth laboratory, and a grant to AD for a prevention trial to evaluate the use of indole-3-carbinol to clear chronic HPV infections.

REFERENCES

1. Parkin DM, Pisani P, Ferlay J. Estimates of the worldwide incidence of 25 major cancers in 1990. Int J Cancer 1999;80:827–841.

2. Greenlee RT, Hill-Harmon MB, Murray T et al. Cancer statistics, 2001. CA: Cancer J 2001;51(1): 15–36.
3. Vizcaino AP, Moreno V, Bosch FX et al. International trends in incidence of cervical cancer: II. Squamous-cell carcinoma. Int J Cancer 2000;86:429–435
4. Franco EL, Duarte-Franco E, Ferenczy A. Cervical cancer: epidemiology, prevention and the role of human papillomavirus infection. CMAJ 2001;164:1017–1025
5. Hwang YY, Moon H, Cho SH et al Ten-year survival of patients with locally advanced, stage Ib–IIb cervical cancer after neoadjuvant chemotherapy and radical hysterectomy. Gynecol Oncol 2001;82:88–93
6. Brewster WR, Monk BJ, Ziogas A et al. Intent-to-treat analysis of stage Ib and IIa cervical cancer in the United States: radiotherapy or surgery 1988–1995. Obstet Gynecol 2001;97:248–254
7. Richart RM. A modified terminology for cervical intraepithelial neoplasia. Obstet Gynecol 1990; 75:131–133.
8. National Cancer Institute Workshop. The 1988 Bethesda System for reporting cervical /vaginal cytological diagnosis. JAMA 1989;262:931–934.
9. Naissell K, Roger V, Naissel M. Behaviour of mild cervical dysplasia during long-term follow-up. Obstet Gynecol 1986;67:665–669.
10. Ostor AG. Natural history of cervical intraepithelial neoplasia: a critical review. Int J Gynecol Pathol 1993;12:186–192.
11. Holowaty P, Miller AB, Rohan T, To T. Natural history of dysplasia of the uterine cervix. J Natl Cancer Inst 1999;91:252–258.
12. Naissel K, Naissel M, Vaclavinkova V. Behavior of moderate cervical dysplasia during long-term follow-up. Obstet Gynecol 1983;61:609–614.
13. Schiffman MH, Brinton LA. The epidemiology of cervical carcinogenesis. Cancer 1995;76: 1888–1901.
14. Kjellberg L, Hallmans G, Ahren AM et al. Smoking, diet, pregnancy and oral contraceptive use as risk factors for cervical intra-epithelial neoplasia in relation to human papillomavirus infection. Br J Cancer 2000;82:1332–1338.
15. Lacey JV Jr, Frisch M, Brinton LA et al. Associations between smoking and adenocarcinomas and squamous cell carcinomas of the uterine cervix (United States). Cancer Causes Control 2001;12:153–161.
16. Tjiong MY, Out TA, Ter Schegget T et al. Epidemiologic and mucosal immunologic aspects of HPV infection and HPV-related cervical neoplasia in the lower female genital tract: a review. Int J Gynecol Cancer 2001;1:9–17.
17. Daling JR, Madeleine MM, McKnight B et al. The relationship of human papillomavirus–related cervical tumors to cigarette smoking, oral contraceptive use and prior herpes simplex virus type 2 infection. Cancer Epidemiol Biomarkers Prevent 1996;5:541–548.
18. Schiffman MH, Bauer HM, Hoover RN et al. Epidemiological evidence showing that human papilloma virus infection causes most cervical intraepithelial neoplasia. J Natl Cancer Inst 1993; 85:958–964.
19. Herrero R, Hildesheim A, Bratti C et al. Population-based study of human papillomavirus infection and cervical neoplasia in rural Costa Rica. J Natl Cancer Inst 2000;92:464–474.
20. Ho GY, Bierman R, Beardsley L et al. Natural history of cervicovaginal papillomavirus infection in young women. N Engl J Med 1998;338:423–428.
21. Ngelangel C, Munoz N, Bosch FX et al. Causes of cervical cancer in the Philippines: a case-control study. J Natl Cancer Inst 1998;90:43–49.

22. Woodman CB, Collins S, Winter H et al. Natural history of cervical human papillomavirus infection in young women: a longitudinal cohort study. Lancet 2001;357:1831–1836.

23. Berumen J, Ordonez RM, Lazcano E et al. Asian-American variants of human papillomavirus 16 and risk for cervical cancer: a case-control study. J Natl Cancer Inst 2001;93:1325–1330.

24. Bosch FX, Manos MM, Munoz N et al. Prevalence of human papillomavirus in cervical cancer: a worldwide perspective. International biological study on cervical cancer (IBSCC) Study Group. J Natl Cancer Inst 1995;87:796–802.

25. Rohan T, Mann V, McLaughlin J et al. PCR-detected genital papillomavirus infection: prevalence and association with risk factors for cervical cancer. Int J Cancer 1991;49:1–5.

26. Moscicki AB, Hills N, Shiboski S et al. Risks for incident human papillomavirus infection and low-grade squamous intraepithelial lesion development in young females. JAMA 2001;285: 2995–3002.

27. Bontkes HJ, de Gruijl TD, Walboomers JM et al. Immune responses against human papillomavirus (HPV) type 16 virus-like particles in a cohort study of women with cervical intraepithelial neoplasia: II. Systemic but not local IgA responses correlate with clearance of HPV-16. J Gen Virol 1999;80(2):409–417

28. Sillman F, Stanek A, Sedlis A et al. The relation between human papilloma virus infection and lower genital intraepithelial neoplasia in immunosuppressed women. Am J Obstet Gynecol 1984; 150:300–308.

29. Palefsky JM, Minkoff H, Kalish LA et al. Cervicovaginal human papillomavirus infection in human immunodeficiency virus-1 (HIV)-positive and high-risk HIV- negative women. J Natl Cancer Inst 1999;91:226–236.

30. Schneider A, Oltersdorf T, Schneider V et al. Distribution of human papilloma virus 16 genome in cervical neoplasia by molecular in situ hybridization of tissue sections. Int J Cancer 1987; 39:717–723

31. Meyers C, Wettstern FL. The late region differentially regulates the in vitro transformation by cottontail rabbit papilloma virus DNA in different cell types. Virology 1991;181:637–646.

32. Howley PM, Lowy DR. Papillomaviruses and their replication. In: Knipe DM, Howley PM, eds. Fields Virology, vol 2. Philadelphia: Lippincott Williams & Wilkins, 2001:2197–2229.

33. Wilson WG, Ludes-Meyers J. A bovine papilloma virus E1-related protein binds specifically to bovine papillomavirus DNA. J Virol 1991;65:5314–5322.

34. Wu X, Zial W, Brandsma JL. Papilloma formation by cottontail rabbit virus requires E1 and E2 regulatory genes in addition to E6 and E7 transforming genes. J Virol 1994;68:6097–6102.

35. Scheffner M, Werness BA, Huibregtse JM et al. The E6 oncoprotein encoded by human papillomavirus type s 16 and 18 promotes the degradation of p53. Cell 1990;63:1129–1136.

36. Phillips AC, Vousden KH. Human papillomavirus and cancer: the viral transforming genes. Cancer Surv 1999;33:55–74.

37. Barbosa MS, Vass WC, Lowy DR, Schiller JT. In vitro biological activities of the E6 and E7 genes vary among human papillomaviruses of different oncogenic potential. J Virol 1991;65:292–298.

38. Atkin MB, Baker MC. Nonrandom chromosome changes in carcinoma of the cervix uteri: II. Ten tumors in the triploid-tetraploid range. Cancer Genet Cytogenet 1984;13:18–27.

39. Sverdrup FM, Sheahan LC, Khan SA. Development of human papilloma virus plasmids capable of episomal replication in human cell lines. Gene Ther 1999;6:1317–1321.

40. Fujii T, Brandsma JL, Peng XY et al. Species specific mechanisms of transcriptional regulation by cottontail rabbit papillomavirus and human papillomavirus 16. J Biol Chem 2001;276: 867–874.

41. Foller M, Schottenfeld D. Surrogate end-point biomarkers and their modulation in cervical chemoprevention trials. Cancer 2001;91:1758–1776.

42. Sun CA, Lai HC, Chang CC et al. The significance of human papillomavirus viral load in prediction of histologic severity and size of squamous intraepithelial lesions of uterine cervix. Gynecol Oncol 2001;83:95–99.

43. Hu W, Mitchell MF, Boiko IV et al. Progressive dysregulation of proliferation during cervical carcinogenesis as measured by MPM-2 antibody staining. Cancer Epidemiol Biomarkers Prev 1997;6:711–6718.

44. Shurbaji MS, Brooks SK, Thurmond TS. Proliferating cell nuclear antigen immunoreactivity in cervical intraepithelial neoplasia and benign cervical epithelium. Am J Clin Pathol 1993;100: 22–26.

45. Boiko IV, Mitchell MF, Hu W et al. Epidermal growth factor receptor expression in cervical intraepithelial neoplasia and its modulation during an a-difluoromethylornithine chemoprevention trial. Clin Cancer Res 1998;4:1383–1391.

46. Lai CH, Hsueh S, Tsao KC, Chen HM. DNA aneuploidy in benign tumors and normal tissues of the female genital tract. Int J Gynecol Pathol 1996;15:63–68.

47. Ziegler RG, Brinton LA, Hamman RF et al. Diet and the risk of invasive cervical cancer among white women in the United States. Am J Epidemiol 1990;132:432–445.

48. Potischman N, Brinton LA. Nutrition and cervical neoplasia. Cancer Causes Control 1996;7: 113–126.

49. La Vecchia C, Decarli A, Fasoli M et al. Dietary vitamin A and the risk of intraepithelial and invasive cervical neoplasia. Gynecol Oncol 1988;30:187–195.

50. Giuliano AR, Papenfuss M, Nour M et al. Antioxidant nutrients: association with persistent human papillomavirus infection. Cancer Epidemiol Biomarkers Prev 1997;6:917–923.

51. Wideroff L, Potischman N, Glass AG et al. A nested case-control study of dietary factors and the risk of incident cytological abnormalities of the cervix. Nutr Cancer 1998;30:130–136.

52. Goodman MT, McDuffie K, Hernandez B et al.Case-control study of plasma folate, homocysteine, vitamin B(12), and cysteine as markers of cervical dysplasia. Cancer 2000;89:376–382.

53. Fowler BM, Giuliano AR, Piyathilake C et al. Hypomethylation in cervical tissue: Is there a correlation with folate status? Cancer Epidemiol Biomarkers Prev 1998;7:901–906.

54. Weinstein SJ, Ziegler RG, Frongillo EA Jr et al. Low serum and red blood cell folate are moderately, but insignificantly associated with increased risk of invasive cervical cancer in U.S. women. J Nutr 2001;131:2040–2048.

55. Alberg AJ, Shelhub J, Shah KV et al. The risk of cervical cancer in relation to serum concentrations of folate, vitamin B12 and homocisteine. Cancer Epidemiol Biomarkers Prev 2000;9:761–764.

56. Mason JB, Levesque T. Folate: the effects on carcinogenesis and the potential for cancer chemoprevention. Oncology 1996;10:1727–1742.

57. Butterwoth CE Jr, Hatch KD, Gore H et al. Improvement in cervical dysplasia associated with folic acid therapy in users of oral contraceptives. Am J Clin Nutr 1982;35:73–82.

58. Butterwoth CE Jr, Hatch KD, Soong Sf et al. Oral folic supplementation for cervical dysplasia: a clinical intervention trial Am J Obstet Gynecol 1992;166:803–809.

59. Weinstein SJ, Ziegler RG, Frongillo EA Jr et al. Low serum and red blood cell folate are moderately, but insignificantly associated with increased risk of invasive cervical cancer in U.S. women. J Nutr 2001;131:2040–2048.

60. Childers JM, Chu J, Voigt LF et al. Chemoprevention of cervical cancer with folic acid: a phase II Southwest Oncology Group Intergroup study. Cancer Epidemiol Biomarkers Prev 1995;4: 155–159.

61. Rock CL, Michael CW, Reynolds RK, Ruffin MT. Prevention of cervix cancer. Crit Rev Oncol Hematol 2000;33:169–185.

62. Gossage C, Deyhim M, Moser-Veillon PB et al. Effect of beta-carotene supplementation and lactation on carotenoid metabolism and mitogenic T lymphocyte proliferation. Am J Clin Nutr 2000;71:950–955.

63. Schiff MA, Patterson RE, Baumgartner RN et al. Serum carotenoids and risk of cervical intraepithelial neoplasia in southwestern American Indian women. Cancer Epidemiol Biomarkers Prev 2001; 10:1219–1222

64. Palan PR, Mikhail MS, Goldberg GL et al. Plasma levels of beta-carotene, lycopene, canthaxanthin, retinol, and alpha- and tau-tocopherol in cervical intraepithelial neoplasia and cancer. Clin Cancer Res 1996;2:181–185.

65. Giuliano AR, Papenfuss M, Nour M et al. Antioxidant nutrients: association with persistent human papillomavirus infection. Cancer Epidemiol Biomarkers Prev 1997;6:917–923.

66. Tabrizi SN, Fairley CK, Chen S et al. Epidemiological characteristics of women with high grade CIN who do and do not have human papillomavirus. Br J Obstet Gynaecol 1999;106:252–257.

67. Nagata C, Shimizu H, Yoshikawa H et al. Serum carotenoids and vitamins and risk of cervical dysplasia from a case-control study in Japan. Br J Cancer 1999;81:1234–1247

68. de Vet HC, Knipschild PG, Willebrand D et al. The effect of beta-carotene on the regression and progression of cervical dys-plasia: a clinical experiment. J Clin Epidemiol 1991;44:273–283.

69. Fairley CK, Tabrizi SN, Chen S et al. A randomized clinical trial of beta carotene vs placebo for the treatment of cervical HPV infection. Int J Gynecol Cancer 1996;6:225–230.

70. Romney SL, Ho GY, Palan PR et al. Effects of b-carotene and other factors on outcome of cervical dysplasia and human papillomavirus infection. Gynecol Oncol 1997;65:483–492.

71. Mackerras D, Irwig L, Simpson JM et al. Randomized double-blind trial of beta-carotene and vitamin C in women with minor cervical abnormalities. Br J Cancer 1999;79:1448–1453.

72. Keefe KA, Schell MJ, Brewer C et al. A randomized, double blind, phase III trial using oral beta-carotene supplementation for women with high-grade cervical intraepithelial neoplasia. Cancer Epidemiol Biomarkers Prev 2001;10:1029–1035

73. Yokoyama M, Nakao Y, Iwasaka T et al. Retinoic acid and interferon-alpha effects on cell growth and differentiation in cervical carcinoma cell lines. Obstet Gynecol 2001;98:332–340

74. Allenby G, Janoch R, Kazmer S et al. Binding of 9-cis retinoic acid and all-trans retinoic acid to retinoic acid receptor α, β and γ. J Bio Chem 1994;269:16689–16695.

75. Narayanan BA, Holladay EB, Nixon DW, Mauro CT. The effect of all-trans and 9-cis retinoic acid on the steady state level of HPV16 E6/E7 mRNA and cell cycle in cervical carcinoma cells. Life Sci 1998;63:565–573

76. Xu X-C, Ro JY, Lee JS et al. Differential expression of nuclear retinoic acid receptors in normal, premalignant and malignant head and neck tissues. Cancer Res 1994;54:3580–3587.

77. Xu XC, Mitchell MF, Silva E et al. Decreased expression of retinoic acid receptors, transforming growth factor beta, involucrin, and cornifin in cervical intraepithelial neoplasia. Clin Cancer Res 1999;5:1503–1508.

78. Ahn WS, Lee JM, Namkoong SE et al. Effect of retinoic acid on HPV titration and colposcopic changes in Korean patients with dysplasia of the uterine cervix. J Cell Biochem Suppl 1997;28/29:133–139.

79. Creek KE, Jenkins GR, Khan MA et al. Retinoic acid suppresses human papillomavirus type 16 (HPV16)-mediated transformation of human keratinocytes and inhibits the expression of the HPV16 oncogenes. Adv Exp Med Biol 1994;354:19–35

80. Khan MA, Jenkins GR, Tolleson WH et al. Retinoic acid inhibition of human papillomavirus type 16-mediated transformation of human keratinocytes. Cancer Res 1993;53:905–909

81. Nees M, Geoghegan JM, Munson P et al. Human papillomavirus type 16 E6 and E7 proteins inhibit differentiation dependent expression of transforming growth factor β2 cervical keratinocytes. Cancer Res 2000;60:4289–4298.

82. Borger DR, Mi Y, Geslani G et al. Retinoic acid resistance at late stages of human papillomavirus type 16-mediated transformation of human keratinocytes arises despite intact retinoid signaling and is due to a loss of sensitivity to transforming growth factor-beta. Virology 2000;270:397–407

83. Hembree JR, Agarwal C, Beard RL et al. Retinoid X receptor-specific retinoids inhibit the ability of retinoic acid receptor-specific retinoids to increase the level of insulin-like growth factor binding protein-3 in human ectocervical epithelial cells. Cancer Res 1996;56:1794–1799

84. Higo H, Duan C, Clemmons DR, Herman B. Retinoic acid inhibits cell growth in HPV negative cervical carcinoma cells by induction of insulin-like growth factor binding protein-5 (IGFBP-5) secretion. Biochem Biophys Res Commun 1997;239:706–709

85. Meyskens FL Jr, Surwit E, Moon TE et al. Enhancement of regression of cervical intraepithelial neoplasia II (moderate dysplasia) with topically applied all-trans-retinoic acid: a randomized trial. J Natl Cancer Inst 1994;86:539–543.

86. Ruidi C, Aihua D, Peiyu B et al. Chemoprevention of cancer of uterine cervix: a study on chemoprevention of retinamide II from cervical precancerous lesions. J Cell Biochem Suppl 1997;28(29):140–143.

87. Hansen LA, Sigman CC, Andreola F et al. Retinoids in chemoprevention and differentiation therapy. Carcinogenesis 2000;21:1271–1279.

88. National Cancer Institute PDQ. Phase III randomized, double blinded, placebo controlled study of fenretidine in patients with cervical intraepithelial neoplasia (CIN) grade 2–3. (Protocol ID No. NCI-P97-0092). Curr Clin Trials Oncol 2001;

89. Bradlow HL, Michnivicz JJ, Harper M et al. Long term responses of women to indole or a high fiber diet. Cancer Epidemiol Biomarkers Prev 1994;3:591–595.

90. Fong AT, Swanson HI, Dashwood RH et al. Mechanisms of anticarcinogenesis by indole-3-carbinol: studies of enzyme induction, electrophile scavenging, and inhibition of aflatoxin B activation. Biochem Pharmacol 1990;39:19–26.

91. Chen I, Safe S, Bjaldenes L. Indole-3-carbinol and diindolylmethane as aryl hydrocarbon (Ah) receptor agonists and antagonists in T47D human breast cancer cells. Biochem Pharmacol 1996; 51:1069–1076.

92. Michnovicz JJ, Aldercreutz H, Bradlow HL. Changes in levels of urinary estrogen metabolites after oral indole-3-carbinol treatment in humans. J Natl Cancer Inst 1997;89:718–723.

93. Ge XK, Yannai S, Rennert G et al. 3,3′-Diindolylmethane induces apoptosis in human cancer cells. Biochem Biophys Res Commun 1996;228:153–158.

94. Cover CM, Hsieh SJ, Tran SH et al. Indole-3-carbinol inhibits the expression of cyclin-dependent kinase-6 and induces a G1 cell cycle arrest of human breast cancer cells independent of estrogen receptor signaling. J Biol Chem 1998;273:3838–3847.

95. Wu X, Zial W, Brandsma JL. Papilloma formation by cottontail rabbit virus requires E1 and E2 regulatory genes in addition to E6 and E7 transforming genes. J Virol 1994;68:6097–6102.

96. Webster K, Taylor A, Gaston K. Oestrogen and progesterone increase the levels of apoptosis induced by the human papillomavirus type 16 E2 and E7 proteins. J Gen Virol 2001;82(1): 201–213.

97. Jin L, Qi M, Chen D-Z et al. Indole-3-carbinol prevents cervical cancer in human papilloma virus type 16 (HPV16) transgenic mice. Cancer Res 1999;59:3991–3997.

98. Coll DA, Auborn K, Potsic WP, Bradlow HL. Treatment of recurrent respiratory papillomatosis with indole-3-carbinol. Am J Otolaryngol 1997;18:1–4.

99. Rosen CA, Wopodson GE, Thompson JWQ et al. Preliminary results of the use of indole-

3-carbinol for recurrent respiratory papillomatosis. Otolaryngol Head Neck Surg 1998;118: 910–915.

100. Bell MC, Crowley-Nowick P, Brandlow JL et al. Placebo-controlled trial of indole-3-carbinol in the treatment of CIN. Gynecol Oncol 2000;78:123–129.

101. Love RR, Jacoby R, Newton MA et al. A randomized, placebo-controlled trial of low-dose alpha-difluoromethylornithine in individuals at risk for colorectal cancer. Cancer Epidemiol Biomarkers Prev 1998;7:989–992

102. Mitchell MF, Tortolero-Luna G, Lee JJ et al. Phase I dose de-escalation trial of alpha-difluoromethylornithine in patients with grade 3 cervical intraepithelial neoplasia. Clin Cancer Res 1998;4: 303–310.

103. National Cancer Institute PDQ. Phase II randomized study of eflornithine versus placebo in patients with cervical intraepithelial neoplasia grade 2–3. (Protocol ID No. NCI-P00-0149) Current Clinical Trials Oncology 2001.

Chapter 13.2

Prevention of Cervical Cancer: Vaccination

John T. Schiller

Douglas R. Lowy

Cervical cancer is one of the major cancers in women, with an estimated yearly incidence of 450,000 case and 200,000 deaths worldwide. Rates of cervical cancer tend to be highest in developing countries, in large measure because those countries lack resources to institute effective cervical cytology screening programs.[1] Over the last 20 years, compelling evidence has accumulated that sexually transmitted infection by certain types of human papillomaviruses (HPVs) is the central cause of cervical cancer.[2] This finding provides an opportunity to prevent cervical cancer through vaccination against papillomavirus infection. Both the public and the commercial sectors are vigorously pursuing this opportunity. However, unique features of papillomavirus biology and the relationship of HPV infection to cervical cancer sets certain parameters within which HPV vaccine programs to prevent cervical cancer must be developed. There are three classes of HPV vaccines under active development for the prevention of cervical cancer. The first class is strictly prophylactic and is aimed at producing virion antibodies that prevent virus infection. The second class is aimed at inducing regression of premalignant HPV-induced cervical neoplasia by inducing cell-mediated immune responses against virally infected cells. Although prophylactic with respect to cervical cancer, this type of vaccine is usually considered to be therapeutic because its aim is to eliminate established viral infections. The third class consists of combined prophylactic-therapeutic vaccines that aim both to prevent HPV infections and to induce regression of established infections. Encouraging results have been obtained in animal models and, in some cases, in clinical trials for these vaccines.

CAUSAL RELATIONSHIP BETWEEN HPV INFECTION AND CERVICAL CANCER

It has been recognized for decades that cervical cancer had the epidemiological characteristics of a sexually transmitted disease.[3] However, it was not until 1983, with the isolation of HPV16 from a substantial proportion of cervical cancer specimens, that solid evidence implicating HPV as the infectious agent appeared.[4] Since that time, extremely strong support has accumulated for the conclusion that infection with certain types of sexually transmitted HPVs is the major risk factor for cervical cancer. Important criteria for establishing causal inferences between a presumptive risk factor and a disease are strength of association, consistency, specificity, temporality, biologic plausibility, and experimental evidence.[5] All these criteria have been adequately met for the HPV–cervical cancer association.

There is a remarkably strong and consistent association of HPV DNA with cervical cancer. Recently published studies have repeatedly reported risk estimates in the fifty- to one hundredfold range for any HPV DNA and in the one hundred- to nine hundredfold range for specific genotypes, such as HPV16 and HPV18.[6] These are among the highest and most consistent relative risks for a single factor in the cancer literature, higher than the association between lung cancer and smoking.[7] The high risk ratios apply to both squamous cell cancer and adenocarcinoma of the cervix. A recent worldwide survey that carefully evaluated HPV DNA using multiple sensitive detection methods found that 99.7% of technically adequate cervical cancer specimens contained HPV DNA.[8]

There is specificity of association in that only some of the many HPV genotypes isolated from the female genital tract are routinely detected in cervical cancers. On the basis of repeated isolation from cervical cancer specimens, approximately 15 types are generally considered oncogenic, but they are not equally distributed in the cancers. Worldwide, approximately 50% of cervical cancers contain HPV16, and another 10% contain HPV18. Together with three or four additional types that vary somewhat among countries, these viruses account for 80%–95% of HPV-associated cervical cancers worldwide.[9] A different group of genital HPVs, especially HPV6 and HPV11, cause most genital warts but are rarely, if ever, detected in cancers.[9,10]

HPV infection has the temporal relationship to cervical cancer that would be expected for an etiologic agent. Prospective cohort and retrospective studies have found that cervical HPV infection normally proceeds high-grade cervical dysplasia and malignant cancer by years and decades, respectively.[11–14] Persistent oncogenic HPV infection is by far the most important risk factor for the subsequent development of histologically confirmed high-grade dysplasias, the accepted precursor of cervical cancer (Fig. 13.2.1).[11,12] Two viral proteins, E6 and E7, are selectively retained and expressed during malignant progression.[15] As detailed later, these same genes have potent in vitro activities in normal epithelial cells that can be plausibly related to viral carcinogenesis in vivo.

Compelling experimental evidence supports a causal inference as well. E6 and E7 of oncogenic HPVs, but not nononcogenic types, strongly bind and inactive the p53 and pRB tumor suppressor proteins, respectively.[16–18] Inactivation of these genes through mutation or deletion is among the most common genetic alterations in other cancers that are not associated with virus infections. Through the inactivation of pRB and p53 and the interaction with other cell protein targets, E6 and E7 deregulate cell cycle control, induce epithelial cell proliferation, and prevent apoptosis of the abnormally proliferating cells.[19,20] An important event in progression is the dysregulation of the tight control of E6 and E7 expression. Loss of E2 activity, the major viral transcription regulator, is a critical step and most frequently occurs via integration of the viral genome into a host chromosome. The importance of continued E6/E7 expression is exemplified by the finding that cancer-derived cell lines become nontumorigenic when E6/E7 expression is experimentally inhibited.[21] E6 and E7 also induce genetic destabilization of the host cell.[22] The accumulation of random genetic alterations coupled with the induction of telomerase by E6[23] results in the efficient immortalization of normal human epithelial cells.[15] Immortalizing activity is a property of cancer-associated (but not low-risk) HPV types.[18] Additional genetic changes, presumably promoted

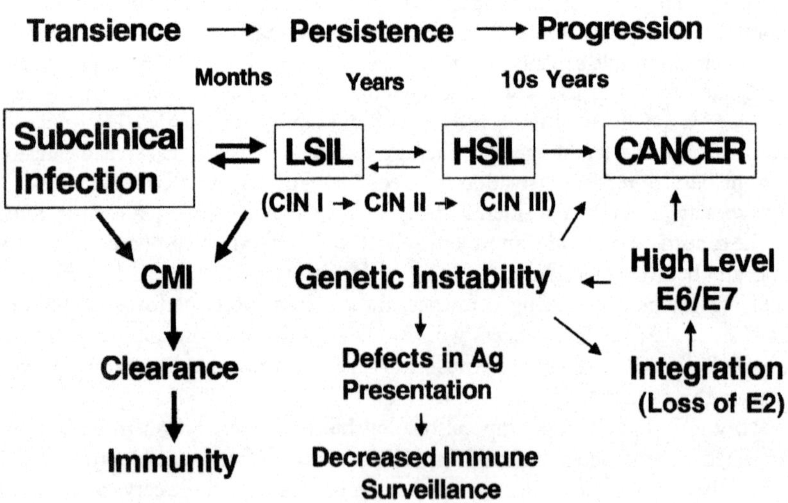

FIGURE 13.2.1 Model for human papillomavirus–induced carcinogenesis. (Ag, antigen; CIN, cervical intraepithelial neoplasia; CMI, cell-mediated immunity; HSIL, high-grade squamous intraepithelial lesion; LSIL, low-grade squamous intraepithelial lesion.)

by the activities of E6 and E7, are thought to be responsible for malignant progression of HPV-immortalized epithelial cells in vivo.[19] A current model of HPV oncogenesis is depicted in Figure 13.2.1.

At present, it is unclear whether HPV negative cervical cancer exists as a distinct biologic entity or whether it is simply a result of misclassification. For practical purposes, HPV infection of the cervix can be considered the first necessary cause of a human cancer to be identified.[8] However, HPV infection is not a sufficient cause of cervical cancer, as most cervical infections by cancer-associated types do not lead to cancer. The usually benign outcome is due to the transient nature of most genital HPV infections and the need for viral persistence for oncogenic progression.[24]

There is also good evidence that HPV infection is causally related to a substantial subset of other anogenital cancers, specifically cancer of the anus, vulva, and vagina.[25,26] In addition, there is increasing evidence that a proportion of head and neck cancers, especially those at oropharyngeal sites, are HPV-induced.[27,28] HPV16 is also the predominant type found in these cancers. This raises the possibility that a vaccine to prevent cervical cancer might also reduce the incidence of these other cancers.

PROPHYLACTIC VACCINES

Prophylactic vaccines against virus infection are among the most successful public health interventions ever devised. They have led to the eradication of small pox and the control of other viral infections, such as polio, measles, and rubella. There is optimism that HPV immunoprophylaxis will ultimately prove to be a potent and cost-effective intervention measure against cervical cancer worldwide. However, none of the successful viral vaccines combat sexually transmitted viruses that locally infect mucosal surfaces. So, without a clear precedence, success of the current candidate HPV vaccines cannot be guaranteed. Prophylactic vaccines based on live viruses, such as the vaccinia-based small pox vaccine, are not a reasonable option for oncogenic HPVs for two reasons. First, the viruses can not be efficiently grown in cultured cells.[29] Second, the viral genome contains the E6 and E7 oncogenes. The presence of these genes would raise the specter of vaccine-induced carcinogenesis even if an attenuated virus that could be efficiently grow in culture were developed. It is doubtful that a vaccine targeting healthy young people could (or should) win regulatory approval if it contained oncogenes.

The HPV prophylactic vaccines under most active development are based on HPV virus–like particles (VLPs).[30] The simplest papillomavirus VLPs consist of well-ordered assemblages of the L1 major virion protein. The VLPs are morphologically and antigenically similar to authentic virions (Fig. 13.2.2). However, they are noninfections, as they are the result of spontaneous self-assembly of L1 in the absence of the viral genome or other viral proteins. High-level expression of L1 leads to VLP production in mammalian cells, insect cells, yeast, and even, to

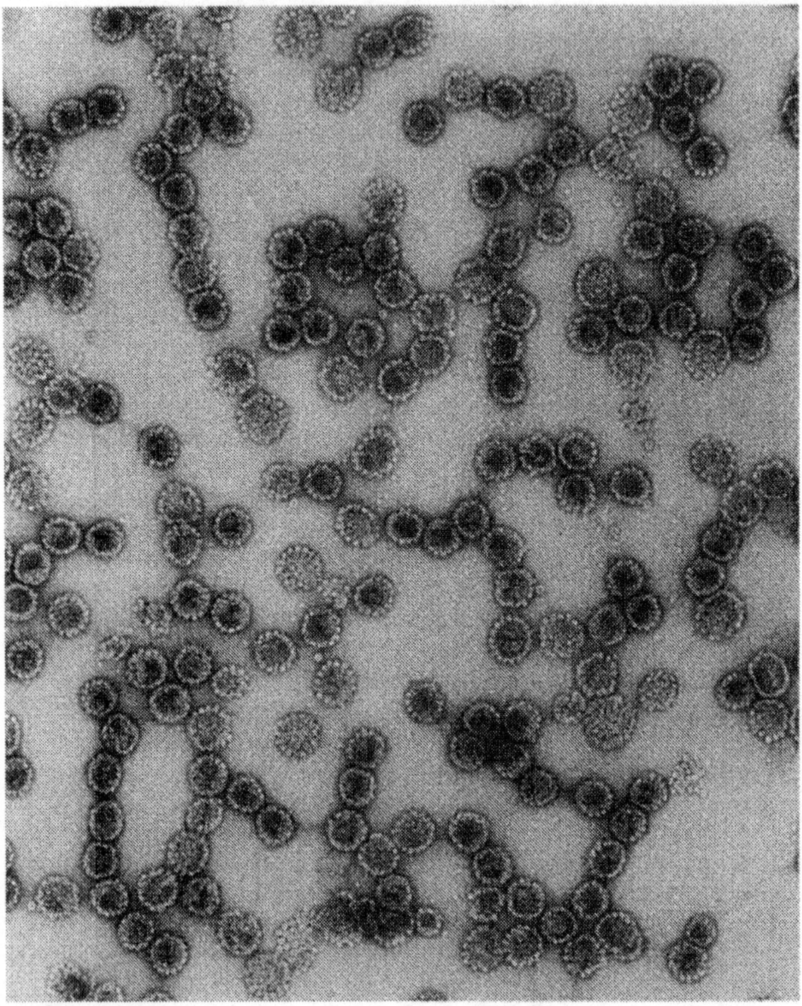

FIGURE 13.2.2 Transmission electron micrograph of HPV16 L1 viruslike particles (original magnification × 36,000).

a limited extent, in bacteria.[31–34] Vaccination of experimental animals with low doses of HPV VLPs induces high titers of virion antibodies that neutralize virus infection of cultured cells.[35–39] A set of studies in animals (rabbits, dogs, and cattle) further determined that VLP vaccination also protects from high-dose experimental challenge with homologous virus.[40–42] Passive transfer studies established that vaccine-induced virion antibodies were sufficient to confer protection from experimental challenge.[40,41] However, papillomavirus infections are remarkably species-restricted, and HPVs do not induce a productive infection or disease in an experimental animal. Consequently, there is no experimental animal model for directly testing prophylactic HPV vaccines. The animal models are also limited by the fact that none involve sexual transmission, the mode by which the HPV infections that cause cervical cancer are transmitted.

Overall, L1 is a highly conserved protein. However, most of the conserved peptides are interior structural elements of the protein.[43] In contrast, the L1 epitopes recognized by neutralizing antibodies are conformation-dependent external loops with variable sequence that are displayed by VLPs but not by denatured L1. As a result, the neutralizing antibodies generated by VLPs (or authentic virions) are predominantly type-specific.[35–37,39] Consequently, it is unlikely that HPV VLPs of one genotype will induce antibody-mediated protection against infection by other genotypes. A possible exception is for very closely related types (e.g., HPV18 and 45; HPV 6 and 11) wherein a limited amount of cross-neutralization has been detected in in vitro neutralization assays.[39,44,45] Although genotypes appear to be distinct serotypes, there is no evidence for multiple serotypes within a genotype. However, this question has been examined only for HPV16.[46] On the basis of the analysis of the HPV DNA in a large set of cervical cancers, it has been estimated that vaccine containing types 16 and 18 VLPs could prevent 70% of cervical cancer in most countries. These types plus HPV31 and HPV45 could prevent more than 80% of cervical cancers.[9]

Vaccination of mice with polypeptides of the L2 minor capsid protein was recently shown to induce cross-neutralizing antisera that were active against distantly related genital HPV types (e.g., between types 16 and 18).[47,48] This was a surprising result, as it was previously found that L1/L2 VLPs, in which L2 is apparently incorporated into its normal context, did not induce broadly cross-neutralizing antibodies.[36] The most likely explanation for this apparent discrepancy is that, in the context of a fully assembled virion or VLP, the cross-neutralizing L2 epitopes either are not well exposed or are subdominant. Consistent with the latter possibility, the titers of neutralizing antibodies induced by L2 peptides are at least one hundredfold lower than the titers induced by L1 VLPs.[47] A challenge for future investigation will be to develop vaccination strategies that are able to induce high titers of L2 cross-neutralizing antibodies.

Several early-phase clinical trials of HPV VLP-based vaccines have been conducted using clinical-grade HPV VLPs produced in L1 recombinant baculovirus–infected insect cells or L1 recombinant yeast. Although there have been many meeting reports, only a few of the studies are published.[49–52] Overall, the results have been encouraging. Intramuscular VLP vaccination, either with alum or without adjuvant, was very well tolerated, with minor local pain the only significant side effect. Three doses of vaccine in the 10- to 50-μg range were sufficient to induce high titers of antibodies. The limited variability in response across subjects and the absence of exceptionally low responders were also encouraging findings. In one study, the mean serum titer induced after vaccination was forty-fold higher than the mean serum titer induced by natural infection.[50] Also, the HPV VLP titers in people were equal to the animal papillomavirus VLP titers that gave good protection from experimental challenge in the animal models. The durability of the antibody response was relatively good, even when the vaccine was administered without adjuvant. Preliminary results from a study sponsored by the National Cancer Institute estimated a mean loss of serum titer of fourfold over the first year (J.T. Schiller, unpublished observations, 2001).

An assessment of cervical mucosal antibodies after parenteral VLP vaccination has also begun. This evaluation is critical, as protection from cervical HPV infection is being sought with these vaccines, and the virus does not induce viremia as a normal part of its life cycle. Preliminary meeting reports indicate that, although parenteral injection does not induce secretory IgA, transudation of VLP-specific serum antibodies is relatively high at the cervix in women vaccinated intramuscularly with VLPs (see *www.IPVSoc.org* for Nineteenth International Papillomavirus Conference Abstract No. O52). In general, the specific immunoglobulin G levels were approximately one order of magnitude lower than that detected in the serum. However, both VLP-specific and total immunoglobulin G dropped approximately tenfold around ovulation in women who were undergoing a normal menstrual cycle. Titers were relatively constant in women taking oral contraceptives. It is difficult to predict whether the drop in titers during ovulation will have an impact on the efficacy of the vaccine, as there is no animal model to evaluate the levels of local antibodies needed to prevent cervical infection by sexually transmitted virus.

Large scale prophylactic efficacy trials of VLP vaccines are being planned by Glaxo/SmithKline, Merck, and the National Cancer Institute[53] (also see *www.IPVSoc.org* for recent presentations at the Nineteenth International Papillomavirus Conference). Indications are that Glaxo/SmithKline is developing a vaccine consisting of baculovirus-derived HPV16 L1 and HPV18 L1 VLPs. Merck has reported on a tetravalent vaccine consisting of yeast derived L1 VLPs of types 16, 18, 6, and 11 in Alum. The planned National Cancer Institute trial will involve intramuscular injection of a baculovirus-derived HPV16 L1 VLPs without adjuvant. It will take place in Guanacaste, Costa Rica, in collaboration with the Costa Rican government. This site was chosen in part because it is the site of a long-term study of genital HPV natural history.[54] The trial will be population-based and placebo-controlled and will involve following up approximately 5000 young women per arm for 4 years. The study will use persistent cervical HPV16 DNA and HPV16-positive low-grade squamous intraepithelial lesions (LSILs) as the primary virologic and clinical endpoints, respectively.[55]

An important question is what endpoints regulatory agencies will require in a pivotal Phase III trial for licensure of HPV prophylactic vaccines. For ethical reasons, cervical cancer can obviously not be used in a study with active follow up. HSIL (or the corresponding histologic designation of cervical intraepithelial neoplasia, grade 3) is accepted as the immediate precursor to cervical cancer. It is also the stage of cervical neoplasia at which ablative treatment of the lesion normally occurs. However, only a few percent of incident oncogenic HPV infections result in HSIL, and it usually takes many years for this degree of dysplasia to develop.[56] Using HSIL as a primary endpoint could necessitate a prohibitively large or long-term trial. LSIL would seem the logical choice for a clinical endpoint in an efficacy trial as it is the frequent outcome of persistent infection by oncogenic types. However, most LSIL regresses spontaneously, and the reliability and interlaboratory consistency of an LSIL diagnosis may be problematic.[57] Also, there is a controversy in the literature over what percent of HSIL (and by implication cancers) develop rapidly from HPV infections without going through a low-grade intermediate.[58] In contrast, persistent type-specific HPV DNA can be reliably and consistently determined, and viral DNA persistence is necessary for the development of high-grade cervical dysplasias and cancers.[11,12] Persistent viral DNA has, therefore, been proposed as a primary virologic endpoint for efficacy trials. However, the length of time that distinguishes low-risk transient infections from persistent infection with a high potential for progression remains somewhat unclear.[24] For practical purposes, it is likely that detection of the same type of HPV DNA in cervical samples taken at an interval of at least 1 year will be operationally defined as persistent infection.

An ad hoc hypothesis that has been raised states that perhaps a prophylactic vaccine could protect against the infections that lead to the majority of LSILs that spontaneously regress but not protect against the minority that persist and progress to HSIL or not protect from the HSILs that arise de novo. Such a vaccine would not reduce the incidence of cervical cancer. Although this possibility cannot be formally excluded, there is also no reason to believe that virion-neutralizing antibodies will be differentially effective in preventing HPV infections that are destined to have different pathological potentials. There is also no reason to expect that the subset of women who fail to clear their cervical infections spontaneously will be the same subset who fail to be protected by the vaccine. This is because most women who develop cervical cancer do not have obvious immune deficiencies, and the immune effector mechanisms involved in the two processes are believed to be distinct. Regression of viral lesions is almost certainly mediated by local mucosal cell-mediated immunity (CMI) responses, whereas vaccine-induced protection will presumably be mediated by systemic B-cell responses.[59,60]

Second-generation prophylactic vaccines have been under extensive preclinical development but are only beginning to be tested in human trials. Most of these alternative strategies also seek to generate high titers of L1-neutralizing antibodies but with vaccines that are potentially more effective, less expensive to manufacture, or easier to distribute than is the prototype. Many strategies address more than one of the preceding issues (Table 13.2.1). Attempts to increase vaccine effectiveness have mostly focused on mucosal application of a VLP-based vaccine to induce secretory IgA in cervical mucosa in addition to systemic antibodies. In

TABLE 13.2.1 Strategies for Second-Generation Prophylactic Human Papillomavirus Vaccines Tested in Animal Models: Potential Advantages Over Injection of VLPs

Strategy	Increased Effectiveness	Lower Production Costs	Lower Distribution Costs	Study
Naked L1 DNA	No	Yes	Yes	101–103
Pentameric L1 fusion protein	No	Yes	No	104
Mucosal delivery of VLPs[a]	Yes	No	Yes	105–108
Live L1 recombinant virus	Yes	No	Yes	109
Live L1 recombinant bacteria	Yes	Yes	Yes	34,110

VLP, viruslike particle.
[a]Intranasal or oral.

animal models, this can be accomplished by direct application of VLPs to a mucosal surface or indirectly via mucosatropic live virus or bacterial vectors (see Table 13.2.1). Because immune responses induced at one mucosal site generate effector responses at other mucosal sites, the vaccine might be delivered to the upper respiratory or gastrointestinal tract rather than to the genital tract. These alternative routes for mucosal vaccination would be easier to administer and will probably be more acceptable to more young women. They would also allow both men and women to be vaccinated in the same way.

Expense and distribution issues are likely to be critical to vaccination programs, especially in developing countries, where the vaccine is most needed. Different strategies address these issues to varying extents. For instance, some live recombinant virus vaccines might be easily administered to a mucosal surface. However, they would probably be relatively expensive to manufacture because they require mammalian cell culture and might require a cold chain. A vaccine based on injection of bacterial plasmid DNA would be inexpensive to produce and could probably be distributed without a cold chain but would still require relatively costly administration with a syringe or gene gun. A vaccine involving oral delivery of VLPs in a crude yeast or plant extract, or involving a recombinant mucosatropic bacteria, could generate both secretory IgA and IgG and be inexpensively produced and distributed in many developing countries. Key questions remain for each of these strategies, most prominently the demonstration of safety and consistent immunogenicity in humans. If the first generation of vaccines proves effective in the upcoming trials, an important question will be whether investment in second-generation vaccines will continue. It may prove especially difficult to secure the funds to conduct large-scale efficacy trials of alternative vaccine candidates in developing countries, if there is the perception that they are not needed in industrialized countries.

Alternative vaccine strategies may be important to maximize coverage in HPV prophylactic vaccine programs in developed countries as well. A vaccination program using the current purified VLP candidates is expected to involve clinic visits by preadolescents for a series of three intramuscular injections. Such a program would require that parents and pediatricians be actively committed to the vaccination of their children against a sexually transmitted disease. It is possible that coverage rates would increase substantially if the vaccine could be administered by a noninjectable means in a school setting.

THERAPEUTIC VACCINES

Vaccines aimed at reducing regression of HPV-induced premalignant neoplasia of the cervix and other anogenital sites are therapeutic with respect to virus infection. However, they are prophylactic with respect to cancer prevention. Therefore, they fall within the scope of this chapter. From the viewpoint of therapeutic vaccine development, it is important to note that women with impairments in CMI (but not humoral immunity) have an increased incidence of high-grade premalignant HPV lesions and cervical cancer.[59,60] This implies that clearing of HPV infections requires cell-mediated immune mechanisms. However, neither the antigenic targets nor effector mechanisms involved in spontaneous immune-mediated regression have been clearly delineated for any papillomavirus infection. The lack of a suitable mouse model has significantly hampered research in this area.

Despite the limited knowledge of the parameters that define an effective immune response to HPV infection, HPV-induced premalignant cervical neoplasia represents an attractive target for immunotherapy for several reasons. First, the E6 and E7 viral oncogenes are selectively retained and expressed throughout the course of malignant progression.[19] Consequently, they provide non-self tumor antigens to which the immune system will not have developed embryologic tolerance. Second, development of cancer from HPV-induced low-grade cervical dysplasias generally takes decades.[61] This period provides a long window of opportunity in which to intervene therapeutically. Third, premalignant disease is common and routinely diagnosed in cervical cytology (e.g., Papanicolaou) screening programs (at least in most developed countries).[62] Fourth, the state of the lesions can be readily monitored noninvasively by colposcopy. Therefore, it is relatively easy to evaluate the effectiveness of immunotherapeutic interventions. Fifth, there are acceptable and usually definitive ablative therapies for premalignant cervical lesions.[63] Consequently, patients who fail to respond successfully to vaccination should not be placed at undue risk of subsequently developing cervical cancer.

Many of the therapeutic vaccine strategies developed to induce CMI against other viral and cancer antigens have been shown to induce anti-tumor immunity to the HPV oncoproteins (mostly HPV16 E7) in animal models (Table 13.2.2). It is beyond the scope of this chapter to describe the individual strategies in detail (see references 64 and 65 for more comprehensive recent reviews). Most models involve protection of mice from subcutaneous challenge with a syngeneic tumor expressing E6 and E7. Many of the approaches have also been shown to work therapeutically (i.e., to induce regression of established tumors). Cytotoxic T-lymphocytes are the main effectors in these models. However, the transplanted mouse tumors bear little resemblance biologically to cervical neoplasia developing in situ. Therefore, although these studies are critical preludes to clinical trials, their value in predicting their comparative effectiveness in inducing regression of HPV-induced anogenital dysplasias is unclear.

A smaller number of immunotherapeutic vaccines targeting E6 or E7 (or both) have been tested in clinical trials. Most have involved advanced cervical cancer patients. The vaccines were either HPV16 E7 peptides[66–68] or an HPV16 and HPV18 E6/E7 expressing vaccinia virus.[69,70] Not unexpectedly, these trials have achieved limited clinical success. Many cancer patients have general immunodeficiencies, and cervical cancer cells often have specific defects in class I antigen

TABLE 13.2.2 Therapeutic Human Papillomavirus Vaccine Studies in Mouse Tumor Models

Vaccine Strategy	Study
Peptide	
Mouse class I–specific 16 E7	111
Human class I–specific 16 E7	112
Protein	
GST-16 E7	113
M. bovis Hsp65-16 E7	114
16 L2-E6-E7	115
Naked DNA	
Mutated 16 E7	116
Sig-Lamp1-16 E7	117
M. bovis Hsp70-16 E7	118
"Shuffled" 16 E7	91
Calreticulin-16 E7	119
Viral vectors	
Vaccinia 16 E6/E7	120,121
Adenovirus 16 E7 peptides	122
Adenovirus 16 E6 + E7	123
AAV 16 E7 peptide	124
Bacterial vectors	
Streptococcus gordonii 16 E7	125
M. bovis 16 E7	110
Listeria 16 E7	126
Cell-based	
Dendritic cells 16 E7 peptide	127
Dendritic cells 16 E7 protein	128
Dendritic cells 16 E7 gene	129,130
E6/E7 tumor cells + IL-2 gene	131
E6/E7 tumor cells + IL-12 gene	132

presentation that are likely to make them refractory to normal cytotoxic T-lymphocyte responses.[71–73] In contrast, most women with premalignant cervical and other HPV-induced anogenital lesions are immunocompetent. The extent to which these patients are specifically tolerant to E6 and E7, and whether a substantial proportion of premalignant lesions already have defects in antigen presentation, are important questions that are under investigation.[74,75] Two vaccine strategies have been tested in early phase studies of immunotherapy of high-grade HPV-induced anogenital dysplasia. One trial involved vaccination of patients positive for HPV16 high-grade cervical and vulvar dysplasia with HPV16 E7 peptide-based vaccines.[76] The other approach involved vaccination of cervical and anal dysplasia patients with a mycobacteria heat shock protein 65-HPV16 E7 fusion protein (see *stressgen.com/news/pr-011129-PhaseIIData.pdf* for a summary of the unpublished results). The vaccines in both studies generated measurable cell-mediated responses to E7, and clinical responses were noted in a proportion of the vaccinees. Additional clinical trials of these and other therapeutic vaccine candidates are likely to follow.

There may be a greater immediate need for effective immunotherapy of anal dysplasias than for that of cervical dysplasias because clinical management of anal lesions can be more difficult.[77] However, most studies in the near future will probably focus on cervical lesions. This is because the natural history and treatment outcomes of cervical disease are better understood and because the large number of routine diagnoses of cervical neoplasias will facilitate patient accrual. Most studies will probably concentrate on high-grade dysplasias (high-grade squamous intraepithelial lesions and cervical intraepithelial neoplasia, grade 3) because they normally persist and are surgically treated.[61,63] In contrast, most low-grade dysplasias (low-grade squamous intraepithelial lesions and cervical intraepithelial neoplasia, grade 1) spontaneously regress within 1 year and are not routinely treated.

COMBINED PROPHYLACTIC AND THERAPEUTIC VACCINES

A vaccine that both prevented initial genital HPV infection and induced regression of established HPV lesions would be more attractive than a solely prophylactic or solely therapeutic vaccine in most settings. Such a combined prophylactic-therapeutic vaccine would be particularly advantageous in developing countries. Strictly therapeutic vaccines would have limited potential in low-resource settings, unless they are effective against advanced cancers, because women with premalignant disease or early-stage cancers are not routinely identified. VLP-based prophylactic vaccines would be relatively expensive seen in the light of health care resources in many developing countries, even if alternative manufacturing and distribution strategies were developed. This would prevent their rapid dissemination to the poorest subset of young women most in need of them. In addition, premalignant cervical HPV disease is asymptomatic and so is not in itself a public health concern. It might be easier to convince public health officials to initiate a relatively expensive vaccination program if it had the potential for short-term benefit than if the program would not be expected to provide a visible health benefit for decades (the mean time from initial infection to the development of cancer). A combined prophylactic-therapeutic vaccine that both prevented initial infection and induced regression of at least a proportion of established HPV anogenital lesions would have the most potential for short-term impact and long-term effectiveness.

It is possible that a vaccine capable of generating potent cell-mediated immune responses to nonstructural (early) viral antigens could both prevent the appearance of detectable virus infections and induce the regression of established lesions. This approach has generated some promising results in the cottontail rabbit papillomavirus (CRPV) cutaneous wart model in rabbits.[78–80] However, as previously successful vaccines appear to be largely dependent on the induction of neutralizing antibodies,[81] it is widely believed that an HPV prophylactic vaccine that also induces neutralizing antibodies has the greatest chances for success.

In addition to generating neutralizing antibodies, HPV L1 VLPs are known to activate dendritic cells as professional antigen cells[82,83] and to induce potent CMI to L1 in both animal models and in human T cells ex vivo.[84–88] However, it is unlikely that these CMI responses will induce regression of established HPV lesions. This is because L1 is not detectably expressed in the basal cells of the stratified squamous epithelium in which the infection is normally maintained.[89] L1 is expressed only in the terminally differentiated cells in the upper layers. This is presumably an adaptation to escape host immune surveillance.[59,60] Additionally, high-grade dysplasias and cancers are sufficiently dedifferentiated to preclude detectable L1 expression anywhere in these lesions.[90] Although some bystander killing of proliferating HPV-positive cells might result from CMI directed against neighboring differentiated cells that express the virion proteins, it is unlikely that this mechanism will consistently clear established lesions.

In theory, a combined vaccine could be produced by mixing separately manufactured VLPs and E6 or E7 proteins or by mixing L1 DNA with DNA encoding E6/E7 peptides. Presumably, DNAs encoding short E6/E7 peptides or scrambled peptide sequences would be used to avoid the theoretical possibility of vaccine-induced carcinogenesis.[91] However, most efforts have been devoted to generating a single VLP-based product that could induce both neutralizing antibodies and CMI to viral early proteins. The most advanced approach involves the incorporation of polypeptides from early proteins into VLPs as fusion proteins with L1 or L2 to form chimeric VLPs.

The prototype L1 chimeric VLPs incorporate 50 or fewer amino acids of HPV16 E7 as a C-terminal fusion of L1.[92,93] The prototype L1/L2 chimeric VLP has full-length HPV16 E7 (100 amino acids) linked to the C-terminus of HPV16 L2.[94] A similar chimera linking full-length E7 and full-length E2 (370 amino acids) to L2 has been generated (J.T. Schiller, unpublished results, 2000). The L1 chimeras have the theoretical advantage of incorporating 360 copies of the target polypeptide, compared with an estimated 12 copies for L1/L2 chimeras. The L1/L2 chimeras have the theoretical advantage of incorporating full-length proteins, whereas L1 chimeras appear to have an upper limit of approximately 60 amino acids for the inserted peptide, and insertion of some smaller peptides were incompatible with L1 self assembly.[92] Both types of E7 chimeras retained the ability to induce virion-neutralizing antibodies. However, they also induced protection from E7-expressing tumor challenge in transplantable mouse tumor models after vaccination with low doses of VLPs in the absence of adjuvant.[94,95] The induction of effective anti-tumor CMI in the absence of adjuvant, and also without T help,[94] probably results from the VLPs ability to bind tightly and activate dendritic cells.[82,83]

Clinical-grade HPV16 L1-E7 chimeric VLPs have been generated and are being tested in therapeutic trials of patients with high-grade cervical dysplasia.[64] Similar trials with an HPV16 L1/L2 chimera are likely to follow. The National Cancer Institute is also considering testing the HPV16 L1/L2-E7-E2 chimera as a third arm in the Costa Rican prophylactic vaccine trial. It is possible that CMI to the inserted proteins will induce early regression of subclinical infections that break through in the vaccinated women, despite the presence of neutralizing antibodies, and will induce regression in women who have clinical lesions at enrollment.

HPV pseudovirions might be effective alternatives to chimeric VLPs for a combined prophylactic-therapeutic vaccine. This approach involves use of the papillomavirus VLPs to deliver into cells DNA molecules expressing the target antigen, in this case peptides of nonstructural viral proteins. This is an attractive approach, as it would use the VLPs as a gene transfer vehicle, as well as an inducer of neutralizing antibodies and activator of dendritic cells. It theory, genetic immunization might lead to longer term exposure of the immune system to target antigens than would be achieved with protein based immunization. Perhaps this would result in a more robust and durable cell mediated immune response. Successful mucosal gene transfer and cytotoxic T-lymphocyte induction in mice has been demonstrated after oral delivery of HPV pseudovirions.[96]

Several strategies for generating HPV pseudovirions have been developed. Except for the study previously noted, these pseudovirions have been used to evaluate antibody mediated virus neutralization in vitro, rather than as vaccines. Some involve encapsidation of the target plasmid within mammalian cells[36,37] or yeast cells.[97] Other methods depend on disassembly-reassembly of the capsids in the presence of the pseudogenome in a test tube.[98,99] An alternative strategy involves linking the target DNA to the exterior of the VLPs.[100] However, none of these approaches is efficient at generating VLPs, and it is unlikely that any can be adapted for large-scale production of a vaccine. In addition to further characterization of papillomavirus pseudovirions as vaccine vehicles, a challenge for the future will be to devise a method of making HPV pseudovirions by a scaleable process.

FUTURE CONSIDERATIONS

There has been an explosion in the development of vaccines to prevent HPV-induced anogenital malignancies over the last decade. The driving forces behind this development were the conclusive evidence that HPV infection is the overwhelmingly important etiologic agent in cervical cancer and, simultaneously, a series of technical advances that produced promising vaccines candidates. There are currently many attractive vaccine candidates, both prophylactic and therapeutic, that have gone through preclinical evaluation in animal models. Additional candidates are likely to continue to emerge in the coming years. However, none of the animal models closely resembles genital tract HPV infection in humans.

Thus, it will be difficult to determine in advance which of these strategies is most likely to be successful against HPV-induced neoplasia in humans. Therefore, the most critical question currently is, Which candidates will or should be chosen for expensive clinical trials. The prophylactic efficacy of the most basic L1 VLP vaccines will almost certainly be determined. The results should provide insights into the degree to which systemically induced neutralizing antibodies can prevent genital HPV disease. If they fail to produce adequate protection, will there be resources available to test alternatives that might be more effective? If they succeed, will there be the resources to test second generation vaccines that might dramatically increase the vaccine utilization in the low resource settings where it is most needed? There are even more therapeutic HPV vaccine candidates competing for limited clinical trial resources. Which of those goes on to definitive clinical trials will largely depend on which ones are championed by corporate sponsors. Public sector resources might be used in conducting early-phase comparative trials of a number of the therapeutic vaccine candidates. Perhaps these trials could not only provide important insights for developing effective vaccines against HPV-induced neoplasia but could establish general principles that could be applied to vaccines against other human cancers as well.

REFERENCES

1. Parkin DM, Pisani P, Ferlay J. Estimates of worldwide incidence from 25 cancers in 1990. Int J Cancer 1999;80: 827–841.
2. Munoz N. Human papillomavirus and cancer: the epidemiological evidence. Journal of Clinical Virology 2000;19: 1–5.
3. Brinton LA. Epidemiology of cervical cancer—overview. In: Munoz N, Bosch FX, Shah KV, Meheus A, eds. The Epidemiology of Human Papillomavirus and Cervical Cancer. Lyon: International Agency of Research on Cancer, 1992.
4. Dürst M, Gissmann L, Ikenberg H, zur Hausen H. A papillomavirus DNA from a cervical carcinoma and its prevalence in cancer biopsy samples from different geographic regions. Proc Natl Acad Sci USA 1983;80:3812–3815.
5. Rothman KJ. Causal inference in epidemiology. In: Rothman KJ, ed. Modern Epidemiology. Boston: Little, Brown, 1986:7–23.
6. Bosch FX, Rohan T, Schneider A et al. Papillomavirus research update: highlights of the Barcelona HPV 2000 international papillomavirus conference. J Clin Pathol 2001;54:163–175.
7. Burk RD. Pernicious papillomavirus infection. N Engl J Med 1999;341:1687–1688.
8. Walboomers JM, Jacobs MC, Manos MM et al. Human papillomavirus is a necessary cause of invasive cervical cancer worldwide. J Pathol 1999;189:12–19.
9. Bosch FX, Manos MM, Munoz N et al. Prevalence of human papillomavirus in cervical cancer: a worldwide prospective. J Natl Cancer Inst 1995;87:796–802.
10. Greer CE, Wheeeler CM, Lander MB et al. Human papillomavirus (HPV) type distribution and serological response to HPV 6 virus-like particle in patients with genital warts. J Clin Microb 1995;33:2058–2063.
11. Ho GY, Bierman R, Beardsley L et al. Natural history of cervicovaginal papillomavirus infection in young women. N Engl J Med 1998;338:423-428.

12. Nobbenhuis MA, Walboomers JM, Helmerhorst TJ et al. Relation of human papillomavirus status to cervical lesions and consequences for cervical-cancer screening: a prospective study. Lancet 1999;354:20–25.

13. Dillner J, Lehtinen M, Bjorge T et al. Prospective seroepidemiologic study of human papillomavirus infection as a risk factor for invasive cervical cancer. J Natl Cancer Inst 1997;89:1293–1299.

14. Wallin KL, Wiklund F, Angstrom T et al. Type-specific persistence of human papillomavirus DNA before the development of invasive cervical cancer. N Engl J Med 1999;341:1633–1638.

15. zur Hausen H. Immortalization of human cells and their malignant conversion by high risk human papillomavirus genotypes. Semin Cancer Biol 1999;9:405–411.

16. Werness BA, Levine AJ, Howley PM. Association of human papillomavirus types 16 and 18 E6 proteins with p53. Science 1990;248:76–79.

17. Dyson N, Howley PM, Munger K, Harlow E. The human papillomavirus-16 E7 oncoprotein is able to bind the retinoblastoma gene product. Science 1989;243:934–937.

18. Barbosa MS, Vass WC, Lowy DR, Schiller JT. In vitro biological activities of the E6 and E7 genes vary among human papillomaviruses of different oncogenic potential. J Virol 1991;65:292–298.

19. zur Hausen H. Papillomaviruses causing cancer: evasion from host-cell control in early events in carcinogenesis. J Natl Cancer Inst 2000;92:690–698.

20. McMurray HR, Nguyen D, Westbrook TF, McCance DJ. Biology of human papillomaviruses. Int J Exp Pathol 2001;82:15–33.

21. von Knebel Doeberitz M, Rittmuller C, zur Hausen H, Dürst M. Inhibition of tumorigenicity of cervical cancer cells in nude mice by HPV E6-E7 anti-sense RNA. Int J Cancer 1992;51:831–834.

22. Duensing S, Munger K. Centrosome abnormalities, genomic instability and carcinogenic progression. Biochim Biophys Acta 2001;2:81–88.

23. Klingelhutz AJ, Foster SA, McDougall JK. Telomerase activation by the E6 gene product of human papillomavirus type 16. Nature 1996;380:79–82.

24. Einstein MH, Burk RD. Persistent human papillomavirus infection: definitions and clinical implications. Papillomavirus Rep 2001;12:119–123.

25. Frisch M, Glimelius B, van den Brule AJ et al. Sexually transmitted infection as a cause of anal cancer. N Engl J Med 1997;337:1350–1358.

26. Pinto AP, Signorello LB, Crum CP et al. Squamous cell carcinoma of the vulva in Brazil: prognostic importance of host and viral variables. Gynecol Oncol 1999;74:61–67.

27. Frisch M, Biggar RJ. Aetiological parallel between tonsillar and anogenital squamous-cell carcinomas. Lancet 1999;354:1442–1443.

28. Gillison ML, Koch WM, Capone RB et al. Evidence for a causal association between human papillomavirus and a subset of head and neck cancers. J Natl Cancer Inst 2000;92:709–720.

29. Hagensee M, Galloway D. Growing human papillomaviruses and virus-like particles in the laboratory. Papillomavirus Rep 1993;4:121–124.

30. Schiller JT. Papillomavirus-like particle vaccines for cervical cancer. Mol Med Today 1999;5: 209–215.

31. Kirnbauer R, Booy F, Cheng N et al. Papillomavirus L1 major capsid protein self-assembles into virus-like particles that are highly immunogenic. Proc Natl Acad Sci USA 1992;89:12180–12184.

32. Hagensee ME, Yaegashi N, Galloway DA. Self-assembly of human papillomavirus type 1 capsids by expression of the L1 protein alone or by coexpression of the L1 and L2 capsid proteins. J Virol 1993;67:315–322.

33. Hofmann K, Cook J, Joyce J et al. Sequence determination of human papillomavirus 6a and assembly of virus-like particles in *Saccharomyces cerevisiae*. Virology 1995;209:506–518.

34. Nardelli-Haefliger D, Roden RBS, Benyacoub J et al. Human papillomavirus type 16 virus-like particles expressed in attenuated *Salmonella typhimurium* elicit mucosal and systemic neutralizing antibodies in mice. Infect Immun 1997;65:3328–3336.

35. Christensen ND, Kirnbauer R, Schiller JT et al. Human papillomavirus types 6 and 11 have antigenically distinct strongly immunogenic conformationally dependent neutralizing epitopes. Virology 1994;205:329–335.

36. Roden RBS, Greenstone HL, Kirnbauer R et al. In vitro generation and type-specific neutralization of a human papillomavirus type 16 virion pseudotype. J Virol 1996;70:5875–5883.

37. Unckell F, Streeck RE, Sapp M. Generation and neutralization of pseudovirions of human papillomavirus type 33. J Virol 1997;71:2934–2939.

38. Lowe RS, Brown DR, Bryan JT et al. Human papillomavirus type 11 (HPV11) neutralizing antibodies in the serum and genital mucosal secretions of African green monkeys immunized with HPV-11 virus-like particles expressed in yeast. J Infect Dis 1997;176:1141–1145.

39. White WI, Wilson SD, Bonnez W et al. In vitro infection and type-restricted antibody-mediated neutralization of authentic human papillomavirus type 16. J Virol 1998;72:959–964.

40. Breitburd F, Kirnbauer R, Hubbert NL et al. Immunization with virus-like particles from cottontail rabbit papillomavirus (CRPV) can protect against experimental CRPV infection. J Virol 1995; 69:3959–3963.

41. Suzich JA, Ghim S, Palmer-Hill FJ et al. Systemic immunization with papillomavirus L1 protein completely prevents the development of viral mucosal papillomas. Proc Natl Acad Sci USA 1995; 92:11553–11557.

42. Kirnbauer R, Chandrachud L, O'Neil B et al. Virus-like particles of bovine papillomavirus type 4 in prophylactic and therapeutic immunization. Virology 1996;219:37–44.

43. Chen XS, Garcea RL, Goldberg I et al. Structure of small virus-like particles assembled from the L1 protein of human papillomavirus 16. Mol Cells 2000;5:557–567.

44. Christensen ND, Hopfl R, DiAngelo SL et al. Assembled baculovirus-expressed human papillomavirus type 11 L1 capsid protein virus-like particles are recognized by neutralizing monoclonal antibodies and induce high titres of neutralizing antibodies. J Gen Virol 1994;75:2271–2276.

45. Roden RBS, Hubbert NL, Kirnbauer R et al. Assessment of the serological relatedness of genital human papillomaviruses by hemagglutination inhibition. J Virol 1996;70:3298–3301.

46. Pastrana DV, Vass WC, Lowy DR, Schiller JT. An HPV16 VLP vaccine induces human antibodies that neutralize divergent variants of HPV16. Virology 2001;279:361–369.

47. Roden RB, Yutzy WI, Fallon R et al. Minor capsid protein of human genital papillomaviruses contains subdominant, cross-neutralizing epitopes. Virology 2000;270:254–257.

48. Kawana K, Kawana Y, Yoshikawa H et al. Nasal immunization of mice with peptide having a cross-neutralization epitope on minor capsid protein L2 of human papillomavirus type 16 elicit systemic and mucosal antibodies. Vaccine 2001;19:1496–1502.

49. Zhang LF, Zhou J, Chen S et al. HPV6b virus like particles are potent immunogens without adjuvant in man. Vaccine 2000;18:1051–1058.

50. Harro CD, Pang YY, Roden RB et al. Safety and immunogenicity trial in adult volunteers of a human papillomavirus 16 L1 virus-like particle vaccine. J Natl Cancer Inst 2001;93:284–292.

51. Evans TG, Bonnez W, Rose RC et al. A phase 1 study of a recombinant virus-like particle vaccine against human papillomavirus type 11 in healthy adult volunteers. J Infect Dis 2001;183: 1485–1493.

52. Brown DR, Bryan JT, Schroeder JM et al. Neutralization of human papillomavirus type 11 (HPV-11) by serum from women vaccinated with yeast-derived HPV-11 L1 virus-like particles: correlation with competitive radioimmunoassay titer. J Infect Dis 2001;184:1183–1186.

53. Connett H. HPV vaccine moves into late stage trials. Nat Med 2001;7:388.

54. Herrero R, Hildesheim A, Bratti C et al. A population-based study of human papillomavirus infection and cervical neoplasia in rural Costa Rica. J Natl Cancer Inst 2000;92:464–474.

55. Schiller JT, Hildesheim A. Developing HPV virus-like particle vaccines to prevent cervical cancer: a progress report. J Clin Virol 2000;19:67–74.

56. Schiffman MH, Burk RD. Human papillomaviruses. In: Evans AS, Kaslow R, eds. Viral Infections in Humans. New York: Plenum Medical Book Co, 1997:983–1023.

57. Stoler MH, Schiffman M. Interobserver reproducibility of cervical cytologic and histologic interpretations: realistic estimates from the ASCUS-LSIL Triage Study. JAMA 2001;285:1500–1505.

58. Kiviat NB, Koutsky LA. Do our current cervical cancer control strategies still make sense? J Natl Cancer Inst 1996;88:317–318.

59. Stern PL, Brown M, Stacey SN et al. Natural HPV immunity and vaccination strategies. J Clin Virol 2000;19:57–66.

60. Konya J, Dillner J. Immunity to oncogenic human papillomaviruses. Adv Cancer Res 2001;82: 205–238.

61. Schiffman MH, Brinton LA. The epidemiology of cervical carcinogenesis. Cancer 1995;76: 1888–1901.

62. Koss LG. The Papanicolaou test for cervical cancer detection: a triumph and a tragedy. JAMA 1989;261:737–743.

63. Montz FJ. Management of high-grade cervical intraepithelial neoplasia and low- grade squamous intraepithelial lesion and potential complications. Clin Obstet Gynecol 2000;43:394–409.

64. Gissmann L, Osen W, Muller M, Jochmus I. Therapeutic vaccines for human papillomaviruses. Intervirology 2001;44:167–175.

65. Da Silva DM, Eiben GL, Fausch SC et al. Cervical cancer vaccines: emerging concepts and developments. J Cell Physiol 2001;186:169–182.

66. Steller MA, Gurski KJ, Murakami M et al. Cell-mediated immunological responses in cervical and vaginal cancer patients immunized with a lipidated epitope of human papillomavirus type 16 E7. Clin Cancer Res 1998;4:2103–2109.

67. van Driel WJ, Ressing ME, Kenter GG et al. Vaccination with HPV16 peptides of patients with advanced cervical carcinoma: clinical evaluation of a phase I-II trial. Eur J Cancer 1999;35: 946–952.

68. Ressing ME, van Driel WJ, Brandt RM et al. Detection of T helper responses, but not of human papillomavirus–specific cytotoxic T lymphocyte responses, after peptide vaccination of patients with cervical carcinoma. J Immunother 2000;23:255–266.

69. Borysiewicz LK, Fiander A, Nimako M et al. A recombinant vaccinia virus encoding human papillomavirus types 16 and 18, E6 and E7 proteins as immunotherapy for cervical cancer. Lancet 1996;347:1523–1527.

70. Adams M, Borysiewicz L, Fiander A et al. Clinical studies of human papilloma vaccines in pre-invasive and invasive cancer. Vaccine 2001;19:2549–2556.

71. Connor ME, Stern PL. Loss of MHC class-1 expression in cervical carcinomas. Int J Cancer 1990;46:1029–1034.

72. Brady CS, Bartholomew JS, Burt DJ et al. Multiple mechanisms underlie HLA dysregulation in cervical cancer. Tissue Antigens 2000;55:401–411.

73. Evans M, Borysiewicz LK, Evans AS et al. Antigen processing defects in cervical carcinomas limit the presentation of a CTL epitope from human papillomavirus 16 E6. J Immunol 2001;167: 5420–5428.

74. Doan T, Herd K, Street M et al. Human papillomavirus type 16 E7 oncoprotein expressed in peripheral epithelium tolerizes E7-directed cytotoxic T-lymphocyte precursors restricted through human (and mouse) major histocompatibility complex class I alleles. J Virol 1999;73:6166–6170.

75. Abdel-Hady ES, Martin-Hirsch P, Duggan-Keen M et al. Immunological and viral factors associated with the response of vulval intraepithelial neoplasia to photodynamic therapy. Cancer Res 2001; 61:192–196.

76. Muderspach L, Wilczynski S, Roman L et al. A phase I trial of a human papillomavirus (HPV) peptide vaccine for women with high-grade cervical and vulvar intraepithelial neoplasia who are HPV 16 positive. Clin Cancer Res 2000;6:3406–3416.

77. Palefsky JM. Anal squamous intraepithelial lesions in human immunodeficiency virus–positive men and women. Semin Oncol 2000;27:471–479.

78. Leachman SA, Tigelaar RE, Shlyankevich M et al. Granulocyte-macrophage colony-stimulating factor priming plus papillomavirus E6 DNA vaccination: effects on papilloma formation and regression in the cottontail rabbit papillomavirus–rabbit model. J Virol 2000;74:8700–8708.

79. Han R, Reed CA, Cladel NM, Christensen ND. Immunization of rabbits with cottontail rabbit papillomavirus E1 and E2 genes: protective immunity induced by gene gun-mediated intracutaneous delivery but not by intramuscular injection. Vaccine 2000;18:2937–2944.

80. Han R, Cladel NM, Reed CA et al. DNA vaccination prevents and/or delays carcinoma development of papillomavirus-induced skin papillomas on rabbits. J Virol 2000;74:9712–9716.

81. Robbins JB, Schneerson R, Szu SC. Hypothesis: serum IgG antibody is sufficient to confer protection against infectious diseases by inactivating the inoculum. J Infect Dis 1995;171: 1387–1398.

82. Rudolf MP, Fausch SC, Da Silva DM, Kast WM. Human dendritic cells are activated by chimeric human papillomavirus type-16 virus-like particles and induce epitope-specific human T cell responses in vitro. J Immunol 2001;166:5917–5924.

83. Lenz P, Day PM, Pang YS et al. Papillomavirus-like particles induce acute activation of dendtritic cells. J Immunol 2001;166:5346–5355.

84. Dupuy C, Buzoni-Gatel D, Touze A et al. Cell mediated immunity induced in mice by HPV16 L1 virus-like particles. Microb Pathog 1997;22:219–225.

85. De Bruijn MLH, Greenstone HL, Vermeulen H et al. L1-specific protection from tumor challenge elicited by HPV16 virus-like particles. Virology 1998;250:371–376.

86. Rudolf MP, Nieland JD, DaSilva DM et al. Induction of HPV16 capsid protein-specific human T cell responses by virus-like particles. Biol Chem 1999;380:335–340.

87. Kaufmann AM, Nieland J, Schinz M et al. HPV16 L1E7 chimeric virus-like particles induce specific HLA-restricted T cells in humans after in vitro vaccination. Int J Cancer 2001;92: 285–293.

88. Palker TJ, Monteiro JM, Martin MM et al. Antibody, cytokine and cytotoxic T lymphocyte responses in chimpanzees immunized with human papillomavirus virus-like particles. Vaccine 2001;19:3733–3743.

89. Stubenrauch F, Laimins LA. Human papillomavirus life cycle: active and latent phases. Semin Cancer Biol 1999;9:379–386.

90. Stoler MH, Rhodes MH, Witbeck A et al. Human papillomavirus type 16 and 18 gene expression in cervical neoplasias. Hum Pathol 1992;23:117–128.

91. Osen W, Peiler T, Ohlschlager P et al. A DNA vaccine based on a shuffled E7 oncogene of the human papillomavirus type 16 (HPV 16) induces E7-specific cytotoxic T cells but lacks transforming activity. Vaccine 2001;19:4276–4286.

92. Muller M, Zhou J, Reed TD et al. Chimeric papillomavirus-like particles. Virology 1997;234: 93–111.

93. Peng S, Frazer IH, Fernando GJ, Zhou J. Papillomavirus virus-like particles can deliver defined CTL epitopes to the MHC class I pathway. Virology 1998;240:147–157.

94. Greenstone HL, Nieland JD, de Visser KE et al. Chimeric papillomavirus virus-like particles elicit antitumor immunity against the E7 oncoprotein in an HPV16 tumor model. Proc Natl Acad Sci USA 1998;95:1800–1805.

95. Jochmus I, Schafer K, Faath S et al. Chimeric virus-like particles of the human papillomavirus type 16 (HPV 16) as a prophylactic and therapeutic vaccine. Arch Med Res 1999;30:269–274.

96. Shi W, Liu J, Huang Y, Qiao L. Papillomavirus pseudovirus: a novel vaccine to induce mucosal and systemic cytotoxic T-lymphocyte responses. J Virol 2001;75:10139–10148.

97. Rossi JL, Gissmann L, Jansen K, Muller M. Assembly of human papillomavirus type 16 pseudovirions in *Saccharomyces cerevisiae*. Hum Gene Ther 2000;11:1165–1176.

98. Kawana K, Yoshikawa H, Taketani Y et al. In vitro construction of pseudovirions of human papillomavirus type 16: incorporation of plasmid DNA into reassembled L1/L2 capsids. J Virol 1998;72:10298–10300.

99. Touze A, Coursaget P. In vitro gene transfer using human papillomavirus-like particles. Nucleic Acids Res 1998;26:1317–1323.

100. Yeager MD, Aste-Amezaga M, Brown DR et al. Neutralization of human papillomavirus (HPV) pseudovirions: a novel and efficient approach to detect and characterize HPV neutralizing antibodies. Virology 2000;278:570–577.

101. Donnelly JJ, Martinez D, Jansen KU et al. Protection against papillomavirus with a polynucleotide vaccine. J Infect Dis 1996;173:314–320.

102. Leder C, Kleinschmidt JA, Wiethe C, Muller M. Enhancement of capsid gene expression: preparing the human papillomavirus type 16 major structural gene L1 for DNA vaccination purposes. J Virol 2001;75:9201–9209.

103. Liu WJ, Zhao KN, Gao FG et al. Polynucleotide viral vaccines: codon optimisation and ubiquitin conjugation enhances prophylactic and therapeutic efficacy. Vaccine 2001;20:862–869.

104. Yuan H, Estes PA, Chen Y et al. Immunization with a pentameric L1 fusion protein protects against papillomavirus infection. J Virol 2001;75:7848–7853.

105. Bamelli C, Roden R, Potts A et al. Nasal immunization of mice with human papillomavirus type 16 virus-like particles elicits neutralizing antibodies in mucosal secretions. J. Virol 1998: 8220–8229.

106. Dupuy C, Buzoni-Gatel D, Touze A et al. Nasal immunization of mice with human papillomavirus type 16 (HPV-16) virus-like particles or with the HPV-16 L1 gene elicits specific cytotoxic T lymphocytes in vaginal draining lymph nodes. J Virol 1999;73:9063–9071.

107. Greer CE, Petracca R, Buonamassa DT et al. The comparison of the effect of LTR72 and MF59 adjuvants on mouse humoral response to intranasal immunisation with human papillomavirus type 6b (HPV-6b) virus-like particles. Vaccine 2000;19:1008–1012.

108. Gerber S, Lane C, Brown DM et al. Human papillomavirus virus–like particles are efficient oral immunogens when coadministered with *Escherichia coli* heat-labile enterotoxin mutant R192G or CpG DNA. J Virol 2001;75:4752–4760.

109. Kowalczyk DW, Wlazlo AP, Shane S, Ertl HC. Vaccine regimen for prevention of sexually transmitted infections with human papillomavirus type 16. Vaccine 2001;19:3583–3590.

110. Jabbar IA, Fernando GJ, Saunders N et al. Immune responses induced by BCG recombinant for human papillomavirus L1 and E7 proteins. Vaccine 2000;18:2444–2453.

111. Feltkamp MC, Smits HL, Vierboom MP et al. Vaccination with cytotoxic T lymphocyte epitope–containing peptide protects against a tumor induced by human papillomavirus type 16-transformed cells. Eur J Immunol 1993;23:2242–2249.

112. Ressing ME, Sette A, Brandt RM et al. Human CTL epitopes encoded by human papillomavirus type 16 E6 and E7 identified through in vivo and in vitro immunogenicity studies of HLA-A*0201-binding peptides. J Immunol 1995;154:5934–5943.

113. Fernando GJ, Murray B, Zhou J, Frazer IH. Expression, purification and immunological characterization of the transforming protein E7, from cervical cancer-associated human papillomavirus type 16. Clin Exp Immunol 1999;115:397–403.

114. Chu NR, Wu HB, Wu T et al. Immunotherapy of a human papillomavirus (HPV) type 16 E7-expressing tumour by administration of fusion protein comprising Mycobacterium bovis bacille Calmette-Guerin (BCG) hsp65 and HPV16 E7. Clin Exp Immunol 2000;121:216–225.

115. van der Burg SH, Kwappenberg KM, O'Neill T et al. Pre-clinical safety and efficacy of TA-CIN, a recombinant HPV16 L2E6E7 fusion protein vaccine, in homologous and heterologous prime-boost regimens. Vaccine 2001;19:3652–3660.

116. Shi W, Bu P, Liu J et al. Human papillomavirus type 16 E7 DNA vaccine: mutation in the open reading frame of E7 enhances specific cytotoxic T-lymphocyte induction and antitumor activity. J Virol 1999;73:7877–7881.

117. Ji H, Wang TL, Chen CH et al. Targeting human papillomavirus type 16 E7 to the endosomal/lysosomal compartment enhances the antitumor immunity of DNA vaccines against murine human papillomavirus type 16 E7-expressing tumors. Hum Gene Ther 1999;10:2727–2740.

118. Chen CH, Wang TL, Hung CF et al. Enhancement of DNA vaccine potency by linkage of antigen gene to an HSP70 gene. Cancer Res 2000;60:1035–1042.

119. Cheng WF, Hung CF, Chai CY et al. Tumor-specific immunity and antiangiogenesis generated by a DNA vaccine encoding calreticulin linked to a tumor antigen. J Clin Invest 2001;108: 669–678.

120. Chen L, Thomas EK, Hu SL et al. Human papillomavirus type 16 nucleoprotein E7 is a tumor rejection antigen. Proc Natl Acad Sci USA 1991;88:110–114.

121. Meneguzzi G, Cerni C, Kieny MP, Lathes R. Immunization against human papillomavirus type 16 tumor cells with recombinant vaccinia virus expressing E6 and E7. Virology 1991;181:62–69.

122. Toes RE, Hoeben RC, van der Voort EI et al. Protective anti-tumor immunity induced by vaccination with recombinant adenoviruses encoding multiple tumor-associated cytotoxic T lymphocyte epitopes in a string-of-beads fashion. Proc Natl Acad Sci USA 1997;94:14660–14665.

123. He Z, Wlazlo AP, Kowalczyk DW et al. Viral recombinant vaccines to the E6 and E7 antigens of HPV-16. Virology 2000;270:146–161.

124. Liu DW, Tsao YP, Kung JT et al. Recombinant adeno-associated virus expressing human papillomavirus type 16 E7 peptide DNA fused with heat shock protein DNA as a potential vaccine for cervical cancer. J Virol 2000;74:2888–2894.

125. Di Fabio S, Medaglini D, Rush CM et al. Vaginal immunization of Cynomolgus monkeys with *Streptococcus gordonii* expressing HIV-1 and HPV 16 antigens. Vaccine 1998;16:485–492.

126. Gunn GR, Zubair A, Peters C et al. Two *Listeria monocytogenes* vaccine vectors that express different molecular forms of human papilloma virus-16 (HPV-16) E7 induce qualitatively different t cell immunity that correlates with their ability to induce regression of established tumors immortalized by HPV-16. J Immunol 2001;167:6471–6479.

127. Mayordomo JI, Zorina T, Storkus WJ et al. Bone marrow–derived dendritic cells pulsed with synthetic tumour peptides elicit protective and therapeutic antitumour immunity. Nat Med 1995; 1:1297–1302.

128. De Bruijn ML, Schuurhuis DH, Vierboom MP et al. Immunization with human papillomavirus type 16 (HPV16) oncoprotein-loaded dendritic cells as well as protein in adjuvant induces MHC class I-restricted protection to HPV16-induced tumor cells. Cancer Res 1998;58:724–731.

129. Tuting T, DeLeo AB, Lotze MT, Storkus WJ. Genetically modified bone marrow–derived dendritic cells expressing tumor-associated viral or "self" antigens induce antitumor immunity in vivo. Eur J Immunol 1997;27:2702–2707.

130. Wang TL, Ling M, Shih IM et al. Intramuscular administration of E7-transfected dendritic cells generates the most potent E7-specific anti-tumor immunity. Gene Ther 2000;7:726–733.

131. Bubenik J, Simova J, Hajkova R et al. Interleukin 2 gene therapy of residual disease in mice carrying tumours induced by HPV 16. Int J Oncol 1999;14:593–597.

132. Hallez S, Detremmerie O, Giannouli C et al. Interleukin-12-secreting human papillomavirus type 16-transformed cells provide a potent cancer vaccine that generates E7-directed immunity. Int J Cancer 1999;81:428–437.

Chapter 14

Smoking Cessation Strategies

Glen Morgan

Patricia L. Fiero

Eva Matthews

Scott Leischow

The importance of the oncologist's role in intervening with patients who smoke cannot be underestimated. Approximately 48 million adult Americans, representing 25% of the population, smoke, and 30% of all cancer mortality is attributable to tobacco use.[1,2] Thus, there is tremendous opportunity for oncologists to intervene with their patients who smoke. Consequently, the Public Health Service of the U.S. Department of Health and Human Services developed a guideline that recommends that all patients be assessed for smoking status at every encounter and that those who smoke be advised to stop and be offered assistance with their attempt.[3] Furthermore, the National Cancer Institute (NCI) Lung Cancer Progress Review Group recently recommended that "smoking cessation advice should be a routine part of any clinical trial involving smokers."[4] This chapter first describes the epidemiology and etiology of smoking, follows that with a description of treatment approaches, and finally outlines guidelines for intervening with smokers in general and in populations and settings for which special considerations may apply.

EPIDEMIOLOGY

Cigarette smoking remains firmly entrenched in American society today, although the demographics of smokers vary from those 30 years ago. The prevalence of smoking among adults declined steadily through the 1970s and 1980s and has remained relatively stable in the last decade.[1,3,5] Smoking prevalence and the trajectory of tobacco use initiation among America's youth, however, are alarming. During a 6-year period in the last decade, reports of youth smoking increased by 32%.[6] This is particularly noteworthy given the increased policies concerning smoking, litigation concerning the tobacco industry, and (presumably) heightened public awareness of the negative health consequences of smoking. Worldwide, it is estimated that there are more than 1 billion smokers.[7]

Smoking is more prevalent among men (27.6%) than among women (22.1%) and more prevalent among American Indians and Alaska natives (34.1%) than among blacks (26.7%), whites (25.3%), and Hispanics (20.4%).[1,2] When viewed collectively, Asian Americans and Pacific Islanders have relatively low rates of smoking (16.9%). These aggregated figures obscure, however, significant variation among individual ethnic groups. For example, 55% of Southeast Asian men living in the United States smoke.[8] The consequences and costs of tobacco use are significant and severe. Smoking has been the chief preventable cause of illness and death in the United States for more than three decades and is responsible for 20% of all-cause mortality (i.e., > 400,000 deaths annually). Smoking is a leading cause of death from coronary heart disease, chronic obstructive pulmonary disease, stroke, and lung cancer. Thirty percent of all cancers in the United States are attributable to smoking.[4] Specifically, smoking has been implicated in cancers of the lung, larynx, oral cavity, esophagus, bladder, kidney, other urinary areas, and pancreas.[9] The attributable risk from smoking for oral, pharyngeal, and esophageal cancers is substantial, although less than that for lung cancer.[10,11]

Smoking accounts for almost 90% of lung cancer cases; no other cluster of risk factors, including genetic and biologic factors, lifestyle factors, and environmental factors, has as high an association with lung cancer.[4] The NCI's Lung Cancer Progress Review Group stated that "the greatest impact on deaths from lung cancer in the United States will result from efforts to prevent smoking and from helping smokers to quit."[4] Lung cancer is the largest single cause of cancer-associated mortality and is the most common cause of smoking-related mortality in the United States.[12] Worldwide, tobacco causes more than 3 million deaths every year[13,14] and is the largest preventable cause of death.[15]

Beyond the emotional and physical toll on patients and families from tobacco-related disease and death, there are broader societal and economic consequences. The cost of medical care attributable to smoking was estimated at more than $50 billion in 1993. Smoking-related illness and disability caused $47 billion in lost productivity and forfeited earnings.[3] Subsequent to the U.S. Surgeon General's warning about the hazards of smoking, cessation efforts have increased dramatically in the last three decades. The number of former smokers is nearly equal to the number of smokers in the United States.[1] This is encouraging in light of the difficulty of stopping smoking; approximately 6% of adults who were daily smokers 1 year earlier reported abstinence for at least the previous month in 1991.[1]

ETIOLOGY

Habitual smoking is determined by a multitude of factors stemming from behavioral, social, environmental, psychological, and biologic influences.[16–19] In addition, behavioral and molecular genetics studies have demonstrated that there is a heritable component to the acquisition and persistence of smoking behavior.[18,20] These individual factors do not, however, operate independently of one another, and their interaction must be considered dynamic and flexible[21] over the entire "career" of a smoker.[16]

Researchers have generally been in agreement with the notion that smoking acquisition and persistence follow a series of stages,[16,21,22] yet have outlined them somewhat differently from one another. Common across most have been the following stages: (1) preparation, (2) initial trying or initiation, (3) regular use, and (4) established smoking, daily use or nicotine dependence.[16,21,23] Often, studies have aggregated the later stages under the more general heading of "regular" use.[21] It should be noted that conceptualizing the smoking experience in this way does not attempt to explain behavior but rather to describe it and potentially to assist in the development of cessation interventions.[21] Although specific timelines for the evolution of a smoker have been posited,[23] research suggests that the progression from smoking initiation to persistence is not necessarily linear and that the duration of stages may vary between smokers.[21,24]

It has been established that smoking initiation most often begins before the age of 18[23] and that smoking during adolescence is a strong predictor of continued use during adulthood.[6] Questions remain: What influences young people to begin smoking? Why do many continue and escalate their smoking? What influences them, as adults, to quit and perhaps relapse?

Social, environmental, psychological, and biologic and genetic factors have been found to influence smoking initiation and cessation. Smoking status has been linked in both youth and adulthood with lower income and education levels.[23,25] Additionally, initiation in youth has been associated with problem behavior, family history of smoking, and peer smoking.[23] Environmental factors, such as exposure to aggressive marketing and advertising of tobacco products, have contributed to normative expectations, increasing the likelihood of initiation and often acting as barriers to quitting.[18,23,25]

Psychological determinants of smoking, such as personality factors, susceptibility to stress, perceived self-efficacy and risk, and depression and other psychiatric comorbidities have been associated with smoking onset and persistence and with relapse.[16,18,19,26] It is important to note that these "psychological" determinants are not purely psychological but illustrate the interplay of psychological, environmental, and biologic factors.

Evidence of nicotine dependence among adult smokers has been well established and is believed to play a significant role in smoking persistence and relapse. Features of dependence include a distinct withdrawal syndrome after cessation, comprised of irritability, frustration, anger, anxiety, difficulty in concentrating, restlessness, decreased heart rate, and increased appetite.[27] Also within the characterization of dependence are cravings, compulsive use, tolerance, and a dose-dependent physiologic response.[19]

Finally, behavioral and molecular genetic studies have shown evidence for the heritability of smoking. Studies of twins have implicated specific genetic factors that explain most of the variability in vulnerability to smoking (initiation) and persistence.[19] Additionally, candidate genes potentially playing a role in the "natural history of the smoking experience" have been identified and are under investigation.[28]

TREATMENT APPROACHES

The Public Health Service guideline, *Treating Tobacco Use and Dependence*,[3] is the most comprehensive, empirically based, smoking cessation guideline currently available and was developed by a consortium panel consisting of experts from the federal government, universities, and private foundations. The Guideline's recommendations reflect the group's consensus after a systematic review and meta-analysis of more than 6,000 scientific publications, each meeting stiff inclusion criteria for methodological rigor. The recommendations reflect a pooling of studies, each rated from A (strongest) to C for strength of evidence. With its clear and unequivocal analytic outcomes, this Guideline serves as the gold standard for all health care providers and as a mandate that all smokers should be offered effective treatments for tobacco dependence. The Guideline is an excellent resource for clinicians and health care administrators and is strongly endorsed by the authors of this chapter.

The Guideline provides solid evidence that tobacco dependence can be effectively treated with medications and behavioral approaches and that all health providers can improve the chances that a smoker will successfully quit. Treatment approaches can be placed into two main categories: behavioral and pharmacological.

Behavioral Treatment

Behavioral approaches range from nonspecific self-help approaches to very specific, clinically driven counseling. For those approaches that have been shown to be effective, there is essentially a dose-response relationship between the intensity and amount of treatment and treatment outcome.[3] Thus, when effective behavioral treatments are intensified or combined, they increase the likelihood that a particular cessation attempt will be successful. Tables 14.1 and 14.2, derived from the Guideline,[3] demonstrate that several behavioral treatment formats are effective for nicotine dependence and demonstrate the impact of combining multiple approaches.

As Tables 14.1 and 14.2 demonstrate, even self-help approaches can result in

TABLE 14.1 Meta-Analysis: Efficacy of and Estimated Abstinence Rates for Various Types of Formats[a]

Format	No. Arms	Estimated Odds Ratio (95% C.I.)	Estimated Abstinence Rate (95% C.I.)
No format	20	1.0	10.8
Self-help	93	1.2 (1.02, 1.3)	12.3 (10.9, 13.6)
Proactive telephone counseling	26	1.2 (1.1, 1.4)	13.1 (11.4, 14.8)
Group counseling	52	1.3 (1.1, 1.6)	13.9 (11.6, 16.1)
Individual counseling	67	1.7 (1.4, 2.0)	16.8 (14.7, 19.1)

CI, confidence interval.

[a]N = 58 studies.

Reprinted with permission from reference 3.

TABLE 14.2 Meta-Analysis: Efficacy of and Estimated Abstinence Rates for Number of Formats[a]

No. of Formats[b]	No. Arms	Estimated Odds Ratio (95% C.I.)	Estimated Abstinence Rate (95% C.I.)
No format	20	1.0	10.8
One format	51	1.5 (1.2, 1.8)	15.1 (12.8, 17.4)
Two formats	55	1.9 (1.6, 2.2)	18.5 (15.8, 21.1)
Three or four formats	19	2.5 (2.1, 3.0)	23.2 (19.9, 26.6)

CI, confidence interval.

[a]N = 54 studies.

[b]Formats included self-help, proactive telephone counseling, group, or individual counseling.

Reprinted with permission from reference 3.

slight but significant increases in cessation rates relative to no treatment. Proactive telephone counseling, group counseling, and individual counseling increase quit rates achieved with self-help. Thus, all smokers can benefit from even the simplest of interventions, but it is strongly recommended that they combine formats to maximize their chances of quitting successfully.

Although nonspecific counseling can be effective, there are differences in the efficacy of counseling and behavioral treatment approaches. As Table 14.3 demonstrates, social support, problem solving, and aversive approaches (such as rapid smoking) are effective, whereas such approaches as relaxation, breathing exercises, cigarette fading, and weight management are not effective by themselves for smoking cessation. These data suggest that smokers planning to quit should develop social support systems with other smokers trying to quit or with family, friends, and coworkers who might be able to provide encouragement. Aversive approaches, such as rapid smoking, reflect what many parents did when they caught their child smoking: Smoke a cigarette at a rapid pace to create nausea and thus break the cycle of smoking and pleasure. Although it can be effective, it is not generally recommended because nicotine toxicity, and hence vomiting, can occur with the rapid intake of nicotine. Approaches that have not been demonstrated to be effective include hypnosis and acupuncture.

Pharmacological Treatment

Since 1984, when nicotine gum was approved by the U.S. Food and Drug Administration (FDA) as an effective smoking cessation treatment, the nicotine patch, nicotine nasal spray, nicotine inhaler, and bupropion SR (sustained release) have been approved by the FDA for smoking cessation. These medications have been identified by the Guideline as first-line treatments. Although each of the medications have been proven effective in controlled studies, the meta-analyses also indicated that combining the nicotine patch with either nicotine gum or nicotine nasal spray increases quit rates over either one alone. Table 14.4 provides the odds ratios for each of the FDA-approved medications.[3]

Similarly, the meta-analyses found that the nicotine patch is moderately effective as an over-the-counter medication. Nicotine gum is also approved as an over-the-counter medication, but there have not been a sufficient number of published studies demonstrating its effectiveness. Those using any pharmacological treatment, prescription, or over-the-counter medication are strongly encouraged to use an adjunctive behavioral support program because such a combination increases quit rates.

Two other medications, clonidine and nortriptyline, were identified by the Guideline meta-analyses as effective but designated as second-line medications because they are not FDA-approved for smoking cessation. Table 14.5 demonstrates the odds ratios found for each of these medications.[3] The Guideline recommends that all patients be encouraged to use effective medications for

TABLE 14.3 Meta-Analysis: Efficacy of and Estimated Abstinence Rates for Various Types of Counseling and Behavioral Therapies[a]

Type of Counseling and Behavioral Therapy	No. Arms	Estimated Odds Ratio (95% C.I.)	Estimated Abstinence Rate (95% C.I.)
No counseling/behavioral therapy	35	1.0	11.2
Relaxation/breathing	31	1.0 (0.7, 1.3)	10.8 (7.9, 13.8)
Contingency contracting	22	1.0 (0.7, 1.4)	11.2 (7.8, 14.6)
Weight/diet	19	1.0 (0.8, 1.3)	11.2 (8.5, 14.0)
Cigarette fading	25	1.1 (0.8, 1.5)	11.8 (8.4, 15.3)
Negative affect	8	1.2 (0.8, 1.9)	13.6 (8.7, 18.5)
Intra-treatment social support	50	1.3 (1.1, 1.6)	14.4 (12.3, 16.5)
Extra-treatment social support	19	1.5 (1.1, 2.1)	16.2 (11.8, 20.6)
General – (problem solving)	104	1.5 (1.3, 1.8)	16.2 (14.0, 18.5)
Other aversive smoking	19	1.7 (1.04, 2.8)	17.7 (11.2, 24.9)
Rapid smoking	19	2.0 (1.1, 3.5)	19.9 (11.2, 29.0)

CI, confidence interval.

[a]N = 62 studies.

Reprinted with permission from reference 3.

TABLE 14.4 Meta-Analyses: Efficacy of U.S. Food and Drug Administration–Approved Smoking Cessation Medications

Pharmacotherapy	No. Studies[a]	Estimated Odds Ratio[b] (95% CI)
Bupropion SR	2	2.1 (1.5, 3.0)
Nicotine gum	13	1.5 (1.3, 1.8)
Nicotine inhaler	4	2.5 (1.7, 3.6)
Nicotine nasal spray	3	2.7 (1.8, 4.1)
Nicotine patch	27	1.9 (1.7, 2.2)
Two NRTs	3	1.9 (1.3, 2.6)

CI, confidence interval; SR, sustained release.
[a]Number of studies included in each meta-analysis.
[b]Odds ratios when compared with placebo.
Reprinted with permission from reference 3.

TABLE 14.5 Meta-Analyses: Efficacy of Clonidine and Nortriptyline for Smoking Cessation

Pharmacotherapy	No. Studies[a]	Estimated Odds Ratio[b] (95% CI)
Clonidine	5	2.1 (1.4, 3.2)
Nortriptyline	2	3.2 (1.8, 5.7)

CI, confidence interval.
[a]Number of studies included in each meta-analysis.
[b]Odds ratios when compared with placebo.
Reprinted with permission from reference 3.

smoking cessation whenever medically feasible. Because data are insufficient to indicate which patients do better with which medication, choice of medication should be based on a combination of patient preference, review of risk potential for each patient, and cost.

TREATMENT DELIVERY

Treatment delivery, as distinguished from treatment approaches, addresses the parameters that characterize provision of smoking cessation interventions. These include intensity and duration of treatment, provider type, and intervention steps.

Brief Versus Intensive

The Guideline organizes clinical interventions into two categories: brief and intensive. Brief interventions are defined as those requiring 3 minutes or less of clinician time during a patient encounter. They are designed to be integrated into a routine office visit with relative ease. Even the most minimal intervention, such as a clinician's repeated advice to quit, can foster smoking cessation.[1] There is substantial evidence to suggest that the percentage of people who are successful at quitting smoking improves as the duration and frequency of appointments increases.[3]

Team Approach

All health care professionals across disciplines (nurses, physicians, pharmacists, physician assistants, nurse practitioners, psychologists, etc.) have roles in providing smoking cessation interventions. They may individually and (most important) collectively as a team be integral in delivering an intervention and promoting cessation in cancer patients. Some research, in fact, points to greater efficacy with multiple clinicians.[29]

The Guideline characterizes the brief clinician-delivered smoking cessation intervention as the "Five *A*'s approach". Originally developed and promulgated by scientists at the NCI, it has seen several iterations and modifications.[3,30,31]

The Five *A*'s are outlined in Table 14.6. This approach has been associated with abstinence rates of 5%–8%.[1,29] Screening ("*Ask*") for smoking status has been shown to increase rates of clinician intervention significantly.[3] Such practice can be systematized by expanding the vital-signs assessment to include smoking status or by using chart stickers or computerized prompts.

The Guideline recommends that all clinicians (and especially all physicians) strongly *Advise* every tobacco using patient to quit. Substantial evidence demonstrates the impact of physician advice on patients' smoking abstinence rates.[3] Advice should be clear, strong, and personalized.

The third strategy, *Assess*, has been added to the original NCI model, which included only four *A*'s. Clinicians should ask smokers whether they are willing to make a quit attempt within the next 30 days. Clinicians should provide motivational messages (Table 14.7, The Five *R*'s) to those patients who are unwilling to make an immediate quit attempt.

The *Assist* phase of intervention has multiple components. These are described in significant detail in the Guideline.[3] Clinicians should assist patients ready to quit in setting a quit date and suggesting that they enlist the support of their social network in their efforts. Quit dates that are established provide both enough preparation time and relatively immediate action (i.e., between 1 and 2 weeks). Patients should be instructed to strive for total abstinence and to develop an action plan for how to respond to triggers or challenges in their upcoming attempt. It is prudent for smokers to refrain from or limit alcohol intake while quitting because it can trigger a relapse. Support from the health care team and patients' friends and family is associated with increased abstinence.[1,3] The Guideline also lists sources for supplementary materials that might help patients in their quit

TABLE 14.6 The Five *A*'s for Smoking Interventions in Oncology Care

Ask about smoking	Identify and document smoking status for every patient
Advise to quit	Urge every smoker to quit in a clear, strong, and personalized manner
Assess willingness to make a quit attempt	Is the smoker ready to make a quit attempt in the next month?
Assist in quit attempt	Provide counseling and pharmacotherapy for patients willing to make a quit attempt
Arrange follow-up	Schedule follow-up contact (initially within the first week of the quit date).

Reprinted with permission from Reference 3.

TABLE 14.7 Enhancing Motivation to Quit Smoking: The Five R's

Relevance	How quitting is personally relevant to each patient (e.g., disease status)
Risks	Acute and long-term risks, personalized to be relevant to each patient. These might include impact on cancer treatment and prospects for recovery (and recurrence)
Rewards	Potential benefits of smoking cessation (e.g., cancer and other disease risk reduction, monetary savings, improved health)
Roadblocks	Possible barriers to quitting and abstinence (e.g., withdrawal, fear of failure, poor support, pessimism, depression)
Repetition	Motivational intervention repeated every time an unmotivated patient is seen by a member of the oncology care team (including, for smokers who have previously failed, a reminder that most people make repeated quit attempts before achieving success)

Reprinted with permission from Reference 3.

efforts. The Guideline strongly recommends that first-line medications be provided to all patients, unless contraindicated. Pharmacotherapy should be delivered in combination with the strategies outlined earlier.

Smoking is a persistent problem and therefore requires persistence on the part of the physician in treating patients who smoke. Not only should the health care provider routinely *ask* every patient at every visit whether they smoke but, because the rate of relapse for smoking is very high (i.e., under the best circumstances, only 30% of those attempting to quit succeed on any given attempt), it also means that they should *arrange* for follow-up care for all patients attempting to quit. Ex-smokers average seven or more quit attempts before they maintain their abstinence for 1 year or longer. Quitting can then be viewed not as an "all-or-none" phenomenon but as a *process* in which people learn how to quit. It also means that physicians should persist in their offers to help patients to quit, despite the fact that the patient may have quit and relapsed back to smoking numerous times before. The percentage of people who succeed at their quit attempts is greatly enhanced by providing follow-up visits, with a greater number of visits associated with better quit rates. It is especially critical that follow up be provided during the first 2 weeks after a quit date, as the vast majority of smokers who relapse are prone to do so at this time.

APPLIED SETTINGS AND POPULATIONS

Although the foregoing treatment strategies are useful for smokers in general, there are circumstances that call for modification of procedures. In this section, factors relevant to tobacco use and its treatment are discussed for subgroups of smokers for whom tailored approaches may be indicated and who are likely to be encountered by the oncologist (i.e., hospitalized or cancer patients, the elderly, women, ethnic minorities, and depressed patients). Adolescents, patients who are abusing substances, and pregnant smokers may also benefit from tailored interventions, and these are covered in brief. *Tailoring* refers to modifying treatment program to suit the intended audience. For example, written materials can be modified on the basis of language, reading level, ethnicity, or age. It may be appropriate to refer smokers from any category to community-based or workplace interventions, so a brief description on how to contact local community resources is provided.

Hospitalized Smokers, Cancer Patients, Cancer Survivors

A hospital stay or serious illness often presents a "window of opportunity" for intervening with a smoker. Feelings of personal vulnerability are high, increasing motivation to quit, especially among those with smoking-related diagnoses, such as cancer.[32] Despite the obvious health incentives to quit, 23%–35% of head and neck cancer patients[33–37] and 13%–20% of lung cancer patients[38–40] continue to smoke after cancer treatment, which puts them at increased risk for poorer treatment outcomes and treatment complications[41] and reduced effectiveness of radiotherapy.[42] Patients may not be fully aware of the relationship between smoking and their health status, and those facing surgery should be rendered aware that even passive smoking has adverse effects on anesthesia.[43] Surgery patients should be advised to quit 8 weeks prior to surgery for maximum benefit, but even quitting at least for 24 hours prior to surgery is beneficial.[43]

Intervening with patients during active treatment or hospitalization may be especially effective for several reasons. First, patients are essentially a "captive audience." Moreover, opportunities to smoke in hospital settings are greatly reduced, if not eliminated. Perhaps most importantly, smokers are removed from smoking cues present in their home environment, allowing them to experience physiologic withdrawal prior to and separate from encounters with the psychosocial factors in their natural environment that maintain their addiction. Abstinence rates as high as 70% have been reported in post–myocardial infarction patients receiving cessation intervention.[44]

Treatment components that have been proven efficacious for hospitalized and cancer patients are the same as those that have been shown to work with smokers in general and are discussed in detail in previous sections.[45] Intensive initial interventions that are followed by relapse prevention are advocated, as they are associated with greater long-term abstinence rates.[46]

Depression and Smoking

A cancer diagnosis can precipitate clinically significant depressive symptoms and a pessimistic outlook,[47] and treating the cancer patient for smoking cessation calls for an approach tailored to this population. Thirty percent of smokers who seek treatment have a history of depression,[48] and depressed smokers are more likely to relapse to smoking after a quit attempt.[49–52] Moreover, quitting smoking may exacerbate depression and increase vulnerability to a new depressive episode.[52–55]

Bupropion may be the best pharmacotherapy for depressed smokers provided that its use is not contraindicated by existing medications.[3] Stopping smoking may affect the pharmacokinetics of certain psychiatric medications[56] and should be considered when advising medicated patients to quit.

Geriatric Smokers

The health benefits of quitting smoking are substantial, even among older smokers who constitute the majority of patients seen by most oncologists. Reduced risk of myocardial infarction, of death from coronary artery disease, and of lung cancer is one of the health benefits. Quitting smoking can also reduce time to recuperate from illnesses that are exacerbated by smoking and can improve cerebral circulation.[57] Interventions that have proven effective with the general population have also benefited geriatric smokers.[3] *Clear Horizons*[58] is a self-help quitting smoking program designed specifically for individuals older than age 50 and has been shown to double abstinence rates when delivered in the context of a physician-assisted intervention that includes pharmacotherapy for appropriate individuals.[59,60] Tailored programs for older adults should include personalized feedback linking smoking to symptoms, information about health benefits of quitting and consequences of continued smoking for older smokers, and problem-solving counseling. Written materials should be easily understood and feature examples of smokers in the patients' age group.[59]

Women

When it comes to quitting smoking, it is clear that women are different from men. For example, women report weight gain as a deterrent to quitting smoking more often than do men and have been observed to alter their smoking habits in response to fluctuations in hormonal cycles.[61] Moreover, as compared to the results for men, nicotine replacement therapy is less effective in helping women to quit smoking,[62,63] which has led some to speculate that women smoke more for the nonphysiologic effects of smoking (i.e., social pressures, taste, psychological reasons, habit). However, treatment implications based on these observations are not yet well developed. Given that premise, it is reasonable to expect that women would benefit from gender-specific cessation programs; however, thus far there is no empirical evidence to support this idea. With the foregoing exception of nicotine replacement therapy, women seem to be equally responsive to the same types of interventions that are effective with men.

High-Risk Ethnic Groups

Various ethnic groups have greater rates of smoking and are at higher risk of developing tobacco-related cancers; this is especially true for smokers of lower socioeconomic status. Little empirical evidence currently exists suggesting interventions that are effective on the basis of a smoker's ethnicity. There is some suggestion that church-based programs may provide an effective location for cessation programs, but little else is known.[64]

Special Concern Groups: Pregnant Smokers, Adolescents, and Substances Abusers

Pregnant smokers may experience increased motivation to quit and yet may be afraid to disclose their smoking for fear of being rebuked. They may rationalize their behavior by minimizing the adverse effects on the fetus. Because of the potential teratogenic effects of any pharmacotherapy, pregnant smokers should be urged to quit via behavioral interventions alone, before receiving medication.[3] When nicotine replacement is used, blood nicotine levels should be monitored, lower doses of nicotine should be used, and intermittent (gum, inhaler, spray) versus continuous (patch) forms of nicotine replacement should be used to minimize health risk to the fetus.[3] Follow-up care is vitally important, as rates of relapse to smoking after delivery are high even in those who quit for many months.

Tobacco use among preadolescent and adolescent cancer survivors appears to be low,[65] yet 90% of adult smokers begin smoking before age 17. Efforts to discover effective, empirically validated treatments for tobacco use in adolescents are ongoing,[66,67] In the meantime, all adolescents should be screened for tobacco use and offered assistance with quitting using treatment materials that have been modified to developmentally appropriate levels.[3] As recommended for adult smokers, bupropion or nicotine replacement therapy should be considered when there is evidence of dependence, although there is some evidence to suggest that the nicotine patch may be ineffective for teenage smokers.[66]

More than 70% of people with alcohol or other substance dependencies smoke cigarettes.[68–70] Smoking cessation treatment does not appear to interfere with concurrent substance abuse treatment. Therefore, smokers with other chemical dependencies should receive concurrent, coordinated, treatment for all their addictions.[3]

Community-based cessation programs (Table 14.8) can be very effective for those willing to take advantage of them. The American Lung Association offers adult (Freedom From Smoking) and adolescent (Not-On-Tobacco) cessation programs in 8 or 10 sessions in face-to-face group formats or those for adults only; as self-help programs delivered online; or via written materials, audio cassette, or videotape. The American Cancer Society has educational material about quitting smoking on their Web site, along with links to other organizations offering

TABLE 14.8 Community-Based Cessation Programs: Contact Information

Organization	Web Ssite	Phone
American Lung Association	*lungusa.org*	212-315-8700
American Cancer Society	*www.cancer.org*	800-ACS-2345
NCI Cancer Information Service	*cis.nci.nih.gov*	800-4-CANCER (800-422-6237)

NCI, National Cancer Institute.

cessation programs. The American Cancer Society often has local cessation groups (interested individuals can call to find out). The NCI's Cancer Information Service offers a free telephone-based quit-line and offers a Web site with information and advice for smokers trying to quit. Workplace-based interventions can also be effective, and smokers who have access to them should be urged to take advantage of them.

SUMMARY

Smoking is the chief, single, preventable cause of death in the United States and the leading cause of cancer. Approximately 25% of U.S. adults smoke. The path from experimentation to regular smoking is complex and is determined by multiple factors, including behavioral, social, environmental, psychological, physiologic, and genetic factors.

Treating Tobacco Use and Dependence is the most comprehensive, empirically based guideline for smoking cessation issued to date. It is published by the U.S. Public Health Service and is available by calling the NCI Cancer Information Line at 1-800-4CANCER (1-800-422-6237).

The Guideline recommends treating smokers with both behavioral and pharmacological approaches. The most effective, palatable behavioral approaches are problem solving and social support. Greater frequency and intensity of interventions yield better outcomes. First-line pharmacotherapies include bupropion and nicotine replacement therapies.

Brief interventions (as short as 3 minutes) have been shown to be effective, as summarized in the Guideline's recommendations to health care practitioners. Many patients may benefit from tailored approaches to quitting. Discussed were hospitalized and cancer patients, adolescents, the elderly, women, ethnic minorities, depressed patients, patients with chemical dependencies, and pregnant smokers. Community and workplace resources for quitting smoking are available from the American Lung Association, the American Cancer Society, and the NCI.

REFERENCES

1. Department of Health and Human Services. Reducing Tobacco Use. A Report of the Surgeon General. Atlanta: US Department of Health and Human Services, Centers for Disease Control and

Prevention, National Center for Chronic Disease Prevention and Health Promotion, Office on Smoking and Health, 2000.

2. Centers for Disease Control and Prevention. Cigarette smoking among adultsUnited States, 1997. Morb Mortal Wkly Rep 1999a;48(43):993–996.

3. Fiore MC, Bailey WC, Cohen SJ et al. Treating Tobacco Use and Dependence. Clinical Practice Guideline. Rockville, MD: U.S. Department of Health and Human Services, Public Health Service, 2000.

4. National Cancer Institute. Report of the Lung Cancer Progress Review Group (August, 2001), National Institutes of Health, *http://osp.nci.nih.gov/prg_assess/prg/lungprg/lung_rpt.htm#priority-b*

5. Husten CG, Shelton DM, Chrismon JH et al. Cigarette smoking and smoking cessation among older adults: United States. 1965–95. Tob Control 1997;6(3):175–180.

6. Centers for Disease Control and Prevention. Tobacco Use Among High School Students—United States, 1997. Morb Mortal Wkly Rep 1998;47(12):229–233.

7. World Health Organization. The tobacco epidemic: a global public health emergency. Tobacco Alert. April 1998. *www.who.int/archives/tobalert/apr96/fulltext.htm.*

8. U.S. Department of Health and Human Services. Public Health Service. Healthy People 2000: National health promotion and disease prevention objectives. Washington, DC: US Department of Health and Human Services, Public Health Service. DHHS Publication No. (PHS) 91-50212, 1991.

9. National Cancer Institute. Changes in Cigarette-Related Disease Risks and Their Implications for Prevention and Control. Smoking and Tobacco Control Monograph No. 8. Bethesda, MD: National Cancer Institute. NIH Publication No. 97-4213, February 1997.

10. Day GL, Blot WJ, Austin DF et al. Racial differences in risk of oral and pharyngeal cancer: alcohol, tobacco, and other determinants. J Natl Cancer Inst 1993:85(6):465–473.

11. Gammon MD, Schoenberg JB, Ahsan H et al. Tobacco, alcohol, and socioeconomic status and adenocarcinomas of the esophagus and gastric cardia. J Natl Cancer Inst 1997:89(17):1277–1284.

12. Shopland DR, Eyre HJ, Pechacek TF. Smoking-attributable cancer mortality in 1991: Is lung cancer now the leading cause of death among smokers in the United States? J Natl Cancer Inst 1991;83:1142–1148.

13. Peto R, Lopez AD, Boreham J et al. Mortality from tobacco in developed countries: indirect estimation from national vital statistics. Lancet 1992:339(8804):1268–1278.

14. National Cancer Institute. The Nation's Investment in Cancer Research. A Plan and Budget Proposal for Fiscal Year 2002. National Institutes of Health. NIH Publication No. 00-4373, October 2000.

15. Engstrom PE, Clapper M, Schnoll RA et al. Prevention of tobacco-related cancers. In: Holland JF, Frie E, eds. Cancer Medicine, 5th ed. Hamilton, Ontario, Canada: BC Decker, 2000:127–140.

16. Haire-Joshu D, Morgan G, Fisher EB. Determinants of cigarette smoking. Clin Chest Med 1991; 12(4):711–725.

17. Jarvis M. A profile of tobacco smoking. Addiction 1994;89(11):1371–1381.

18. Bergen AW, Caparaso N. Cigarette smoking. J Natl Cancer Inst 1999;91(16):1365–1375.

19. Shadel WG, Shiffman S, Niaura R et al. Current models of nicotine dependence: what is known and what is needed to advance understanding of tobacco etiology among youth. Drug Alcohol Depend 2000;59[suppl 1]:S9–S21.

20. Munafo M, Johnstone E, Murphy M et al. New directions in the genetic mechanisms underlying nicotine addiction. Addict Biol 2001;6(2):109–117.

21. Mayhew KP, Flay BR, Mott JA. Stages in the development of adolescent smoking. Drug Alcohol Depend 2000;59[suppl 1]:S61–S81.

22. Chassin L, Presson C, Rose J et al. The natural history of smoking form adolescence to adulthood: demographic predictors of continuity and change. Health Psychol 1996;15(6):478–484.

23. U.S. Department of Health and Human Services. Preventing Tobacco Use Among Young People: A Report of the Surgeon General. Washington, DC: Public Health Service, 1994. Publication No. S/N 017-001-00491-0.

24. Benowitz N. The nature of nicotine addiction. In: Lynch BS, Bonnie, RJ, eds. Growing Up Tobacco Free: Preventing Nicotine Addiction in Children and Youths. Washington, DC: National Academy Press, 1994:29–68.

25. U.S. Department of Health and Human Services. Tobacco Use Among U.S. Racial/Ethnic Minority Groups—African Americans, American Indians and Alaska Natives, Asian Americans and Pacific Islanders, and Hispanics: A Report of the Surgeon General. Atlanta: U.S. Department of Health and Human Services, Centers for Disease Control and Prevention, National Center for Chronic Disease Prevention and Health Promotion, Office on Smoking and Health, 1998.

26. Romer D, Jamieson P. The role of perceived risk in starting and stopping smoking. In: Slovic P, ed. Smoking: Risk, Perception, and Policy. Thousand Oaks, CA: Sage Publications, Inc, American Academy of Political and Social Science, 2001:64–80.

27. Hughes JR, Higgins ST, Hatsukami DK. Effects of abstinence from tobacco. In: Kozlowski L, Annis HM, Cappell HD et al, eds. Recent Advances in Alcohol and Drug Problems. New York: Plenum, 1990:317–398.

28. Lerman C, Caporaso NE, Audrain J et al. Evidence suggesting the role of specific genetic factors in cigarette smoking. Health Psychol 1999;18(1):14–20.

29. Kottke TE, Battista RN, DeFriese GH et al. Attributes of successful smoking cessation interventions in medical practice: a meta-analysis of 39 controlled trials. JAMA 1988;259(19):2882–2889.

30. Glynn TJ, Manley MW. How to Help Your Patients Stop Smoking: A National Cancer Institute Manual for Physicians. Bethesda, MD: US Department of Health and Human Services, Public Health Service, National Institutes of Health, National Cancer Institute, 1993. NIH Publication No. 93-3064.

31. Fiore MC, Bailey WC, Cohen SJ et al. Smoking Cessation. Clinical Practice Guideline No. 18. Rockville, MD: US Department of Health and Human Services, Public Health Service, Agency for Health Care Policy and Research, 1996. AHCPR Publication No. 96-0692.

32. Halpern MT, Schmier JK, Ward KD et al. Smoking cessation in hospitalized patients. Respir Care 2000;45(3):330–336.

33. Gritz ER, Schacherer C, Koehly L et al. Smoking withdrawal and relapse in head and neck cancer patients. Head Neck 1999;21(5):420–427.

34. Ostroff JS, Jacobsen PB, Moadel AB et al. Prevalence and predictors of continued tobacco use after treatment of patients with head and neck cancer. Cancer 1995;75(2):569–576.

35. Spitz MR, Fueger JJ, Chamberlain RM et al. Cigarette smoking patterns in patients after treatment of upper aerodigestive tract cancers. J Cancer Educ 1990;5(2):109–113.

36. Vander Ark W, DiNardo LJ, Oliver DS. Factors affecting smoking cessation in patients with head and neck cancer. Laryngoscope 1997;107(7):888–892.

37. Passik SD, Ricketts PL, Moadel AB et al. Psychological issues related to site of cancer. In: Holland JC, ed. Psycho-Oncology. New York: Oxford University Press, 1998:303–433.

38. Dresler CM, Bailey M, Roper CR et al. Smoking cessation and lung cancer resection. Chest 1996; 110(5):1199–1202.

39. Sridhar KS, Raub WA. Present and past smoking history and other predisposing factors in 100 lung cancer patients. Chest 1992;101(1):19–25.

40. Sarna L. Lung cancer. In: Holland JC, ed. Psycho-Oncology. New York: Oxford University Press, 1998:340–348.

41. Cinciripini PM, Gritz ER, Tsho JY et al. Psychological and behavioral factors in cancer risk. In: Holland JC, ed. Psycho-Oncology. New York: Oxford University Press, 1998:27–143.

42. Browman GP, Wong G, Hodson I et al. Influence of cigarette smoking on the efficacy of radiation therapy in head and neck cancer. N Engl J Med 1993; 328(3):159–163.

43. Rodrigo C. The effects of cigarette smoking on anesthesia. Anesth Prog 2000;47(4):143–150.

44. Frid D, Ockene IS, Ockene JK et al. Severity of angiographically proven coronary artery disease predicts smoking cessation. Am J Prev Med 1991;7(3):131–135.

45. Schnoll RA, Miller SM. Smoking cessation initiatives for cancer patients. Prim Care Cancer 2000; 20:1–19.

46. France EK, Glasgow RE, Marcus AC. Smoking cessation interventions among hospitalized patients: What have we learned? Prev Med 2001;32(4):376–388.

47. Schnoll RA, Malstrom M, James C et al. Correlates of tobacco use among smokers and recent quitters diagnosed with cancer. Patient Educ Couns 2002;46:137–145.

48. Anda RF, Williamson DF, Escobedo LG et al. Depression and the dynamics of smoking. A national perspective. JAMA 1990;264(12):1541–1545.

49. Gilbert DG, Crauthers DM, Mooney DK et al. Effects of monetary contingencies on smoking relapse: influences of trait depression, personality, and habitual nicotine intake. Exp Clin Psychopharmacol 1999;7(2):174–181.

50. Brandon TH. Negative affect as motivation to smoke. Curr Psychol Res Rev 1990;3(33):33–37.

51. Hall SM, Munoz RF, Reus VI et al. Nicotine, negative affect, and depression. J Consult Clin Psychol 1993;61(5):761–767.

52. Glassman AH, Covey LS, Dalack GW et al. Smoking cessation, clonidine, and vulnerability to nicotine among dependent smokers. Clin Pharmacol Ther 1993;54(6):670–679.

53. Covey LS, Glassman AH, Stetner F. Cigarette smoking and major depression. J Addict Dis 1998; 17(1):35–46.

54. Ginsberg JP, Klesges RC, Johnson KC et al. The relationship between a history of depression and adherence to a multicomponent smoking-cessation program. Addict Behav 1997;22(6):783–787.

55. Glassman AH. Cigarette smoking: implications for psychiatric illness. Am J Psychiatry 1993; 150(4):546–553.

56. Hughes JR. Pharmacotherapy for smoking cessation: unvalidated assumptions, anomalies, and suggestions for future research. J Consult Clin Pscyhol 1993;61(5):751–760.

57. Hermanson B, Omenn GS, Kronmal RA et al. Beneficial six-year outcome of smoking cessation in older men and women with coronary artery disease. Results from the CASS registry. N Engl J Med 1988;319(21):1365–1369.

58. Orleans CT, Rimer BK, Fleisher L. Clear horizons: a quit smoking guide especially for those 50 and over. Philadelphia: Fox Chase Cancer Center, 1989.

59. Morgan GD, Noll EL, Orleans CT et al. Reaching midlife and older smokers: tailored interventions for routine medical care. Prev Med 1996;25(3):346–354.

60. Rimer BK, Orleans CT, Fleisher L et al. Does tailoring matter? The impact of a tailored guide on ratings and short-term smoking-related outcomes for older smokers. Health Educ Res 1994;9(1): 69–84.

61. Gritz ER, Nielsen IR, Brooks LA. Smoking cessation and gender: the influence of physiological, psychological, and behavioral factors. J Am Med Womens Assoc 1996;51(1–2):35–42.

62. Perkins KA. Sex differences in nicotine versus nonnicotine reinforcement as determinants of tobacco smoking. Exp Clin Psychopharmacol 1996;4(2):166–177.

63. Wetter DW, Kenford SL, Smith SS et al. Gender differences in smoking cessation. J Consult Clin Psych 1999;67(4):555–562.

64. Pederson LL, Ahluwalia JS, Harris KJ et al. Smoking cessation among African Americans: what we know and do not know about interventions and self-quitting. Prev Med 2000;31(1):23–38.

65. Tyc VL, Hadley W, Crockett G. Prediction of health behaviors in pediatric cancer survivors. Med Pediatr Oncol 2001;37(1):42–46.

66. Backinger CL, Leischow SJ. Advancing the science of adolescent tobacco use cessation. Am J Health Behav 2001;25(3):183–190.

67. Patel DR, Greydanus DE. Office interventions for adolescent smokers. Adolesc Med 2000;11(3): 577–588.

68. Budney AJ, Higgins ST, Hughes JR et al. Nicotine and caffeine use in cocaine-dependent individuals. J Subst Abuse 1993;5(2):117–130.

69. Clemmey P, Brooner R, Chutuape MA et al. Smoking habits and attitudes in a methadone maintenance treatment population. Drug Alcohol Depend 1997;44(2–3):123–32.

70. DiFranza JR, Guerrera MP. Alcoholism and smoking. J Stud Alcohol 1990;51(2):130–135.

Chapter 15

Smoking Cessation Strategies: Targeting Populations

James O. Prochaska

In the United States, approximately 50,000,000 Americans continue to smoke, with nearly 500,000 deaths per year attributed to smoking.[1] Approximately 30% of all U.S. cancer deaths each year are due to smoking. Globally, the problem promises to be catastrophic. Of the people alive in the world today, 500 million are expected to die from this single behavior, losing approximately 5 billion years of life to tobacco use.[2]

Smoking cessation clinics have little impact on the problem. When offered for free by health maintenance organizations in the United States, such clinics recruit only approximately 1% of subscribers who smoke.[3] For such behavior, medicine services simply cannot make much difference if they treat such a small percentage of the problem.

Startled by such statistics, behavioral scientists took health promotion programs into communities and work sites. The results in the largest trials ever attempted were discouraging. In the Minnesota Heart Health project, for example, $40 million was spent, with 5 years of intervention in four communities, totaling 400,000 people. However, there were no significant differences between treatment and control communities in smoking, diet, cholesterol, weight, blood pressure, and overall risks for cardiovascular disease.[4]

What went wrong? The investigators speculated that they may have diluted their programs by targeting multiple behaviors. However, the Community Intervention Trial for Smoking Cessation had no effects with its primary target of heavy smokers and only a small effect with light smokers.[5] Similarly, the largest work site cessation programs produced no significant effects.[6]

A closer look at participation rates can probably account for some of the disappointing data. In the Minnesota study, nearly 90% of smokers in both the treatment and control communities had processed media information about smoking in the last year.[7] However, only approximately 10% had physicians intervene, and only 3% participated in the most powerful behavioral programs, such as individualized and interactive clinics, classes, and contests. Prevention programs cannot have much impact on the health of communities if they interact with only a small percentage of populations with the highest risk behavior.

A NEW PARADIGM FOR PREVENTION STRATEGIES

There is an old interventionist rule that reads, "If we don't like how our clients or our communities are acting, we need to change our behavior." Behavior medicine cannot continue to offer only action-oriented cessation programs and expect the results to be better. A shift has to be made from an action paradigm to a stage paradigm if behavior medicine is to interact effectively with a much higher percentage of populations at risk. The action paradigm equates behavior change with taking action, such as quitting smoking. The stage paradigm, however, construes behavior change as a process that unfolds over time and involves progress through six stages: precontemplation, contemplation, preparation, action, maintenance, and termination. Action is seen as one of the six stages, and it becomes integrated as part of a more comprehensive approach to individual, community, or population change.

Precontemplation is the stage in which people are not intending to take action in the foreseeable future, usually measured as the next 6 months. People may be in this stage because they are uninformed or underinformed about the consequences of their behavior. Also, they may have tried to change a number of times and have become demoralized about their abilities to change, as do many smokers. These groups tend to avoid reading, talking, or thinking about their smoking. They are often characterized in other theories as noncompliant, resistant, or unmotivated or as not ready for treatment. The fact is that traditional action-oriented behavior medicine programs were not ready for such individuals and were not motivated to match their needs.

People in precontemplation underestimate the benefits of changing and overestimate the costs. However, they typically are unaware that they are making such mistakes. If they are not conscious of making such mistakes, it will be difficult for them to change. So many remain stuck in the precontemplation stage for years, doing considerable damage to themselves and others. We have found no inherent motivation for people to progress from one stage to the next. These are not like stages of human development, in which children have inherent motivation to progress from crawling to walking even though crawling works very well and even though learning to walk can be painful and embarrassing.

Two major forces that have been identified can move people to progress. The first is developmental events. In our research, the *mean* age of smokers who finally quit and reach longer-term maintenance is 39 years. Those of us who have gone through age 39 know that it is a mean age. It is an age to reevaluate how we have been living and whether we want to die from the way we have been living or whether we want to enhance the quality and quantity of the second half of our lives.

The other naturally occurring force is environmental events. One example is a couple, both heavy smokers, whom we followed up for 2 years. Their dog of many years died of lung cancer. This eventually moved the wife to quit smoking. The husband bought a new dog. So, even the same events can be processed differently by different people.

There has been a common belief that people with addictions must "hit bottom" before they will be motivated to change. So family, friends, and physicians wait helplessly for a crisis to occur. However, how often do people become 39 or have a dog die? When people show the first signs of cancer, others around them can become mobilized to help them to seek early intervention. We know that early interventions are often life-saving, and we would not wait for such patients to hit bottom. We shall see that we have created a third force to help troubled patients and populations in precontemplation to progress. It is called *stage-matched interventions*.

Contemplation

Contemplation is the stage in which people are intending to take action in the next 6 months. They are more aware of the "pros" of changing but are also acutely aware of the "cons." When people begin seriously to contemplate giving up their long-term favorite substances, their awareness of the costs of changing can increase. There is no free change. This balance between the costs and benefits of changing can produce profound ambivalence. This profound ambivalence can reflect a type of love-hate relationship with an addictive substance, for example, and it can keep people stuck in this stage for long periods. We often characterize this phenomenon as chronic contemplation or behavioral procrastination. These folks are not ready for traditional action oriented programs.

Preparation

Preparation is the stage in which people are intending to take action in the immediate future, usually measured as the next month. They have typically taken some significant action in the last year. These individuals have a plan of action, such as talking to their physician, consulting a counselor, buying a self-help book, or relying on a self-change approach. These are the patients who should be recruited for action-oriented cessation programs.

Action

Action is the stage in which people have made specific overt modifications in their lifestyles within the last 6 months. Because action is observable, behavior change often has been equated with action. Not all modifications of behavior count as action in the stage model. People must attain a criterion that scientists and professionals agree is sufficient to reduce risks for disease or other self-defeating or self-destructive consequences. In smoking, for example, only total abstinence counts. With alcoholism and alcohol abuse, there are many who believe that only total abstinence can be effective, whereas there are those who accept controlled drinking as effective action.

Maintenance

Maintenance is the stage in which people are working to prevent relapse but do not apply change processes as frequently as do people in the action stage. They are less tempted to relapse and increasingly more confident that they can continue their changes. On the basis of temptation and self-efficacy data, we estimated that maintenance lasts from 6 months to approximately 5 years.

One of the common reasons why people relapse early in action is that they are not well prepared for the prolonged effort needed to progress to maintenance. Many think the worst will be over in a few weeks or a few months. If they ease up on their efforts too early, they are at great risk for relapse.

To prepare people for what is to come, we encourage them to think of overcoming a chronic problem, such as running a marathon rather than a sprint. They may have wanted to enter the 100th running of the Boston Marathon, but if they had little or no preparation, they know that they would not succeed, so they would not enter the race. If they had done some preparation, they might last for several miles before failing to finish the race. Only those well prepared could maintain their efforts mile after mile.

In the Boston Marathon metaphor, runners know they have to be well prepared if they are to survive Heartbreak Hill, an obstacle that occurs after some 20 miles. What is the behavioral equivalent of Heartbreak Hill? The best evidence we have across chronic problems is that the majority of relapses occur at times of emotional distress. Times of depression, anxiety, anger, boredom, loneliness, stress, and distress are the times during which we are at our emotional and psychological weakest.

How does the average American cope with such troubling times? The average American drinks more, eats more, smokes more, and uses more drugs to cope with such distressing times.[8] Not surprising, therefore, is that people struggling to overcome smoking will be at greatest risk of relapse when they face distress without their substance of choice. We cannot prevent emotional distress from occurring, but we can help to prevent relapse if our patients have been prepared for how to cope with distress without falling back on addictive substances or other self-defeating behaviors.

If so many Americans rely on oral consumptive behavior as a way to manage their emotions, what is the healthiest oral behavior they could use? Talking with others about one's distress is a means of seeking support that can help to prevent relapse. Acute distress is the number one reason why people seek psychotherapy, so that they can have someone supportive and helpful with whom to talk.[9] Exercise is another healthy alternative on which large numbers of people can rely. Not only does such physical activity help to manage moods, stress, and distress but for 60 minutes a week, clients can receive more than 50 physical and mental health benefits.[10] Exercise should be prescribed to all sedentary patients with addictions as the bargain basement of behaviors. A third healthy alternative is some form of deep relaxation, such as meditation, yoga, prayer, massage, or deep-muscle relaxation. Letting the stress and distress drift away from one's muscles and one's mind helps patients to keep progressing at the most tempting of times.

As is now well known, most people taking action to modify such chronic conditions as smoking do not successfully maintain their gains on their first attempt. With smoking, successful self-changers make an average of five to six action attempts before they become long-term maintainers.[10] Many New Year's resolvers report 3 or more years of consecutive pledges before maintaining the behavioral goal for at least 6 months.[11] Relapse and recycling through the stages occur fairly frequently as individuals attempt to modify or cease addictive behaviors. Variations of the stage model are being used increasingly by behavior-change specialists to investigate the dynamics of relapse.[12,13]

As relapse is the rule rather than the exception with such problems as smoking, we found that we needed to modify our original stage model. Initially, we conceptualized change as a linear progression through the stages: People were supposed to progress simply and discretely through each step. Linear progression is a possible but relatively rare phenomenon with many chronic conditions, such as smoking.

A spiral pattern better reflects how many people actually move through the stages of change. In a spiral pattern, people can progress from contemplation to preparation to action to maintenance, but many individuals will relapse. During relapse, individuals regress to an earlier stage. Some relapsers feel like failures: embarrassed, ashamed, and guilty. These individuals become demoralized and resist thinking about behavior change. As a result, they return to the precontemplation stage and can remain there for various periods. Approximately 15% of smokers who relapsed in our self-change research regressed back to the precontemplation stage.[14]

Fortunately, this research indicates that the 85% of smokers recycle back to the contemplation or preparation stages.[11,15] They begin to consider plans for their next action attempt while trying to learn from their recent efforts. To take another example, fully 60% of unsuccessful New Year's resolvers make the same pledge the next year.[11–15] The spiral model suggests that most relapsers do not revolve endlessly in circles and that they do not regress all the way back to where they began. Instead, each time relapsers recycle through the stages, they potentially learn from their mistakes and try something different the next time around.[16]

On any trial, successful behavior change is limited in the absolute numbers of individuals who are able to achieve maintenance.[10,17] Nevertheless, analysis of a cohort of individuals reveals that the number of successes continues to increase gradually over time. However, a large number of individuals remain in contemplation and precontemplation stages. Ordinarily, the more action taken, the better the prognosis. We need much more research to distinguish better between those who benefit from recycling and those who end up spinning their wheels.

Termination

Termination is the stage in which individuals have zero temptation and 100% self-efficacy. Regardless of whether they are depressed, anxious, bored, lonely, angry, or stressed, they are sure that they will not return to their old unhealthy habit as a way of coping. It is as though they never acquired the habit in the first place. In a study of former smokers and alcoholics, we found that approximately 20% of each group had reached the criteria of no temptation and total self-efficacy.[18] Although our ideal goal is to be cured or totally recovered, we recognize that for many people, the best we can do is a lifetime of maintenance.

Outreach

Research on stage distributions in the United States shows that approximately 40% of smokers are in precontemplation, 40% in contemplation, and only 20% in preparation.[19] These data suggest that action-oriented interventions match the needs of fewer than 20% of smokers. If cessation programs are to match the needs of entire populations, interventions are needed for the 40% in precontemplation and the 40% in contemplation.

To reach entire populations requires a shift from a passive-reactive to a proactive approach to practice. Most professionals have been trained to be passive-reactive: to wait passively for patients to seek services and then react. The biggest problem with this approach is that the majority of people with behavior risks never seek services.

Offering stage-matched interventions and applying proactive or outreach recruitment methods, we have been able to motivate 80%–90% of smokers to enter our treatment programs in a series of large-scale clinical trials.[20–22] This is a quantum increase over the 1%–4% participation rates found in earlier studies.

What happens if professionals change only one practice and proactively recruit entire populations into action-oriented clinics? This experiment has been tried in one of the largest U.S. managed care organizations.[3] Physicians spent time with all smokers to recruit them for a state-of-the-art, action-oriented, clinic-based smoking cessation program. If that did not work, nurses spent up to 10 minutes to get them to sign up, followed by 12 minutes of health education and a counselor call to the home. This intensive recruitment protocol motivated 35% of smokers in the precontemplation stage to sign up. However, only 3% showed up, 2% finished up, and 0% ended up better off. Sixty-five percent of individuals in the contemplation and preparation stages signed up, but 15% showed up, 11% finished up, and some percent ended up better off.

Continuation

What motivates patients to continue with treatment? Conversely, what moves patients to terminate treatment quickly and prematurely? A meta-analysis of 125 studies found that nearly 50% of clients drop out of behavior medicine programs.[23] These rates of dropout from behavior medicine are remarkably similar to the 50% discontinuation rates found across most categories of biologic medicines.[24]

One excellent predictor of premature dropout from treatment is the client's stage of change at intake.[25,26] Professionals should not treat patients in the precontemplation stage as though they were in the action stage and expect them to continue therapy. Health professionals try to pressure patients to take action when they are not prepared, driving them away and then blaming patients for not complying with action-oriented treatments.

With smokers who enter therapy in the action stage, relapse prevention strategies are appropriate. However, would relapse prevention make any sense with the 40% of patients in precontemplation? What might be a good match here? We recommend a dropout prevention approach, as we know that these patients are likely to drop out early if we do not help them to continue.

We now have four studies that examine program retention rates of individuals receiving stage-matched interventions.[20–22,27] What is clear is that when treatment is matched to stage of change, people in precontemplation continue at the same high rates as those who started in the preparation stage. This result held when participants were recruited proactively (we reached out to them to offer help) and when they were recruited reactively (they called us for help).

Progress

What moves people to progress in treatment and to continue to progress after treatment has ended? The *stage effect* predicts that the amount of successful action taken during treatment and after treatment is directly related to the stage in which people are at the start of treatment.[25] Smokers in preparation are twice as likely to be abstinent at 6 months after treatment as contemplators, who in turn are twice as likely to be abstinent as precontemplators.[16] A single brief intervention that helps individuals to advance only one stage can double their chances of taking effective action in the near future.[28] If we help them to progress two stages, we can triple or quadruple their chances of taking effective action.[28]

A realistic goal for brief interventions is to use stage-matched interventions to help patients to progress one stage. For patients who move relatively quickly, we can aim for two stages.

Six thousand British health professionals who were trained proactively in this approach experienced a dramatic increase in morale. They were able to see progress with the majority of their patients, where they once saw failure when immediate action was the only criterion of success. They are much more confident that they can match the needs of all their patients rather than just the 20% or so who were prepared to take immediate action (H.M. Waring, personal communication).

Process

If health professionals are to help patients progress from one stage to the next, they will need to know principles and processes of change that can produce such progress.

Principle 1 The pros of changing must increase for people to progress from precontemplation. We found that in 12 of 12 studies, the pros were higher in contemplation than in precontemplation.[29] This pattern held true across 12 problem behaviors: quitting cocaine, delinquency, consistent condom use, safer sex, sedentary life styles, high fat diets, obesity, sun exposure, smoking, radon testing, mammography screening, and physicians not practicing behavior medicine.

Here is a technique for raising the pros. Ask smokers in precontemplation to list all the benefits or pros of quitting smoking. They typically can list three of four. Let them know that there are 10 to 14 times that number. Challenge them to double or triple their lists for the next meeting. As their list grows, they will be progressing to contemplation.

Principle 2 The cons of changing must decrease for people to progress from contemplation to action. In 12 of 12 studies, we found that the cons of changing were lower in action than in contemplation.[29]

Outcomes and Impacts

What happens when we combine 12 principles and processes of change to help patients and entire populations to progress toward action? What are the outcomes that can be produced with groups of patients, and what are the impacts on entire populations when stage-matched interventions are proactively delivered to entire populations? We examine a series of clinical trials applying stage-matched interventions to see what lessons we might learn about the future of behavior medicine and cancer prevention.

In the first large-scale clinical trial, we compared four treatments: (1) one of the best home-based action-oriented cessation programs (standardized), (2) stage-matched manuals (individualized), (3) expert system computer reports plus manuals (interactive), and (4) counselors plus computers and manuals (personalized). We randomly assigned by stage 739 smokers to one of the four treatments.[27] In the computer condition, participants completed by mail or telephone 40 questions that were entered into central computers that generated feedback reports. These reports informed participants about their stage of change, their pros and cons of changing, and their use of change processes appropriate to their stages. At baseline, participants were given positive feedback about what they were doing correctly and guidance in which principles and processes they needed to apply more to progress. In two progress reports delivered over the next 6 months, participants also received positive feedback about any improvement they made in any of the variables relevant to progressing. So, demoralized and defensive smokers could begin progressing without having to quit and without having to work too hard. Smokers in the contemplation stage could begin taking small steps, such as delaying their first cigarette in the morning for an extra 30 minutes. They could choose small steps that would increase their self-efficacy and help them to become better prepared for quitting.

In the personalized condition, smokers received four proactive counselor calls over the 6-month intervention period. Three of the calls were based on the computer reports. Counselors reported much more difficulty in interacting with participants without any progress data. Without scientific assessments, it was much harder for both clients and counselors to tell whether any significant progress had occurred since their last interaction.

Point prevalence abstinence rates were compared for each of the four treatment groups over 18 months, with treatment ending at 6 months. The two self-help manual conditions paralleled each other for 12 months. At 18 months, the stage-matched manuals moved ahead. This is an example of a delayed action effect, which we often observe with stage-matched programs specifically and which others have observed with self-help programs generally. It takes time for participants in early stages to progress all the way to action. Therefore, some treatment effects as measured by action will be observed only after considerable delay. However, it is encouraging to find treatments producing therapeutic effects months and even years after treatment ended.

The computer-alone and computer-plus-counselor conditions paralleled each other for 12 months. Then, the effects of the counselor condition flattened out, whereas the computer condition effects continued to increase. We can only speculate as to the cause of the delayed differences between these two conditions. Participants in the personalized condition may have become somewhat dependent on the social support and social control of the counselor calling. The last call was after the 6-month assessment, and benefits would be observed at 12 months. Termination of the counselors could result in no further progress because of the loss of social support and control. The classic pattern in smoking cessation clinics is rapid relapse beginning as soon as the treatment is terminated. Some of this rapid relapse could well be due to the sudden loss of social support or social control provided by the counselors and other participants in the clinic.

The next test was to demonstrate the efficacy of the expert system when applied to an entire population recruited proactively. With more than 80% of a representative sample of 5170 smokers participating and fewer than 20% in the preparation stage, we demonstrated significant benefit of the expert system at each 6-month follow up.[22] Furthermore, the advantages over proactive assessment alone increased at each follow up for the full 2 years assessed. The implications here are that expert system interventions in a population can continue to demonstrate benefits long after the intervention has ended.

We then showed remarkable replication of the expert system's efficacy in a health maintenance organization (HMO) population of 4000 smokers with 85% participation.[21] In the first population-based study, the expert system was 34% more effective than was assessment alone; in the second, it was 31% more effective. These replicated differences were clinically significant as well. While working on a population basis, we were able to produce the level of success normally found only in intense clinic-based programs with low participation rates of much more selected samples of smokers. The implication is that once expert systems are developed and show effectiveness with one population, they can be transferred at much lower cost and produce replicable changes in new populations.

Enhancing Interactive Interventions

In recent benchmarking research, we have been trying to create enhancements to our expert system to produce even greater outcomes. In the first enhancement in our HMO population, we added a personal hand-held computer designed to bring the behavior under stimulus control.[21] This commercially successful innovation was an action-oriented intervention that did not enhance our expert system program on a population basis. In fact, our expert system alone was twice as effective as the system plus the enhancement. There are two major implications here: More is not necessarily better, and providing interventions that are mismatched to stage can make outcomes markedly worse.

Counselor Enhancements

In our HMO population, counselors plus expert system computers were outperforming expert systems alone at 12 months. However, at 18 months, the counselor enhancement had declined while the computers-alone intervention had increased. Both interventions were producing identical outcomes of 23.2% abstinence, which are excellent for an entire population.[21] Why did the effect of the counselor condition drop after the intervention? Our leading hypothesis is that people can become dependent on counselors for the social support and social monitoring that they provide. Once these social influences are withdrawn, people may do worse. The expert system computers, conversely, may maximize self-reliance. In a current clinical trial, we are fading out counselors over time as a method for dealing with dependency on the counselor. If fading is effective, it will have implications for how counseling should be terminated: gradually over time rather than suddenly.

We believe that the most powerful change programs will combine the personalized benefits of clinicians with the individualized, interactive, and data-based benefits of expert system computers. However, to date we have not been able to demonstrate that the more costly counselors, who had been our most powerful change agents, can actually add value over computers alone. These findings have clear implications for cost-effectiveness of expert systems for entire populations needing behavior medicine programs.

Interactive Versus Noninteractive Interventions

Another important aim of the HMO project was to assess whether interactive interventions (computer-generated expert systems) are more effective than are noninteractive communications (stage-matched self-help manuals) when controlling for number of intervention contacts.[20] At 6, 12, and 18 months for groups of smokers receiving a series of one, two, three, or six interactive versus noninteractive contacts, the interactive interventions (expert system) outperformed the noninteractive manuals in all four comparisons. In three of the comparisons (one, two, and three), the differences at 18 months was at least five percentage points, a difference between treatment conditions assumed to be clinically significant. These results clearly support the hypothesis that interactive interventions will outperform the same number of noninteractive interventions.

These results support our assumption that the most powerful health promotion programs for entire populations will be interactive. In the reactive clinical literature, it is clear that interactive interventions, such as behavioral counseling, produce greater long-term abstinence rates (20%–30%) than do noninteractive interventions, such as self-help manuals (10%–20%). It should be kept in mind that these traditional action-oriented programs were implicitly or explicitly recruiting for populations in the preparation stage. Our results indicate that even with proactively recruited smokers, with fewer than 20% in the preparation stage, the long-term abstinence rates are in the 20%–30% range for the interactive interventions and in the 10%–20% range for the noninteractive interventions. The implications are clear. Providing interactive interventions via computers is likely to produce greater outcomes than relying on noninteractive communications, such as newsletters, media, or self-help manuals.

Proactive Versus Reactive Results

We believe that the future of behavior health programs lies with stage-matched, proactive, and interactive interventions. Much greater impacts can be generated by proactive programs because of much higher participation rates, even if efficacy rates are lower. However, we also believe that proactive programs can produce outcomes comparable to traditional reactive programs. It is counterintuitive to believe that comparable outcomes can be produced with people whom we reach out to help as with people who call us for help, but that is what informal comparisons strongly suggest. A comparison of 18-month follow ups for all subjects who received our three expert system reports in our previous reactive study and in our current proactive study shows the abstinence curves to be remarkably similar.[22,27]

The results with our counseling plus computer conditions were even more impressive. Proactively recruited smokers working with counselors and computers had higher abstinence rates at each follow up than did the smokers who had called for help. One of the differences is that our proactive counseling protocol had been revised and, it is hoped, improved on the basis of previous data and experience. However, the point is that if we reach out and offer people improved behavior change programs that are appropriate for their stage, we probably can produce efficacy or abstinence rates at least equal to those we produce with people who reach out to us for help. Yet, there is no experimental design that could permit us to assign people randomly to proactive versus reactive recruitment programs. We are left with informal but provocative comparisons.

INCREASING IMPACTS

To date, we have been able to demonstrate unprecedented impacts of cessation programs with entire populations of smokers. However, our cessation research over the last decade has failed to enhance impacts further. Impacts equal participation rates times efficacy or abstinence rates. With 80%–90% recruitment rates, a ceiling effect limits any significant increase in participation. In spite of our best efforts, such as adding counselors and nicotine-fading computers and doubling the number of computer interactions, we have not been able to break through an apparent glass ceiling of approximately 25% abstinence at long-term follow up.

An alternative strategy has been to intervene on multiple behavior risks in entire populations. Applying our best practices of proactive recruitment and three stage-matched interventions, the following was accomplished in our first study: Proactively, we were able to recruit 83.6% of available parents of ninth graders who were participating in similar programs at school. The high recruitment rates continued even although this population had to focus on changing multiple behaviors (smoking, diet, and sun exposure) rather than the single behavior of smoking.

The efficacy with smoking fell within the range of results generated in our studies targeting the single behavior of smoking. At 24-month follow up, 22% of the smokers were abstinent. The results with high-fat diets were even better, with 33.5% of the parents having progressed from high-fat to low-fat diets. With sun exposure, 29.7% of the parents had progressed to the action or maintenance stage at 24 months and were practicing safe sun behaviors.[30]

If these results continue to be replicated, smoking cessation programs will be able to produce unprecedented impacts on entire populations. We believe that such unprecedented impacts require scientific and professional shifts:

1. From an action paradigm to a stage paradigm
2. From reactive to proactive recruitment
3. From expecting participants to match the needs of our programs to having our programs match their needs
4. From clinic-based to population-based programs that still apply the field's most powerful individualized and interactive intervention strategies
5. From single behavior change programs to multiple behavior change programs for entire populations

VISION FOR THE FUTURE

If the cancer prevention field makes these paradigm shifts, a future can be envisioned in which behavior medicine programs will receive the emphases that they require. No longer will only a small minority of patients with major health behavior risks be reached. A behavior medicine delivery system will be developed to reach 80% or more of people with behaviors that are major cost drivers and causes of cancer and other chronic diseases.

How can population approaches to cancer prevention be funded? Here are two scenarios. Longitudinal data indicate that in populations with multiple behavior risks, effectively treating two behaviors reduces health care costs by approximately $2000 per year.[31] Population-based behavior medicine is one of the few opportunities for health care systems to increase services that improve health and reduce health care costs. The point is that over time, population-based prevention programs pay for themselves.

Another alternative is to use proactive recruitment in primary care or at home via telephone, mail, or Internet and reimburse physicians for diagnosing behavior risks such as smoking and prescribing the appropriate behavior medicine. With computers and 40,000 behavior medicine counselors competitively paid, we could recruit 80% of smokers in the United States. We could reduce smoking by approximately 20% in 2 years; it has decreased only approximately 1.5% since 1990. We could reduce multiple behavior risks, such as high-fat diets and unsafe sun exposure, by an even greater percentage. Further, we could accomplish all of this for less than 10% of the recent tobacco settlement.

We can envision a health care system in the near future in which stage-matched interactive interventions will be to behavior medicine what pharmaceuticals are to biologic medicine: One of the most cost-effective methods to bring optimal amounts of science to bear on multiple behavior problems in entire populations in a relatively user-friendly manner, but with no known side effects. The science is available, the professionals are available, the technology is available, and the money is available. What is needed is to have the political and health priorities be available.

ACKNOWLEDGMENTS

This study is from the Cancer Prevention Research Center, University of Rhode Island, Kingston, Rhode Island. The research in this chapter was supported by grants CA27281 and CA50087 from the National Cancer Institute.

REFERENCES

1. U.S. Department of Health and Human Services. Healthy People 2010: National Health Promotion and Disease Prevention Objectives—Full Report, with Commentary. Washington, DC: U.S. Department of Health and Human Services, 2000.
2. Peto R, Lopea A. World-wide mortality from current smoking patterns. Durstone B, Jamrogik K, eds. Global War: Proceedings of the Seventh World Conference on Tobacco and Health. 1990: 62–68.
3. Lichtenstein E, Hollis J. Patient referral to smoking cessation programs: Who follows through? J Fam Pract 1992;34:739–744.
4. Luepker RV, Murray DM, Jacobs DR et al. Community education for cardiovascular disease prevention: risk factor changes in the Minnesota Heart Health Program. Am J Public Health 1994; 84:1383–1393.
5. COMMIT Research Group. Community Intervention Trial for Smoking Cessation (COMMMIT): I. Cohort results from a four-year community intervention. Am J Public Health 1995;85:83–192.
6. Glasgow RE, Terborg JR, Hollis JF et al. Take heart: results from the initial phase of a work-site wellness program. Am J Public Health 1995;85:209–216.
7. Lando, HA, Pechacek, TF, Pirie, PL et al. Changes in adult cigarette smoking in the Minnesota Heart Health Program. Am J Public Health 1995;85:201–208.
8. Mellinger GD, Balter MB, Uhlenhuth EH et al. Evaluating a household survey measure of psychic distress. Psych Med 1983;13:607–621.
9. Reed GR, Velicer WF, Prochaska JO et al. What makes a good staging algorithm: examples from regular exercise. Am J Health Promo 1997;12:57–66.
10. Schacter S. Recidivism and self cure of smoking and obesity. Am Psychol 1982;198;436–444.
11. Norcross JC, Vangarell DJ. The resolution solution: longitudinal examination of New Year's change attempts. J Subst Abuse 1989;127–134.
12. Brownell KD, Marlatt GA, Lichtenstein E. Understanding and preventing relapse. Am Psychol 1986;41:765–782.
13. Marlatt GA, Gordon JR, eds. Relapse Prevention: Maintenance Strategies in Addictive Behavior Change. New York: Guilford, 1985.
14. Prochaska JO, DiClemente CC. The Transtheoretical Approach: Crossing Traditional Boundaries of Change. Homewood: Dow Jones Irwin, 1984.

15. Norcross JC, Ratzin AC, Payne D. Ringing in the New Year: the change processes and reported outcomes of resolutions. Addict Behav 1989;14:205–212.

16. Prochaska JO, Norcross JC, DiClemente CC. Changing for Good. New York: Morrow, 1994.

17. Cohen S, Lichtenstein E, Prochaska JO et al. Debunking myths about self-quitting: evidence from ten prospective studies of persons quitting smoking by themselves. Am Psychol 1989;44: 355–1365.

18. Snow MG, Prochaska JO, Rossi JS. Stages of change for smoking cessation among former problem drinkers. J Subst Abuse 1992;4:107–116

19. Velicer WF, Fava JL, Prochaska JO et al. Distribution of smokers by stage in three representative samples. Prev Med 1995;24:401–411.

20. Velicer WF, Prochaska JO, Fava J et al. Interactive versus non-interactive and dose response relationships for stage matched smoking cessation programs in a managed care setting. Health Psychol 1999;18:1–8.

21. Prochaska JO, Velicer WF, Fava J et al. Counselor and stimulus control enhancements of a stage matched expert system for smokers in a managed care setting. Prev Med 2000;32:23–32.

22. Prochaska JO, Velicer WF, Fava JL et al. Evaluating a population-based recruitment approach and a stage-based expert system intervention for smoking cessation. Addict Behav 2001;26:583–602.

23. Wierzbicki M, Pekarik G. A meta-analysis of psychotherapy dropout. Prof Psych Res Pract 1993; 29:190–195.

24. Johnson SS, Grimley DM, Prochaska JO. Prediction of adherence using the transtheoretical model: implications for pharmacy care practice. J Soc Admin Pharm 1999;15(3):135–148.

25. Beitman BD, Beck NC, Deuser W et al. Patient stages of change predict outcome in a panic disorder medication trial. Anxiety 1994;1:64–69.

26. Brogan MM, Prochaska JO, Prochaska JM. Predicting termination and continuation status in psychotherapy by using the transtheoretical model. Psychotherapy 1999;36:105–113.

27. Prochaska JO, Di Clemente CC, Velicer WF, Rossi JS. Standardized, individualized, interactive, and personalized self-help programs for smoking cessation. Health Psychol 1993;12:399–405.

28. Prochaska JO, Di Clemente CC, Norcross J C. In search of how people change: applications to addictive behaviors. Am Psychol 1992;47:1102–1114.

29. Prochaska JO, Velicer WF, Ross, JS et al. Stages of change and decisional balance for twelve problem behaviors. Health Psychol 1994;13:39–46.

30. Prochaska JO, Redding, CA, Velicer, WF, Rossi, JS, Fava, JL, Sun, X, Rossi, SR, Greene, GW, Plummer, BA. Stage-based expert systems to help a population of parents to quit smoking, eat healthier and prevent skin cancer. 2001; submitted for publication.

31. Edington D. Paper presented at the Twelfth Annual Art and Science of Health Promotion Conference. February, 2001; Washington, DC.

Chapter 16

The Utility of Mammography for Women Aged 40 to 50 Years (Pro)

Daniel B. Kopans

I have little doubt that some will read this chapter and complain that it is not an objective review. I would dispute the accusation and would challenge anyone to refute the facts provided here on a scientific basis. Having spent at least the last decade debating this topic, I am repeatedly disappointed at the way data have been manipulated and the rules of scientific and statistical analysis ignored in an effort to suggest that there is no benefit from screening women aged 40–49 for breast cancer. The role of several medical journals in promoting this position has been unconscionable. One of the most prestigious, when criticized for not providing readers with both sides of the issue, went as far as to write an editorial explaining that they saw no reason to provide balanced perspectives on controversial topics.[1]

As is well known, absolutes are uncommon in medicine. Proving a benefit from any intervention can be extremely difficult. Much of what is done in day-to-day medical practice is not based on randomized, controlled trials but on anecdotal experience. In the screening debate, however, there are large bodies of data. The confusion that has been brought to this debate has resulted from the inappropriate analysis of these data. As described later, the unplanned stratification of the trial data by age and its use to provide medical recommendations to women aged 40–49 has never been justified. This use of unplanned, retrospective, subgroup analysis of data that lacked statistical power is a violation of one of the major rules for analyzing these types of data. Despite this, the subgroup data have shown a benefit for screening women in their forties. When the original arguments against recommending screening failed, opponents then developed other nonscientific explanations, such as "age creep," wherein, somehow, cancer realized that the age of 50 had been reached and that screening had become efficacious. Arguments that were proposed by radiologists and were based completely on science were dismissed as emotional and due to greed.[2] Instead of dismissing the summary that follows, the reader, it is hoped, will try to understand the issues. If the facts are incorrect, I would be happy to be corrected.

One of the major issues in modern medicine involved in screening of any type is the cost-benefit ratio of the intervention. A discussion of this is beyond the scope of this chapter, but the reader is directed to an excellent summary of the data and analyses written by R.A. Smith of the American Cancer Society.[3]

INTRODUCTION AND HISTORICAL PERSPECTIVE

One of the major medical debates of the 1990s revolved around whether there was a benefit for screening women aged 40–49 for the earlier detection of breast cancer. The argument that had simmered through the 1970s and 1980s was brought to a head when, in 1993, the National Cancer Institute (NCI) convened a workshop to review the latest data on screening for these younger women. Concerns were expressed about the lack of objectivity in this review. Only 3 speakers were invited to defend screening for women aged 40–49, whereas 17 spoke in opposition. The chairperson of the meeting had already expressed her position that screening should not be recommended for these women,[4] and this was reflected in the report of the workshop.[5] A full minority report was not permitted. At the end of 1993, the NCI withdrew the support that it had given just 4 years earlier[6] and stopped recommending screening for these women. A Congressional review of the 1993 NCI decision revealed a mixture of poor science and health care politics.[7] For the first time in its history, the director of the NCI had ignored the advice of the National Cancer Advisory Board (NCAB), which had voted 13 to 1 that the guidelines supporting screening women aged 40–49 should not be changed. The information and chronology suggest that he ignored the NCAB because the NCI, during 1993, had been advising the new Clinton administration that it was going to change the guidelines by dropping screening for women aged 40–49 and was planning to extend the time interval between screens for women aged 50 and older to every 2 years. By the time the NCAB voted at the end of 1993, the administration's health plan was complete, and it was too late to turn back. When asked, at the Congressional hearing convened to review the decision, why he had ignored the 13–1 NCAB vote, Samuel Broder, the then director at the NCI, could only muster the response, "It wasn't unanimous."[7] The decisions and analyses developed from the 1993 workshop[2] appear to have been adopted by many of those opposed to recommending screening for these women without any critical appraisal, and they continue to be used today.

Experts in breast cancer screening were outraged and pointed out that the NCI had required evidence of benefit that the randomized, controlled trials of screening could not possibly provide because they were not designed to evaluate women aged 40–49 as a separate subgroup. The trials had shown a benefit for screening beginning by the age of 40 (Fig. 16.1).[8] However, breaking out the younger women for unplanned subgroup analysis lost all statistical power and, although a benefit was evident in the data, it did not reach statistical significance

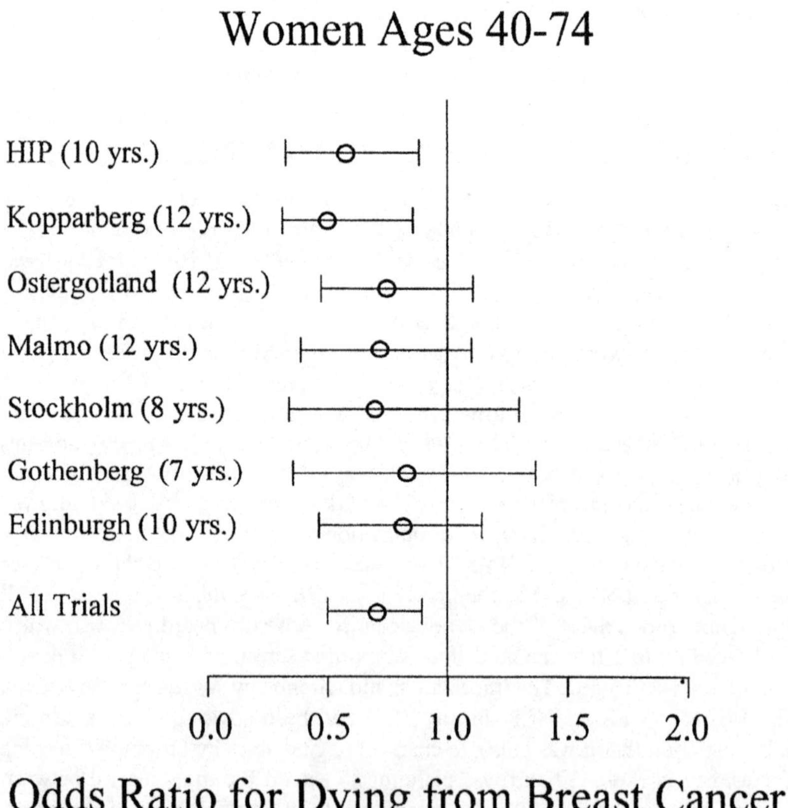

FIGURE 16.1 Odds ratio for dying from breast cancer. When the data are analyzed as the trials were designed, there has always been a benefit for screening women ages 40-49. (HIP, Health Insurance Plan of New York.) (From Shapiro S, Cancer 1994;74:231–238. Reprinted with permission.)

and was dismissed. The workshop summary never addressed the legitimacy of using this type of analysis to guide medical recommendations.[9] This basic issue was ignored by the NCI, and the guidelines were changed.

The confusion persisted and was exacerbated by published studies that reinforced the idea that the age of 50 had some sort of biologic significance,[10] when this was merely an artifact of analyzing data with the age of 50 as the point of analysis. Opposition to recommending screening was reinforced by the spread of misinformation, such as the suggestion that the breast turned to fat at the age of 50, rendering cancer more detectable; that the rate of biopsy changed at the age of 50; that the yield of cancer changed at 50; and that cancer was not a big problem for women younger than age 50 (see Appendix). This occurred in part because a number of the prestigious medical journals printed articles containing fallacious information[11] that opposed screening women in their forties and refused to print analyses that supported screening these women.[12]

In 1997, facing continued pressure and under the leadership of a new director, Richard Klausner, a Consensus Development Conference (CDC) was convened under the auspices of the Office of Medical Applications of Research to review the NCI policy. Concern was expressed that because NCI policy was under review, the CDC had to be objective and not influenced by those at the NCI who had formed the policy that was to be reviewed. However, despite assurances that NCI would have a "hands-off" policy toward the review, the chairman of the Office of Medical Applications of Research organizing committee was from the NCI and was one of the architects of the 1993 decision. Consequently, the panel that was chosen to review the policy had significant biases and conflicts of interest.[13] In addition to the CDC chairman's close collegiality with a major opponent of screening for women aged 40–49, at least three individuals on the review panel were receiving major funding from the NCI. When asked that these conflicts of interest be disclosed, the panel chairman refused.

The CDC convened in January of 1997 and heard testimony from experts on both sides of the issue (the CDC is similar to a trial, with pros and cons of a subject presented to the panel, which acts as a jury). In particular, the trialists from the major randomized, controlled trials in Europe and Scandinavia updated the panel on their latest results (Fig. 16.2). Two of the Swedish trials—Gothenberg and Malmö—by themselves showed statistically significant mortality reductions of 44% and 35%, respectively, from screening women younger than age 50.[14,15] (Although almost everyone agrees that there is a benefit from screening women aged 50 and older, there were actually only two trials, the Health Insurance Plan of New York [HIP] and the Swedish Two County trial, that had shown statistically significant mortality reduction for women aged 50 and older.[8]) When the five Swedish trials were viewed together, they demonstrated a 29% statistically significant mortality reduction.[16] When the seven population-based trials were included in the review, there was a 26%, significant mortality reduction for screening women younger than age 50. Even adding the results from the National Breast

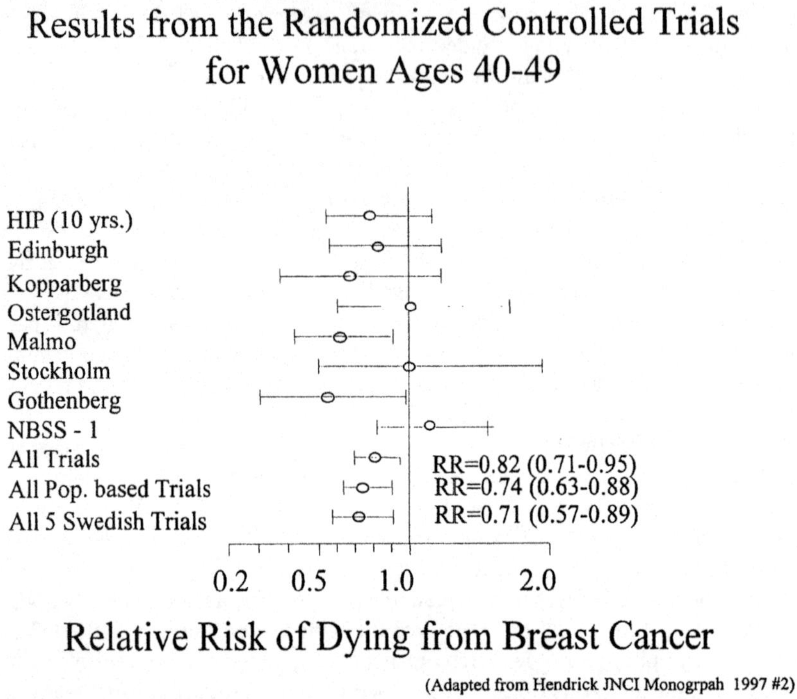

FIGURE 16.2 Relative risk of dying from breast cancer. Even breaking out the younger women, a subgroup analysis that should not have been used for making medical recommendations, there is still significant mortality reduction for screening women aged 40–49. (HIP, Health Insurance Plan of New York; NBSS, National Breast Screening Study.) (From Hendrick RE, Smith RA, Rutledge JH, Smart CR, J Natl Cancer Inst Monogr 1997;22:87–92. Used with permission.)

Screening Study (NBSS) of Canada, which had been severely criticized for being poorly designed and executed[17,18] and in which there were more cancer deaths among the screened women than among the unscreened controls (probably owing to an unblinded randomization process), there was still a statistically significant mortality reduction for screening women aged 49 and younger.

Despite the facts, on January 23, 1997, the CDC Panel, having heard repeatedly that there was a statistically significant benefit for screening women aged 40–49, ignored all the recent data and stated that they could not find any reason to recommend screening to these younger women. Much of the audience was astonished because the CDC's statement appeared to have been written before they had heard the new data. Not only did the panel ignore the new results, they did not even mention them at the press conference where the panel's conclusions were provided to the media and conveyed to the public. Furthermore, they made statements that were factually incorrect.[13] They stated that if there was a benefit for younger women, it was no greater than 30%, ignoring the results from Malmö and Gothenberg. They suggested that any benefit for women aged 40–49 was due to clinical breast examination, completely ignoring the fact that the five Swedish trials did not include any clinical breast examination. Suggestions such as these in the panel statement of January 23, 1997, were so contrary to the facts that they engendered outright anger among many of those present at the meeting. Unfortunately, although the media reported on the great consternation that occurred with the panel pronouncement, they failed to report on the reasons for the consternation, and the opposition was portrayed as due to emotion and greed on the part of radiologists.[2] After the panel had read its decision, the director of the NCI, Richard Klausner, who had heard much of the testimony himself, asked to be asked his opinion. He immediately stated that he disagreed with the panel's conclusions and would ask the NCAB to review the new data.

Because of the significance of the issue, Congress reviewed the CDC results and brought pressure to bear to change the guidelines back to include screening for women aged 40–49. Opponents of screening these women, ignoring Klausner's statement of January 23, have suggested that when the NCI once again supported screening women aged 40–49 on the basis of the NCAB review, it was because the director had given in to pressure from Congress.

By diverting attention from the scientific issues, opponents of screening younger women have been able to continue to ignore the data and avoid defending the inappropriate data analysis that is at the basis of their argument. Approximately 6 months after the CDC and with much less fanfare, the CDC panel published its results.[19] Having realized the validity of the criticisms of their initial report, the panel's final published summary included some of the data that they had ignored in the statement that received widespread media coverage on January 23. The damage had been done by the January 23 release, but the panel covered itself with the final publication, which got little media attention. Although the final published statement provides some of the data showing a benefit (so that the panel cannot be criticized for ignoring it), it disregards its importance and arrives at the same conclusions. In this way, there was great negative impact from the January statement, but the panel was able to claim that they included the data that they had actually excluded in the January statement. Few know that although the panel statement in January was released as unanimous, one of the panel members subsequently resigned in protest and two others wrote a minority report in support of screening younger women.[20]

Those who do not want to understand the facts involved can dismiss the issues by suggesting that experts can look at the same data and disagree on their conclusions. Although this is true, sometimes a group of experts can be wrong (the world is *not* flat). There is no excuse—for those who advise women—for not understanding the reasons for the controversy, and they should understand the available data and how they have been analyzed.

BASIC ISSUES IN BREAST CANCER SCREENING

Superficially, it would seem that finding breast cancer at a smaller size and earlier stage would translate into fewer deaths. However, it is not that simple. Merely showing that the survival time for individuals who are screened is longer than for those who are not screened does not guarantee that there is a benefit from screening. One of the reasons for this is apparent in the following model. Assume that there are two women who are absolutely identical. They will develop a breast cancer in the same breast on the same day, and it will grow at the same rate. The first woman has screening mammograms, and her cancer is detected 5 years after it began. She survives for 10 years from the time of detection and then dies from breast cancer. The second woman is not screened and feels a lump 7 years after the first cell became malignant. She survives 8 years and then dies of breast cancer. If we look only at survival data (date of diagnosis to date of death), it would appear that the first woman benefited by living 2 years more than did the second (10-year survival vs 8 years). However, we know that both actually died 15 years after the cancer began. The first woman only learned about her cancer earlier but derived no benefit from screening because she died at the same time as her unscreened counterpart. This is known as *lead-time bias*. The only way that a benefit from screening could have been shown would have been if the first woman had actually outlived the second.

The only way to prove a benefit from screening, such as with mammography, is to simulate the twin situation. As even identical twins do not have the same cancer course, the simulation is performed using the laws of chance. This is the basis for a randomized, controlled trial (RCT). An RCT works by asking a large number of women to participate. Before anything is known about them, the women are randomly allocated to a group that is offered screening (no one can be forced to be screened) or a group that is not offered screening (unscreened controls). The randomization must be blinded (nothing can be known about the participants), so that the distribution of participants is not unbalanced, thus biasing the trial. If the allocation is truly random and the numbers of participants is large enough, the women in one group will have characteristics identical to those of the women in the other group. There will be the same number of smokers, the same number of women with two children, the same number of women with a college education, and the like. Important for the study is that there will be the same number of women in both groups who, if nothing else is done, will die each year of breast cancer. In effect, every woman in the screened group has a twin in the control group although they cannot be matched ahead of time. Having sufficient numbers of women so that there are "twins" is critical to the success of an RCT.

The study is then conducted, and the women are followed up for years to see whether fewer women die in the screened group. If there are sufficiently fewer deaths among the screened women, such that the differences between deaths among the screened women compared to those in the controls is statistically significant, proof of benefit is shown. One can readily see that the number of participants in these trials has to be very large. Although breast cancer is the most common cancer among women, there are still only approximately 1–5 new cases of breast cancer per 1000 women each year, depending on the age of the women participating. Because only 30%–40% of these will die from their cancers, the number of participants must be very large. The lower the incidence of cancer, the greater the number needed. The lower the benefit from a test, the greater the number needed to prove it. As some women who are offered screening refuse and others who are supposedly unscreened controls obtain mammograms on their own and have their lives saved, even larger numbers are needed to make up for this noncompliance in the screened group and for contamination of the control group.[21]

Once an individual is allocated to one group or the other, she must be counted as having been in the group to which she was allocated so that the results will not be compromised. As a result, screening trials actually underestimate benefit because, for the proper analysis of RCT, women who refuse screening and die of breast cancer must still be counted as having been screened, and women whose lives are saved by having mammography outside the trial are still counted as unscreened controls. In the final analysis, to truly test whether women benefit from screening, there have to be (1) sufficient numbers of women so that they will develop sufficient numbers of breast cancers so that (2) enough of them will die from their breast cancers, such that (3) if there is a benefit from screening, the differences in the number of cancer deaths in the screened group will be lower than that of the deaths in the unscreened control group, such that (4) the difference will be statistically significant.

Although RCTs are difficult to carry out and are very expensive, they are the only way to eliminate lead-time bias, selection bias (the women who participate in screening may be selecting themselves for better or worse cancers), pseudo-disease bias (perhaps the cancers found by the screening test are not lethal and finding them makes screening appear to be effective when it is not), and length bias sampling (periodic screening tends to find slower-growing cancers, whereas the fast-growing, more lethal cancers are missed because they arise between screens).[22] RCTs eliminate all these biases and are the only way, at this time, in which a benefit can be shown.

STATISTICAL SIGNIFICANCE AND STATISTICAL POWER

If a trial showed that 10 women died in the control group whereas only 7 died in the screened group, most would agree that the numbers were so small that the differences could merely be due to chance (even large trials do not have perfectly symmetric distributions). If, however, there were 100 deaths in the control group and only 70 in the screened group, it would be much more likely that the difference was real and not due to chance. Measures of "statistical significance" are mathematical formulas that analyze the likelihood that a result could be real or just due to chance. Most accept as significant a result that has a 5% or less likelihood that it is due to chance. This is expressed as a P value, wherein P is $\leq .05$.

When a trial is being planned, the investigators project the expected benefit that will be gained by screening (the percentage reduction in deaths), then they calculate the number of women needed in the trial so that there will be sufficient cancers and cancer deaths to prove this benefit. This is called the *power calculation*. The smaller the number of participants, the lower the power of the trial to show a benefit. The greater the number, the greater the power of the trial. The power of the data can also be analyzed after the data have been collected to see whether the numbers involved have the ability to demonstrate a benefit. If there are more deaths than expected in the control group, the data have greater power than was planned. If there are fewer deaths, there is less power to show a benefit. Power is influenced by numbers of participants, the number of cancers occurring in the women under study, the number of cancer deaths, the length of the follow up (more deaths occur over time), and the percent mortality reduction. The importance of statistical power has been repeatedly ignored by many in this controversy.

THE HEART OF THE CONTROVERSY

The RCTs were not designed to permit retrospective evaluation of women aged 40–49 as a subgroup. Although there had been close to half a million women who participated in the trials (Table 16.1), there were insufficient numbers of women younger than age 50 to permit the demonstration of a statistically significant benefit in the early (5–7) years of follow up (Table 16.2). The trials lacked the statistical power to show a benefit when women aged 40–49 were analyzed separately. They would have needed close to three times the number of women in these ages for the benefit to have reached statistical significance. Despite the fact that this was clearly demonstrated,[10] the opponents of screening women aged 40–49 have continually ignored this basic scientific issue. Although analysis of the early results did show a benefit, because it did not achieve statistical significance, opponents of screening told women and their physicians that there was no benefit. They failed to tell them that the number of women participating at this age was far too small for there to be a significant benefit. It was mathematically impossible and the result of inappropriate data analysis. When, with longer follow up, the benefit became statistically significant, age creep (discussed in the section Age Creep) was manufactured as a second argument to avoid acknowledging the original mistake.

TABLE 16.1 The Randomized, Controlled Trials of Breast Cancer Screening

	Ages	Interval (months)	Protocol	Follow-up (years)	Invited	Controls
HIP	40–64	12	2 view + CBE	18	30,131	30,585
Kopparberg	40–74	24–33	1 view	12	38,562	18,478
Ostergotland	40–74	24–33	1 view	12	38,405	37,145
Malmo	45–69	18–24	1 or 2 views	12	20,695	20,783
Stockholm	40–64	28	1 view	8	38,525	20,651
Gothenberg	39–59	18	2 views	10	20,724	28,809
Edinburgh	45–64	24	1 or 2 views	10	23,226	21,904
NBSS (Canada)	40–49	12	2 views + CBE	7	25,214	25,216
NBSS (Canada)	50–59	12	2 views + CBE vs CBE	7	19,711	19,694

CBE, clinical breast exam; HIP, Health Insurance Plan of New York; NBSS, National Breast Screening Study.

TABLE 16.2 Number and Percentage of Women in Trials Who Were Aged 49 or Younger at the Time of Allocation

	Total women	% under 50	No. under 50
HIP	62,000	48%	14,000
Kopparberg	57,171	25%	14,595
Ostergotland	75,894	27%	20,835
Malmo	42,000	20%	7,427
Stockholm	60,000	37%	22,342
Gothenberg	49,533	18%	9,000
Edinburgh	65,000	18%	11,723
NBSS	90,000	50%	50,000
Total			**165,922**

HIP, Health Insurance Plan of New York; NBSS, National Breast Screening Study.

Why Age 50?

Women and their physicians have been repeatedly told that the age of 50 represents a point at which screening suddenly begins to work. Opponents of screening younger women neglect to point out that it is actually an arbitrary age, and the data have been analyzed so as to reinforce—inappropriately—its importance. The age of 50 was initially chosen as a surrogate for the age of menopause. As breast cancer is clearly hormonally mediated, analysts sought to determine whether menopause had any influence on the benefit that had shown up in the first RCT of screening performed in the HIP study. Because there were no good data on the actual ages of menopause among those women, the investigators chose the age of 50 as the average age of menopause and broke apart their data, analyzing women aged 40–49 and those aged 50–64. Other trials that followed did the same thing, analyzing women aged 49 and younger and comparing them to those aged 50 and older. This is called *subgroup analysis*. Trials are often designed so that there are enough participants in the subgroups to permit these analyses. In the breast cancer screening trials, however, subgroup analysis of this type was not planned, and there were insufficient numbers of women in the age group 40–49 to permit accurate analysis. The investigators were not deterred, even though many have warned against the fact that this can lead to major misinterpretations of results.[23,24] Even the NBSS, a trial that was touted as being designed to evaluate women aged 40–49, by the investigators' own calculations, could show a benefit of only 40% or greater had the trial evolved as expected[25] (only a 25%–30% reduction had been shown in the trial that preceded theirs). Couple this with the unexpectedly very low death rate among the control group and their levels of noncompliance and contamination and the NBSS was a trial that was grossly underpowered.[10] The NBSS was further compromised by the fact that women with obviously advanced breast cancer were allowed to enter a trial of screening and, owing to a nonblinded allocation that followed a clinical breast examination, there were more women with advanced breast cancer who were allocated to the screened group than the control group. These women were destined to die and could not possibly benefit from screening, and they imbalanced the trial.

When HIP researchers performed their retrospective subgroup analysis, they found that in the first 5 years of follow up, there was no benefit for screening women aged 40–49, whereas there seemed to be an immediate benefit for women aged 50–64. What the investigators ignored was the question as to how a periodic screening test (which is more likely to detect slow- and moderately fast-growing cancers and not the fast-growing cancers) can result in an immediate mortality reduction for anyone. The test would have to find the cancer in the screened women just before it metastasized in the control women (to save the screened women's lives), and the recent metastasis would have to kill the control women almost immediately for a benefit to appear immediately. No one has ever explained how this could occur. Nevertheless, analysts expected that there should be an immediate benefit. They focused on the "delayed" benefit in the younger women (a much more likely result from screening) but were skeptical of the benefit *because* it was "delayed." Although there began to be fewer deaths among the younger screened women than among the controls as the groups were followed out over the years, the difference did not reach statistical significance in the early years of follow up, so it was ignored.

What the analysts failed to appreciate and what opponents of screening younger women have never justified, is the fact that the trials did not have sufficient numbers of women at these ages to permit accurate subgroup analysis. Nevertheless, they unconscionably not only relied on the analysis but used it to make medical recommendations. Opponents ignored the obvious. If retrospective subgroup analysis of data that lacked statistical power could be used to make medical recommendations, RCTs could be made smaller and smaller and, reduced to the absurd, would require only two women. If opponents of screening women aged 40–49 are to have any credibility, they should be required to address this issue.

The reliance on the inappropriate use of subgroup analysis that lacked statistical power in the formulation of medical recommendations was prolonged by a marked imbalance of publications in important medical journals that prevented the issues from being presented to physicians and the public in a balanced and impartial fashion.[13] Physicians were not alerted to the importance of appropriate data analysis. When challenged (i.e., in the author's unpublished letters to the *New England Journal of Medicine*, the *Journal of the American Medical Association*, the *Journal of the National Cancer Institute*, and the *Annals of Internal Medicine*), many journals refused to address the issue.

Age Creep

With longer follow up and despite the fact that the RCTs were not designed, legitimately, to permit medical advice based on retrospective subgroup analysis, the benefit that had been apparent for years for women aged 40–49 (fewer cancer deaths) became statically significant despite the lack of power in the early years of follow up. Confronted with data that had fulfilled their inappropriate requirements,[5] the opponents of screening younger women invoked a new explanation and suggested that the benefit for women aged 40–49 was due to the fact that they had reached the age of 50 during the trials and that screening had suddenly begun to work. Ignoring the fact that there is absolutely no biologic explanation as to how the body and cancers would know that the age of 50 had arrived, the opponents have persisted in this suggestion. They have ignored the warning that RCT analysis requires that the age at allocation is the only safe age to use.[26] Using the age at diagnosis biases the study against showing a benefit for younger women because a woman whose cancer is diagnosed by screening before the age of 50 may have a "twin" in the control group whose cancer is not diagnosed until after the age of 50. If the data are analyzed by the age at diagnosis, there will be no benefit for the screen-detected patient younger than 50. Supporters of age creep point to an analysis of the data by de Konig et al.[27] What they fail to point out is that those authors did not have access to the complete data[28] and that when this was provided to them at the CDC, de Konig recanted his analysis at the CDC meeting in January 1997 and acknowledged that most of the benefit was due to detection of cancers before the age of 50. It is not clear why de Konig has not published this revision.

MISINFORMATION THAT HAS SUSTAINED THE OPPOSITION TO SCREENING OF WOMEN AGES 40-49

Some opponents of screening women younger than age 50 have manipulated data to support the premise that the age of 50 has some significance. They have suggested that the parameters of screening change at the age of 50. They also have argued that breast cancer is not very important among women in their forties.[29] For example, it was argued in 1993 that only 16% of all of the breast cancers diagnosed in that year were among women aged 40–49. It was stressed that we should concentrate on screening the other women because it was among them that 84% of the cancers occurred. What was not pointed out was that this type of analysis compared women in one decade of life with all the other women in the other three decades of life. In fact, the same could have been said for women aged 50–59, among whom "only" 17% of breast cancers occurred in that year. Using the same reasoning, it could be argued that we should concentrate on the other women who accounted for the 83% of cancers diagnosed in that year. The fact is that there was no decade that accounted for more than 25% of the cancers detected in 1993.

This kind of deceptive age grouping has been used repeatedly to mislead women and their physicians. Women aged 40–49 have been considered as a uniform group and are repeatedly compared to women aged 50 and older, as though they too are a uniform group. This type of dichotomous comparison selects data that change gradually with increasing age, such as the incidence of breast cancer, and causes them to appear to change abruptly at the age of 50. I use the term *mislead* purposely because, even after investigators were warned that these dichotomous analyses were leading to inappropriate conclusions, some of them persisted. One study contained data that showed that the cancer detection rates in a screening program increased steadily with increasing age, with no abrupt change at any age,[11] yet by grouping the data and comparing women aged 30–49 to women aged 50–74, the authors concluded that we should concentrate on screening women aged 50 and older because the cancer detection rate among them was 10 per 1000, whereas it was only 2 per 1000 for women aged 49 and younger. Other authors have not even bothered to review the data critically but have merely parroted the results.[30] This has led to a great deal of misinformation that has been used to support the opponents' positions.

Another misuse of age grouping has been an explanation as to why screening might not be as effective in women younger than age 50 as in those aged 50 and older. It has been well established that, although far from ineffective, mammographic screening is more difficult in women who have radiographically dense breast tissues. Opponents have made the incorrect assumption that radiographic density was the same as clinically appreciable firmness. Assuming that premenopausal women have firm breasts, and misreading the literature, they have indirectly argued that because the breast becomes less dense at age 50, this would support their argument.[5] The fact is that there is no correlation between radiographic density and breast firmness. The data clearly show that there is no abrupt change in the percentage of women who have dense tissue and those with fatty tissue (clear on mammography) at any age, and certainly not at the age of 50.[31] The misunderstanding has come because, once again, the data have been analyzed dichotomously, comparing women aged 40–49 with those aged 50 and older. This approach takes changes that occur steadily with increasing age and causes them to appear to occur suddenly at the age of 50.

There are absolutely no data that show that the age of 50 has any biologic significance. None of the parameters of screening change abruptly at the age of 50.[32] The recall rates for an abnormal mammogram reading increase very slowly but steadily with increasing age. The percentage of women for whom a biopsy is recommended on the basis of an abnormal mammogram result is almost exactly the same regardless of age. The cancer detection rate increases steadily with increasing age, merely reflecting the prior probability of breast cancer in the population. None of these parameters changes abruptly at the age of 50 or at any other age.

APPLICATION TO THE GENERAL PUBLIC

Once a screening study has been shown to be efficacious by an RCT, the true test of its effectiveness is whether it can result in decreased deaths in the population in general. In a remarkable review by Tabár et al.,[33] the death rate from breast cancer has been shown to decrease in a population in direct proportion to the number of women being screened. The fact that there was an abrupt increase in cancers detected in the United States in 1983–1985 is a marker for the start of widespread mammographic screening. This was followed by an equally abrupt decrease in cancer deaths beginning 5–7 years later. The abrupt changes in incidence (detection rates) and death rates and the timing of the changes is a strong indication that mammographic screening is effective outside of clinical trials.

CONCLUSION

There has been evidence for years that women can benefit from screening beginning in their forties. Despite the fact that the data should not be analyzed using age subgroups, there is nevertheless, statistically significant "proof" of benefit for screening women in their forties. In the future, analysts should be required to justify their approaches to data analysis. Furthermore, they should stop using the age of 50 as though it has biologic significance. It is, essentially, an arbitrary age when it comes to the parameters of screening. Women aged 40–49 are not a uniform group, just as those aged 50 and older are not uniform. Dichotomous comparisons of these two groups using the age of 50 as a point of analysis should cease.

REFERENCES

1. Kassirer JP, Angell M. Controversial journal editorials. N Engl J Med 1997;337:1460–1461.
2. Fletcher SW. Whither scientific deliberation in health policy recommendations. N Engl J Med 1997;336:1180–1183
3. Smith RA. Breast cancer screening among women younger than age 50: a current assessment of the issues. CA Cancer J Clin 2000;50:312–336.
4. Fletcher SW, Fletcher RH. The breast is close to the heart. Ann Intern Med 1992;117:969—971.
5. Fletcher SW, Black W, Harris R et al. Report of the international workshop on screening for breast cancer. J Natl Cancer Inst 1993;85:1644–1656.
6. National Medical Roundtable on Mammography Screening Guidelines. Washington, DC: National Press Club, June 27, 1989 [press release].
7. House Committee on Government Operations. Misused Science: The National Cancer Institutes elimination of mammography guidelines for women in their forties. Union Calendar No. 480, House Report 103—863, October 20, 1994.
8. Shapiro S. Screening: assessment of current studies. Cancer 1994;74:231–238.
9. Kopans DB, Halpern E, Hulka CA. Statistical power in breast cancer screening trials and mortality reduction among women 40–49 with particular emphasis on the National Breast Screening Study of Canada. Cancer 1994;74:1196–1203.
10. Kerlikowske K, Grady D, Barclay J et al. Positive predictive value of screening mammogrpahy by age and family history of breast cancer. JAMA 1993;270:2444–2450.
11. Lee Davis D, Love SM. Mammographic screening. JAMA 1994;271:152–153.

12. Kopans DB. The breast cancer screening controversy: lessons to be learned. J Surg Oncol 1998; 67:143–150.

13. Kopans DB. The breast cancer screening controversy and the National Institutes of Health Consensus Development Conference on breast cancer screening for women ages 40–49. Radiology 1999; 210:4–9.

14. Bjurstam N, Bjorneld L, Duffy S et al. The Gothenberg breast cancer screening trial: preliminary results on breast cancer mortality for women ages 39–49. J Natl Cancer Inst Monogr 1997;22: 53–55.

15. Andersson I, Janzon L. Reduced breast cancer mortality in women under 50: update from the Malmö Mammographic Screening Program. J Natl Cancer Inst Monogr 1997;22:63–67.

16. Hendrick RE, Smith RA, Rutledge JH, Smart CR. Benefit of screening mammography in women ages 40–49: a new meta-analysis of randomized controlled trials. J Natl Cancer Inst Monogr 1997;22:87–92.

17. Kopans DB, Feig SA. The Canadian National Breast Screening Study: a critical review. Am J Roentgenol AJR 1993;161:755–760.

18. Tarone RE. The excess of patients with advanced breast cancers in young women screened with mammography in the Canadian National Breast Screening Study. Cancer 1995;75:997–1003.

19. National Institutes of Health Consensus Conference on Breast Cancer Screening for Women Ages 40–49. Consensus statement. J Natl Cancer Inst Monogr 1997;22:7–12.

20. National Institutes of Health Consensus Conference on Breast Cancer Screening for Women Ages 40–49. Minority report. J Natl Cancer Inst Monogr 1997;22:12–18.

21. Eyre H, Sondik E, Smith RA, Kessler L. Joint meeting on the feasibility of a study of screening premenopausal women (40–49 years) for breast cancer, April 20–21, 1994. Cancer 1995;75: 1391–1403.

22. Kopans DB. Breast Imaging, 2nd ed. Philadelphia: Lippincott-Raven, 1997.

23. Lachin JM. Introduction to sample size determination and power analysis for clinical trials. Control Clin Trials 1981;2:93–113.

24. Moher D, Dulberg C, Wells GA. Statistical power, sample size, and their reporting in randomized controlled trials. JAMA 1994;272:122–124.

25. Miller AB, Howe GR, Wall C. The National Study of Breast Cancer Screening. Clin Invest Med 1981;4:227–258.

26. Prorok PC, Hankey BF, Bundy BN. Concepts and problems in the evaluation of screening programs. J Chron Dis 1981;34;159–171.

27. De Konig HJ, Boer R, Warmerdam PG et al. Quantitative interpretation of age-specific mortality reductions from the Swedish Breast Cancer Screening Trials. J Natl Cancer Inst 1995;87: 1217–1223.

28. Tabár L, Duffy SW, Chen HH. Re: quantitative interpretation of age-specific mortality reductions from the Swedish breast cancer screening trials. J Natl Cancer Inst 1996;88:52–53.

29. Harris RP, Fletcher SW, Gonzalez JJ et al. Mammography and age: Are we targeting the wrong women? Cancer 1991;67:2010–2014.

30. Sox H. Screening mammography in women younger than 50 years of age. Ann Intern Med 1995; 122:550–552.

31. Stomper PC, D'Souza DJ, DiNitto PA, Arredondo MA. Analysis of parenchymal density on mammograms in 1353 Women 25–79 years old. Am J Roentgenol AJR 1996;167:1261–1265.

32. Kopans DB, Moore RH, McCarthy KA et al. Biasing the interpretation of mammography screening data by age grouping: nothing changes abruptly at age 50. Breast J 1998;4:139–145.

33. Tabár L, Vitak B, Tony HH et al. Beyond randomized controlled trials: organized mammographic screening substantially reduces breast carcinoma mortality. Cancer 2001;5(9):1724–1731.

APPENDIX

Fiction and Facts About Screening for Women Aged 40–49

Fiction

Breast cancer is not an important problem for women aged 40–49.

Fact

Although the incidence of breast cancer increases steadily with increasing age in women (approximately 1 per 1000 in their forties, 2 per 1000 in their fifties, 3 per 1000 in their sixties, and 4 per 1000 in their seventies), because of the large numbers of women in their forties, the total number of women with breast cancer in this decade is approximately the same as the number of those with diagnosed cancer in their fifties. In 1995 and 1996, there were actually more women in their forties with diagnosed breast cancer than there were women in their fifties. No decade accounts for more than 25% of the cancers diagnosed each year. Furthermore, many cancers not diagnosed until women are in their fifties could be found with screening while they are in their forties. Most women would likely find that a risk that goes from 1 per 1000 per year to 5 per 1000 per year is not a major difference.

Fiction

Young women have firm breasts. This means that cancers are more difficult to see on mammograms.

Fact

It is the radiographic density of the breast (the x-ray attenuation of its structures) that can hide cancers. There is no relationship between the physical attributes of the breast and its radiographic density. Radiographic density does not correlate with the size of the breast or its firmness. Very firm breasts can be radiolucent, and cancers can be seen easily. Very soft breasts can be radiodense and hide cancers.

Fiction

The breast tissues are dense in younger women and turn to fat (become less dense) at the age of 50 (with menopause), rendering cancers detectable and curable.

Fact

The radiographic density of the breast is related to age. Approximately 90% of women have radiographically dense breast at the age of 30, but the percentage changes slowly and steadily by approximately 1%–2% per year. There is no abrupt change at any age and no abrupt change at menopause.

Fiction

The percentage of women called back for evaluation of an abnormal mammogram result changes abruptly at the age of 50.

Fact

The rate of call back changes slowly and steadily from age 40 to age 80 but only from approximately 8% to 6%. There is no abrupt change at any age and no abrupt change at the age of 50. The call back rate decreases when women are screened repeatedly, being higher with the first screen and lower with subsequent screens.

Fiction

The percentage of women recommended for a biopsy on the basis of an abnormal mammogram result changes abruptly at the age of 50.

Fact

The percentage of women for whom a biopsy is recommended on the basis of an abnormal mammogram reading is actually virtually the same regardless of age, fluctuating from 0.5% to 2.0%, with no abrupt change at any age.

Fiction

The percentage of women who are diagnosed with breast cancer having undergone a biopsy on the basis of an abnormal mammogram outcome changes abruptly at the age of 50.

Fact

The percentage of women who are diagnosed with breast cancer and having undergone biopsy on the basis of an abnormal mammogram outcome increases steadily with increasing age, with no abrupt change at the age of 50 or at any other age. The yield of cancers is directly related to the prior probability of cancer in the population, which increases steadily with increasing age.

Chapter 17

The Utility of Mammography for Women 40 to 50 Years of Age (Con)

Donald A. Berry

In many countries, mammographic screening for breast cancer is not standard practice. In the United States, such screening is regarded by women and their caregivers to be mandatory for good health. Most U.S. women older than age 40 participate in regular screening programs. I do not address the reasons for these widely disparate attitudes, but I do describe the reasoning and evidence on which the U.S. attitude is based. I argue that the reasoning is faulty and that the evidence is biased and misleading at worst, and not compelling at best.

Politicians in the United States unanimously favor screening, but this is neither surprising nor relevant as to whether it has any benefits. In 1997, the U.S. Senate in effect ruled by a vote of 98–0 that screening mammography is effective for women in their forties. This is both comical and worrisome.[1–3] Politicians are neither trained to interpret scientific evidence nor empowered by the Almighty to change nature!

Screening mammography for women in their forties may reduce breast cancer mortality in comparison with starting at age 50, say, but any incremental benefit is minimal. Also, there are risks associated with screening. Although these risks are modest in severity, taken in toto they are sufficient to render a blanket policy of screening in this age group questionable at best. Women (and their caregivers) need to understand how to interpret the available evidence before they make a decision to initiate a screening program.

There is a substantial literature that concludes that screening mammography is effective. The authors compare the prognosis and survival of women whose cancers were detected by mammography with those of women whose cancers were detected by other means. Although it is very compelling, the enterprise is misguided, and the results are misleading. I show that the biases associated with screening are so profound that comparing outcomes of screened and unscreened patients is meaningless outside the context of randomized controlled trials. My arguments apply as well to observations made in clinical practice—however large the practice and however objective the practitioner. Such observations contain no information about screening's effectiveness. Clinicians are accustomed to learning while doing, but learning is not possible in this case. The only good evidence regarding screening effectiveness is found in the results of the eight randomized trials that compared survival of women assigned to be screened with survival of those assigned to be controls. In this chapter, I focus on the women who entered these trials while in their forties. Concern over the quality of the randomized trials[4,5] and the resulting flurry of debate draw into question any conclusions made from the trials, but I do not engage in this debate. Rather, I argue that even when taking the trial results at face value, the mortality differences are tiny in absolute terms. Therefore, even if screening is assumed to be effective in a population of women, such effectiveness translates into questionable benefit for an individual woman.

On the other hand, the probabilities of false positives and subsequent workups (such as biopsies) are substantial. In addition, the increased likelihood of ductal carcinoma in situ (DCIS) detection and treatment is of uncertain value. The risk-benefit ratio of screening for women in their forties is not clear, but it most assuredly will differ depending on the individual woman, if she is adequately informed. I offer guidelines for women in this age group to help them to decide whether screening is right for them.

SCREENING FOR CANCER AND THE POSSIBILITY OF CURE

Screening for cancer has an enormously compelling intuitive appeal: It *must* be better to find and treat cancer earlier in its development. This attitude is so widely accepted in the United States that an estimated 88% of women between the ages of 45 and 54 have had at least one mammogram, and most of these women had their most recent mammogram within the last two years.[6]

The intuition that screening is beneficial may be correct, depending on the type of cancer, but intuition is frequently wrong when applied to screening. That screening is beneficial is supported by the commonly held but possibly fallacious belief that some cancer patients are cured of their disease. ("Cure" has many different interpretations in cancer, so many that perhaps the word should be avoided. But I use it, giving it a very strict interpretation: Cure can result only by intervening and eliminating the disease from the body, and it applies only when the disease would have been fatal without such intervention. In particular, it is not possible to cure a patient who has DCIS if she died of heart disease and would have died of heart disease in any case.) Also supporting the benefits of screening is the surgeon's claim that "We got it all." It seems reasonable that we are more likely to get it all and thereby cure the patient when the tumor is smaller. However, our knowledge of the biology of cancer is limited, and it is impossible to tell for certain that a particular patient would have died from her disease without treatment. We might get it all and yet not improve the patient's survival. Conversely, as evinced by small node-negative tumors that become metastatic despite optimal therapy, we sometimes only think we got it all. The heterogeneity of cancer and its penchant for spreading render it impossible to conclude that a particular patient has been cured.

Perhaps we can make a general claim that we cure at least some patients of their breast cancer even though we cannot say for sure which ones. However, our ability to infer that available treatments cure a proportion of patients in some larger population is not much better than it is for individual patients. There have been many important advances in breast cancer therapy. Some treatments are unquestionably effective in the sense that they prolong lives. Perhaps the best example is tamoxifen in patients with estrogen receptor (ER)-positive tumors. The available evidence leaves no doubt that tamoxifen prolongs these women's lives.[7] However, prolonging life does not necessarily mean curing the disease. Distinguishing between prolonging life and cure on the basis of empirical evidence is difficult or impossible in primary breast cancer because many patients survive for longer than 20 years.

Figure 17.1 illustrates the difficulty in discriminating between cure and prolonging survival on the basis of empirical evidence. Suppose that a clinical trial is designed to evaluate a new therapy that may improve survival. Suppose further that in the population of interest, the current annual rate of breast cancer mortality is 8%. The corresponding survival is shown by the dashed survival curve labeled *current* in the figure. The implied current median survival is 8.66 years. The goal of the new therapy is to improve this by one-third, to 11.55 years. If this happens, it may be through prolonging everyone's survival by reducing the annual mortality rate to 6% (the curve labeled *prolong*) or by leaving the annual rate unchanged (at 8%) for most of the patients but curing a fraction of them (the curve labeled *cure*). To have the same median (11.55 years) as *prolong* implies a cure rate of 17.1%.

In view of the sampling variability present in empirical survival information, it is impossible to discriminate between the prolong and cure curves shown in Figure 17.1 on the basis of results of even very large clinical trials. Indeed, the critical part of the follow-up period for this discrimination is 20 years and beyond, and few trials have followed up patients for this long. Moreover, information

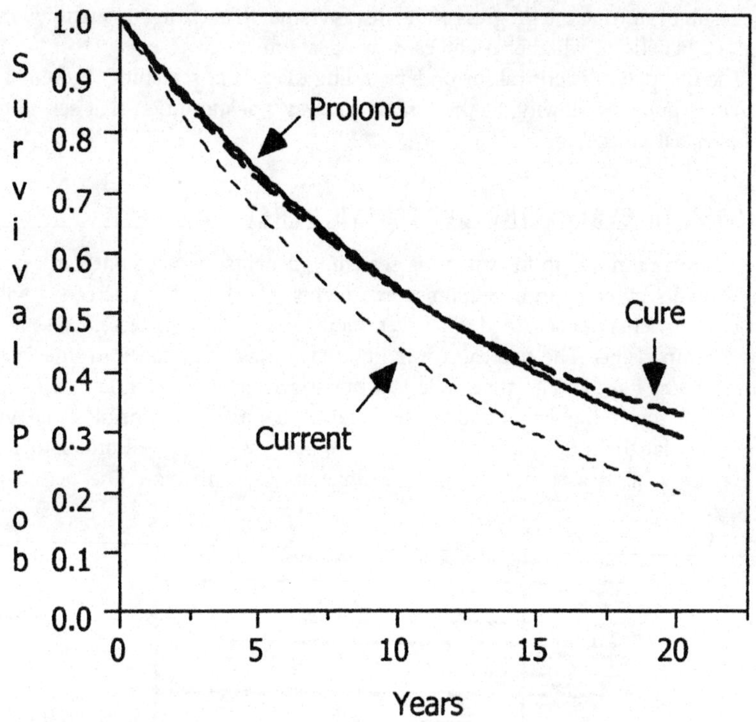

FIGURE 17.1 Difficulty in discriminating between curing disease and prolonging survival. The median survival times of prolong and cure are the same, and both are one-third longer than current.

beyond 20 years is sparse in any case because, by then, earlier events and competing risks (such as cardiovascular disease) have removed patients from the at-risk population. To make matters worse, there is an enormous array of possible curves that are similar to the two shown in the Figure 17.1, with some having cure rates and others not. Finally, the "current" survival distribution assumes that all breast cancer is fatal (although survival times vary). More realistically, some breast cancer (including some invasive as well as in situ breast cancer) will never kill the patient. Deciding whether a new therapy cures some patients is even more difficult if a proportion of patients is assumed to have nonfatal disease.

So, not only is it impossible to verify cure in a particular patient, it is impossible to know that *any* breast cancer patient has been cured. It is entirely conceivable that breast cancers become or do not become lethal in their very early development, before they are detectable on a mammogram. If this is so, early detection may not help, and the observed benefits of therapy, however substantial, may be the result of slowing the progress of the disease rather than curing it. Such slowing may be beneficial, whether it comes early or late in the disease.

The distinction is critical for understanding the role of screening. If there are no cures but only slowing of the disease process, one's intuition that screening is beneficial evaporates.

BIASES IN EVALUATING SCREENING BENEFITS

If intuition cannot help in evaluating screening benefits, perhaps one can assess the benefits by comparing outcomes in patients who have been screened with those in patients not screened. However, there are a number of biases present in such comparisons. The two most important are length bias and lead-time bias. These biases have an enormous effect in breast cancer, so great in fact that they dwarf any screening benefit and render database comparisons worthless. Length bias is by far the more important of the two, but it is not as well understood.

Figure 17.2 is a schematic diagram illustrating length bias. The period of

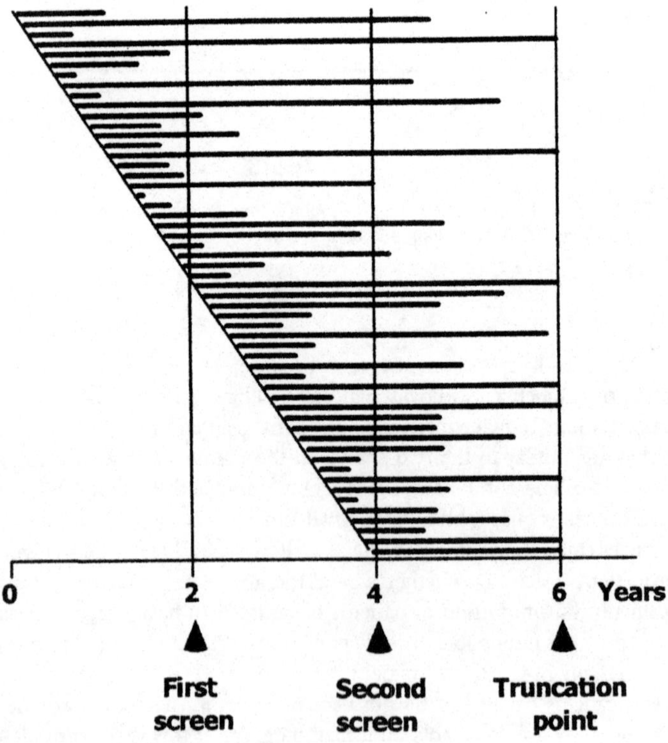

FIGURE 17.2 Illustration of length bias in evaluating screening.

observation is 6 years. The figure allows for considering both possibilities: that the participants are screened and that they are not screened. Each of the 54 horizontal lines corresponds to a tumor. The tumor is detectable at the leftmost endpoint of the line, and it becomes clinically detectable at the rightmost endpoint of the line (except that all lines have been truncated at the end of the observation period). The length of a line is the tumor's *sojourn time*, the period during which the cancer is detectable mammographically but not clinically. The longest sojourn time for the 54 tumors is 8.4 years (for the fourth one from the top). The left endpoints of the lines are staggered to correspond to a uniform distribution of tumor initiations that would be typical in a trial or observational study in which approximately one cancer is initiated every 2 weeks. The tumor is present for a period to the left of its line, when it is not detectable mammographically. To the right of a line, the tumor is detectable by either route, and presumably it has been removed at the right endpoint, regardless of whether the patient has been screened. (Not shown are tumors detectable clinically before they can be detected mammographically.) The lengths of the lines in Figure 17.2 were generated from an exponential distribution having a mean sojourn time of 2 years, which is within the range of claims for mammographic screening.[8]

The vertical lines at years 2 and 4 correspond to screening times. Twelve of the tumors became clinically detectable before the first screen. Nine of the lines start to the right of the first screen and end to the left of the second screen. These correspond to *interval cancers* that are observed between the two screens. The vertical line at year 6 signals the end of observation. The eight horizontal lines intersecting this vertical line have their times of clinical detection beyond the observation period. Eight fewer cancers would be discovered in these 54 women if there were no screenings. (The truncation point is arbitrary in this illustration but, regardless of the truncation point, some unscreened women will die with undetected cancers.)

The crux of length bias is that any vertical line laid down on the horizontal lines will tend to intersect lines that are longer, and the difference can be enormous, depending on the heterogeneity of the tumors. The exponential distribution evinces a modest level of heterogeneity: Its standard deviation is the same as its mean. The average length of all 54 horizontal lines in Figure 17.2 is 2 years, chosen somewhat arbitrarily to be the same as the interval between screens. The 33 lines that intersect the vertical lines ("first screen" and "second screen") correspond to cancers detected mammographically. The 21 lines that do not intersect the vertical lines are cancers detected clinically. Horizontal lines that intersect the vertical lines tend to be long and include many slowly growing cancers. The mean length of the 33 horizontal lines that intersect either of the screening lines is 2.90 years. The mean length of the 21 horizontal lines not intersecting a vertical line (cancers detected only clinically) is 0.58 years. In this example, the sojourn times of mammographically detected tumors are on average five times longer than those of tumors detected clinically. The difference would be even greater if the picture were to extend further to the left and consider those tumors that were mammographically detectable more than 2 years before the first screen, for these tumors will tend to be even more slowly growing than those in the figure.

Because it is not possible to watch a breast tumor grow without doing something about it, tumor growth in humans is not well understood. A tumor may grow slowly at first and then slow down, even with no interventions. A tumor with similar characteristics in another patient may grow more rapidly over time. For this reason and for other reasons, sojourn time is an imperfect predictor of survival time, but the two are almost certainly related. For purposes of illustration, suppose that survival time, ignoring competing risks, is 15 times as large as the sojourn time (i.e., an average of 30 years). Suppose further that all 54 patients in the figure would live an additional 30 years were it not for their cancer. Then those with sojourn times of less than 2 years will die of their disease, and the others will not. In the figure, 13 of 33 (39%) of the women with tumors detected mammographically will die of breast cancer, and 21 of 21 (100%) of those with tumors detected clinically will die of breast cancer. The average survival time in the mammographically detected group is 25.03 years, and that in the unscreened group is 8.67 years. This comparison assumes no therapy in either group; the 65% reduction in breast cancer mortality is spurious and is due to length bias.

The example assumed an exponential distribution of sojourn times, which may or may not be realistic. However, any distribution would show the same effect. The magnitude of length bias may be greater or less than that shown in the example, but all that is required to have such a bias is that some sojourn times are longer than others. Many investigators have fallen prey to the biases present in comparing screened versus unscreened women. Among the many egregious examples is Tabár et al,[9,10] who showed a 63% reduction in breast cancer mortality that is coincidentally fairly similar to that calculated in the foregoing example in which all the reduction is simply an artifact of screening. (Individual investigators may be ignorant of the existence or magnitude of these biases, but journal editorial boards have no excuse for failing to understand the basics of inference or to be unaware of the screening bias traps. Publishers of medical journals embarrass themselves and, by association, the medical profession when they publish such misinformation.)

The role of DCIS is not specifically considered in the preceding discussion or in Figure 17.1. Adding DCIS to the mix of tumors does not fit with the assumption that the mean sojourn time is 2 years. Sojourn times for DCIS tend to be much longer than those for invasive disease, and some part of a sojourn time for DCIS would likely be a period with both invasive and DCIS components. Indeed, some DCIS lesions have sojourn times that are effectively infinite because they would not clinically manifest during the patients' lifetimes. A reasonable approach would be to consider the distribution of sojourn times to be a mixture, with a component for DCIS having greater mean than that for invasive disease. The greater heterogeneity would accentuate all the comparisons made previously. In the example, the

65% reduction in breast cancer mortality for mammographically versus clinically detected cancer (including DCIS) would be even more pronounced. Again, this is pure bias and has nothing to do with any real benefits of mammography.

One could minimize length bias by spacing screenings closer together. However, even daily screening would fail to pick up all cancers. Besides being impractical, frequent screening exacerbates its negative aspects.

Lead-time bias is easier to understand than is length bias. Length bias is a consequence of the heterogeneity in the distribution of sojourn times. Lead-time bias applies even if all tumors have the same sojourn time. Consider the second tumor in Figure 17.2. The patient would receive diagnosis 2.7 years earlier mammographically than clinically. If one starts the clock at the time of diagnosis, this patient would be observed to live 2.7 years longer in the first case than in the second—even with no interventions in either case! For those 33 patients in Figure 17.2 whose tumors were detected mammographically, the average lead time is 2.0 years (which is similar to some estimates from the randomized trials).[8]

The preceding illustration does not consider the possible benefits of therapy. If patients with tumors detected early benefit from the earlier use of therapy, this real benefit of mammography will add to the spurious benefit that is due to bias. However, as suggested by the example, the effects of the biases are so large and the ability to quantify them so remote that it is not possible to identify any real benefit of screening that is separate from the biases or even to decide that screening has a benefit.

The foregoing discussion about length and lead-time biases was couched in terms of comparing databases, but it applies as well to ordinary clinical practice. Clinicians observe that their patients whose tumors were detected mammographically do very well in comparison with their unscreened patients. This is inevitable, even if screening has no benefit. Moreover, the magnitudes of these biases are so great that it is easy to see a difference in the outcomes of the two groups on the basis of a very small number of patients, such as those that one oncologist might treat and follow up over a few years. The unwary clinician may associate the observed benefit with screening, and many do just that. However, as the preceding illustration suggests, any screening benefit is impossible to discern in clinical practice, nor is it possible in the clinic to discriminate a screening benefit from the artificial benefits due to length and lead-time biases. Clinicians who think that they can see a benefit for screening in their practices are fooling themselves. Clinicians are accustomed to learning in the process of practicing medicine. It is difficult for people to accept that there is a circumstance in which learning by observation is not possible!

RANDOMIZED SCREENING TRIALS

So far, in understanding the benefits of screening mammography, we have discounted intuition, clinical experience, and observations from within and across databases. The only mode of inference that remains for deciding whether screening reduces mortality is found in randomized trials. In most circumstances of cancer research (such as in Phase II therapy trials), it is possible to learn without randomizing (although randomization is always preferable). However, for reasons discussed, randomization is essential for evaluating the benefits of screening.

In the simplest randomized screening trial, women who are free of breast cancer are assigned to screening according to some schedule or to no screening. All participants are then followed up for mortality and breast cancer mortality. The two groups are compared with respect to these endpoints. Randomization eliminates bias in the selection process, and because all patients begin observation at a time before any information is available about breast cancer, length and lead-time biases are eliminated.

Despite being the gold standard of medical research and the best way to infer breast-screening benefit, randomized trials are not perfect inferential tools. In particular, they come with their own set of biases: Randomization may fail, and women at higher risk may be preferentially assigned to one group; prevalent disease may be easier to detect in the screened group (and be eliminated from the trial); and assessing whether death is due to breast cancer may be different in the two groups, and the like. The Nordic Cochrane Center[4,11] rated the mammography screening trials and found that all were of poor or medium quality. The Center's criticisms are very serious and render it plausible that the survival benefits attributed to screening in the randomized trials are not real, and this is true for all ages. Indeed, the combined results of the only two trials rated to have medium quality (Canada and Malmö) show no reduction in breast cancer mortality for women who were assigned to screening. However, the Center's arguments are not universally accepted, so the issue is still controversial.[5,12,13] For women in their forties, it matters little who is right and whether the results reported from the trials accurately reflect reality. Even if one takes the results of the trials at face value, the benefit of screening in younger women is limited. In the sequel, I address the estimated benefits and risks for these women.

Only one randomized trial (Canadian National Breast Screening Study I) was designed to include only women in their forties.[14,15] The other randomized trials considered these women as part of a larger population. Considering subsets of patients is wrought with inferential problems, but this subset was identified not because of the results within the subset in comparison with the entire set but because it is a natural one to consider. Therefore, the usual statistical concerns do not apply. Still, taking the trials as a whole, it is not obvious how best to address the effect of age. It may not be appropriate to consider these women in isolation. Breast cancer is not a different disease in younger women than in older women. Whether age is an independent prognostic factor in breast cancer is controversial.[16–22] There is no question that patient age is predictive of some tumor characteristics (notably hormone receptor status),[16–20,23–25] and it may have an impact on recurrence and survival even for fixed tumor characteristics. Such an effect is intuitively appealing. It is well known—and commonly stated—that breast cancer is a heterogeneous disease. More aggressive tumors tend to make themselves known earlier in their development, and hence at an earlier age. However, tumors can be aggressive whenever they develop: Heterogeneity extends across ages, and the age of 50 plays no special role in this regard. Moreover, it is far from clear how or whether any mortality benefit of screening mammography depends on tumor aggressiveness.

Regardless of whether it is predictive of survival in breast cancer, age is not a very strong prognostic factor. In addition, it would be unlikely for mammography to have a differential effect depending on age, unless age were itself predictive of the benefits of chemotherapy or hormonal therapy. There is no evidence for such an interaction. Moreover, menopausal status is not predictive of these benefits.[7] Therefore, if screening mammography is effective in reducing mortality in women older than age 50, it is likely to be effective as well in women younger than 50. Conversely, the magnitude of any benefit may well depend on age. For example, the sensitivity and specificity of mammography vary with age, with greater imaging accuracy achieved for older women.[26–28] Also, the incidence of breast cancer is lower in younger women, with the potential for prolonging or saving lives being correspondingly less. In the opposite direction, younger women have more years of life to save and, in that sense, any benefit of screening is potentially greater in these women.

In sum, the magnitude of any screening benefit may well depend on age and in ways that we do not fully understand. Therefore, it is reasonable to consider the results of the randomized trials restricted to women admitted to those trials while in their forties. Indeed, most other tacks for addressing the role of age cannot be taken because few of the trialists have made their raw data available. Trialists have published results for categories of ages, and all have published summary results for participants younger than 50 at trial entry. I consider these published results, as is standard in meta-analysis, but there are at least two caveats for this approach. First, it is not appropriate to attribute benefits to women screened in their forties because these women started screening at ages up to 49. Therefore, many had some or even most of their trial mammograms in their fifties. Second, a woman who considers screening starting at age 40 would not be interested in the way the results are published but with the benefit she might be expected to achieve in comparison with starting screening at a later age, such as 50. Such comparisons are not possible with the available data. Moreover, it is not possible to say whether comparing results of women who entered the trials in their forties is an overestimate or underestimate of the benefit of starting at age 40 as opposed to age 50. One thing that can be said is that applying an estimate of one quantity to another increases uncertainty.

The characteristics of the eight randomized trials of screening mammography are listed in Table 17.1.[29] (There are only seven randomized trials if Kopparberg and Östergötland are viewed as a single "two-county trial.") The designs of the trials varied. The Canadian trial considered volunteers who consented to be

TABLE 17.1 Characteristics of the Eight Randomized Screening Trials[15,30–32,60–63]

Entry Trial (Label)	Age	Accrual Period	FU (yr)	Rndm Type	No. Mam	Interval (mo)	No. Views	Analysis Type[a]
HIP (H)	40–49	1963–66	18.0	Individ	4	12	2	FU
Kopparberg (K)	40–49	1977–89	15.2	Cluster	4	24	1	Eval
Östergötland (O)	40–49	1978–89	14.2	Cluster	4	24	1	Eval
Malmö (M)	45–49	1977–90	12.7	In	5	18,24	1,2	FU
Edinburgh (E)	45–49	1978–85	14.0	Cluster	4	24	1,2	FU
Göteborg (G)	39–49	1982–84	12.0	Cluster-/Ind[b]	5	18	1,2	Eval
Stockholm (S)	40–49	1981–86	11.4	Cluster	2	28	1	Eval
Canada NBSS-I (C)	40–49	1980–85	10.5	In	4, 5	12	2	FU

Eval, evaluation; FU, follow up; HIP, Health Insurance Plan of New York; ind, individual; mam, mammogram; NBSS-I, National Breast Screening Study; rndm, randomization.

[a]Follow-up analysis considers deaths from breast cancer detected at any time after study entry. Evaluation analysis modifies follow-up analysis by not considering deaths from breast cancer detected after the study screening period.

[b]There was a change in randomization procedure partway through this trial; 82% of the women were randomly assigned individually.

randomly assigned. This trial had full compliance at the first screen, but compliance deteriorated for later screens. The other trials were population-based, with one group invited for screening and the other group not invited. Randomization was either in clusters (clinics, for example) or individually (by date of birth, say). The rate of compliance was not as high as in the Canadian trial because some of the women did not accept the invitation. The number of mammograms and the interval between screenings also varied, as indicated in the table. An important difference is what is termed *analysis type*. Four of the trials ("evaluation analysis") employed a mammogram in the control group. This was timed to coincide with the last mammogram in the "screened" group. Breast cancer deaths were counted only if they resulted from those cancers detected at or before the final study mammogram in the screened group, or at or before the only mammogram in the control group. However, the timetable for the control mammogram slipped in all four studies that used this approach, and the slippage was substantial, typically approximately 1 year. As a consequence, many breast cancers (and therefore many deaths due to breast cancer) detected in the control group would not have been found in the screened group.[29] This bias was substantial. For example, the control group in the Göteborg trial had 12% more breast cancers detected per participant than did the screened group.[30] This is a strange result because mammography is exceptionally good at finding cancer, so looking more often would be expected to find more cancer.

Table 17.1 shows the age ranges for women who were younger than 50 and participated in the randomized trials. Table 17.2 shows the corresponding breast cancer mortality results.[30–32] The overall reduction in breast cancer mortality due to mammography is estimated to be 18%. However, the individual trial estimates range from 45% in Göteborg to an *increase* in mortality of 14% in Canada. There are many possible explanations for the differences in estimated benefits. One is simple statistical variation. Another is that the control groups were different and that the mammographic schedules and procedures were different.

In view of the evident differences in the trials and the widely varying results, it would be wrong to assume that the benefit of screening is the same in all eight trials. Yet, such an assumption is made by the Mantel-Haenszel test, which is the standard statistical test employed by meta-analysts. Roughly speaking, this test supposes that all the participants were in a single large trial with 18% reduction in breast cancer mortality. Figure 17.3A shows the implied distribution of the mean percent reduction in breast cancer mortality. The corresponding 95% confidence interval of 5%–29% does not include 0 (no screening benefit). As a reflection of the implausibility of the homogeneity assumption, this interval contains the reductions of only two of the eight trials, Edinburgh and the Health Insurance Plan of New York.

A more reasonable approach is to allow for the possibility of heterogeneity among the trials. A statistical method that does this is a Bayesian hierarchical model. The eight trials are regarded as having been selected from some larger

TABLE 17.2 Breast Cancer Mortality Results from the Eight Randomized Trials, Restricted to Women Aged 40–49 at Entry[30–32]

	Screening Group			Control Group			
Trial	BC Deaths	Life Years	Mortality Rate[a]	BC Deaths	Life Years	Mortality Rate[a]	Comparison: Mortality Reduct (%)[b]
HIP	49	248,000	19.8	65	253,000	25.7	23
Kopparberg	23	144,000	16.0	18	75,000	24.0	33
Östergötland	27	143,000	18.9	27	147,000	18.4	−3
Malmö	57	166,000	34.3	78	144,000	54.2	38
Edinburgh	47	140,000	33.6	53	126,000	41.9	20
Göteborg	18	138,000	13.0	40	168,000	23.8	45
Stockholm	24	174,000	13.8	12	88,000	13.6	−1
Canada	82	283,000	29.0	72	283,000	25.4	−14
Total	327	1,436,000	22.8	365	1,284,000	28.4	18

BC, breast cancer; mortality reduct, breast cancer morality reduction.

[a]Breast cancer mortality rate: deaths per 100,000 life years.

[b]Observed percent breast cancer mortality reduction is 100 (1- relative risk), where relative risk is the ratio of mortality rates, screening to control. For total, relative risk is calculated using the Mantel-Haenszel statistic.

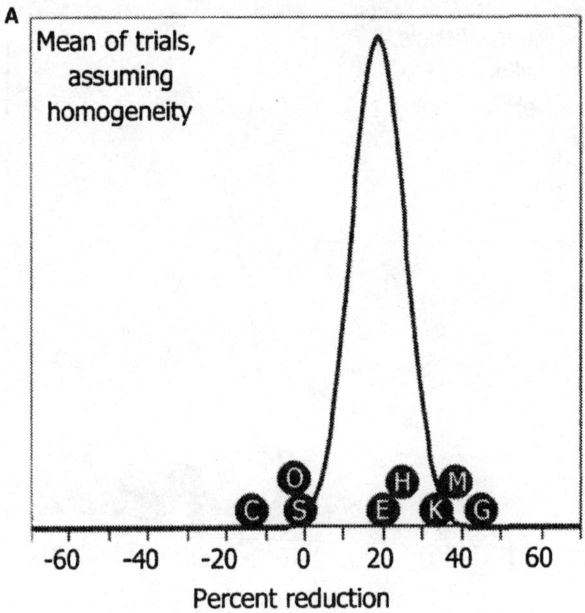

FIGURE 17.3 Distributions of reduction in breast cancer mortality for different assumptions.[29] The horizontal positions of the solid circles indicate the observed mortality reductions (in the horizontal scale) of the eight randomized trials (see Table 17.2); trial labels from Table 17.1. The areas under the curves in (A), (B), and (C) are equal, and the centers of the distributions are similar, approximately 18% in each case. (A) The mean reduction in the population of trials and assuming homogeneity of the trials; precision is high, as indicated by the narrow distribution. (B) Again, the mean reduction in the population of trials, but now allowing for differences in the trials; distribution evinces less precision than in (A). (C) The predictive distribution of breast cancer mortality reduction in a future cohort of women due to choosing screening; the magnitude of any benefit and whether a benefit exists is clearly uncertain.

population of screening trials.[33] There are at least two questions of interest. One is the average reduction over all trials in this larger population. The distribution of this reduction is shown in Figure 17.3B. The 95% probability interval for the mean reduction in the population of trials is from –1% to 36%, which does include 0. The most germane question of interest for a woman entertaining screening is the reduction that will be observed in a future cohort of women. This is most relevant because it refers specifically to women who are now candidates for screening rather than to women in the setting of the trials. Predicting future results entails an extra level of variability.[34] The corresponding distribution is shown in Figure 17.3C. The uncertainty in this distribution is substantial: The 95% probability interval is from –17% to 51%.[29] A cohort of women, all of whom choose screening, has approximately an 85% chance of receiving some benefit.

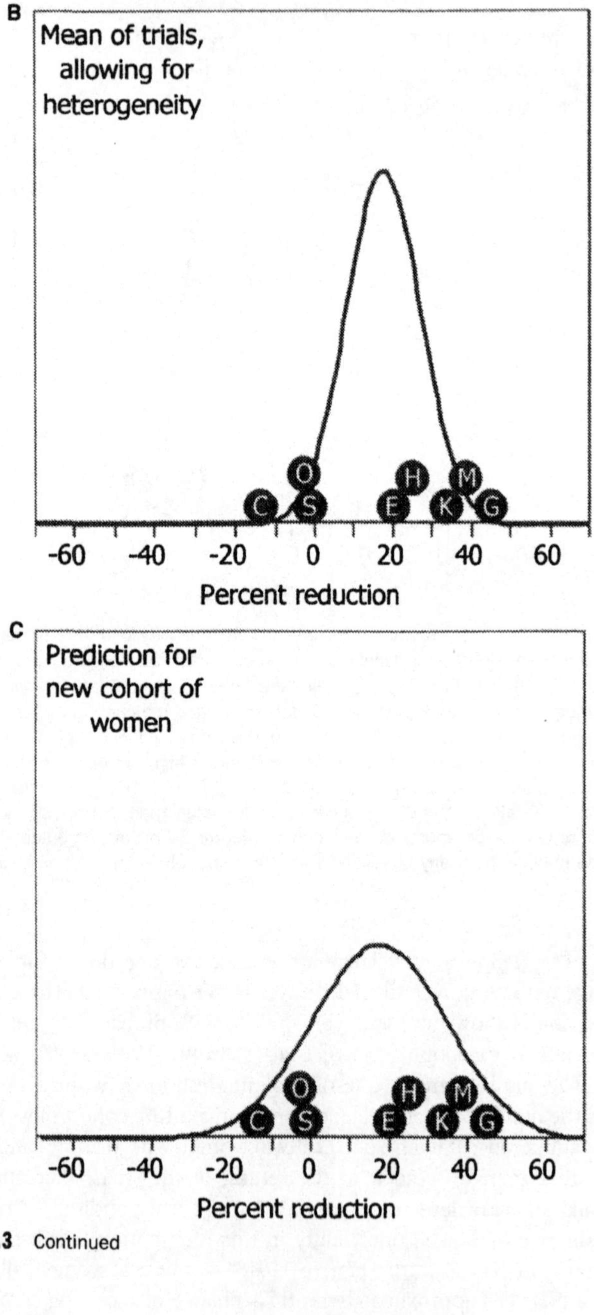

FIGURE 17.3 Continued

(This is the area to the right of 0 under the predictive distribution in Figure 17.3C.) Also, they have approximately a 15% chance of no or negative benefit.

Properly accounting for trial and sampling variability shows that there is enormous uncertainty associated with the point estimate of 18% reduction in breast cancer mortality. However, in the remainder of this chapter, I assume that there indeed is an 18% reduction in breast cancer mortality for women who are screened in their forties.

The estimated reduction of 18% in breast cancer mortality from the randomized trials is *relative risk*, relative in the sense that it compares participants in a screened group with controls. The numeric value of this reduction is difficult to interpret because it depends on the rate of breast cancer mortality in the controls. (To complicate matters, women tend to overestimate greatly their risk of dying of breast cancer,[35] so any reduction seems important.) Suppose that a 65-year-old Iowan could reduce by 18% his risk of getting eaten by a shark in the next 10 years: not worth much. However, suppose he could reduce by 18% his risk of dying of a heart attack in the next 10 years: very worthwhile. The difference is that the *absolute risk* in the latter setting is much higher than in the first setting. The same reduction in relative risk renders the difference much greater. In analyzing trial results, there are good statistical reasons for focusing on relative risk, but relative risk is not appropriate for personal decision making: Decisions should be based on absolute risk. A more appropriate question is, How much savings in life is implied by an 18% reduction in breast cancer mortality?

Any survival benefits due to screening women in their forties accrue gradually. The estimated 18% mortality reduction applies at the end of available follow up in the trials, approximately 15 years after randomization. Figure 17.4 shows the estimated cumulative mortality rates in the two groups over time from randomization out to 15 years.[29] There is not much difference in the two curves until approximately 8 years after randomization. One way to address absolute risk reduction using a metric that everyone understands is to consider the area (shown shaded) between the two mortality curves in Figure 17.4. The units are years per 1000 women. This area is the estimated advantage in life expectancy for screening over control. Out to 15 years, the area is approximately 3.8 years per 1000 women, or 1.4 days per woman. Additional advantage may accrue beyond 15 years. It is unlikely that the advantage would continue to be 18% indefinitely for women who choose to initiate screening in their forties as opposed to starting at, say, age 50. The limited follow up in the randomized trials gives little information about the curves beyond 15 years. For illustration, assume an 18% lifelong reduction in breast cancer mortality and account for competing risks (cardiovascular disease, etc.). Then, the advantage would be an overall life expectancy increase of 5.3 days, owing to screening. Again, this is subject to a great deal of variability, does not rule out the possibility that the true advantage is negative.

The principal endpoint considered by the trialists and by screening meta-analysts is breast cancer mortality. From the perspective of a woman entertaining

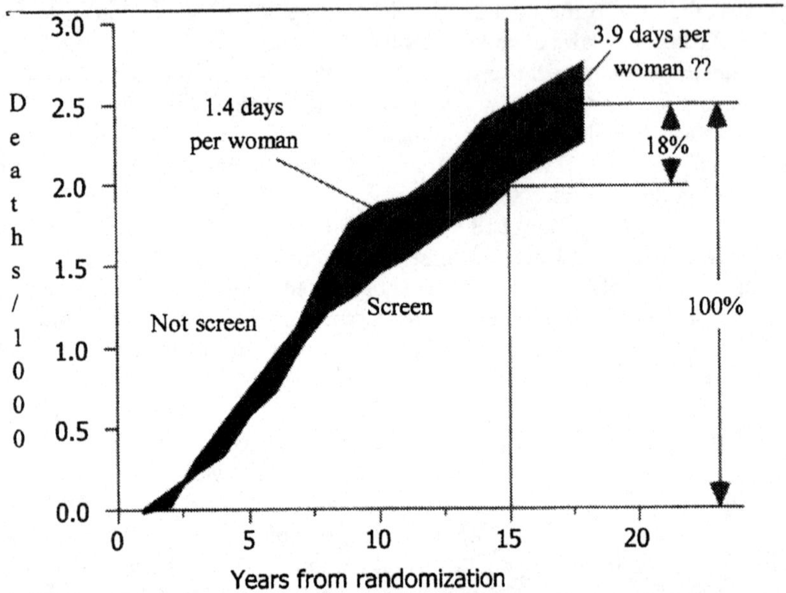

FIGURE 17.4 Cumulative number of deaths per 1000 women for screening and control groups in the randomized trials. Units of shaded areas are expected increases in lifetime per woman due to screening. These are estimates. The curves are sufficiently variable that the true curves may be coincident, so 0 area between them (0 increase in expected lifetime) is not ruled out.

screening, a more appropriate endpoint is death by any cause. This considers any life-threatening effects of screening, including possible deleterious effects of radiation, overtreatment if disease is found or suspected, and motor vehicle accidents while traveling to be screened. However, deaths by other causes swamp those due to breast cancer. So, analysts assume that other causes of death are equal in the two groups. Practically speaking, it would be impossible to power a study to detect a lowering in all-cause mortality, even if millions of women could be randomly allocated. Indeed, in the five Swedish trials combined (considering all ages and not just women in their forties), there was an increased mortality of 4% in the screened group. (After adjusting for an age differential, this dropped to 0%.) So, in spite of a substantial reduction in breast cancer mortality in these trials, there was no difference in all-cause mortality. Any former advantage was erased by random variability. This observation is very important because it highlights the magnitude of the estimated screening advantage in breast cancer mortality (i.e., that any such advantage is so small that it is undetectable against the backdrop of other causes of death).

RISKS OF SCREENING MAMMOGRAPHY

There are several risks associated with screening. If screening has a benefit, these risks may or may not cancel such a benefit. However, they are important and must be considered.

The potential benefit of screening mammography is that it may prolong life, as described. The risks of screening have been extensively described.[36–43] They include false-positive results, inconvenience, pain, and anxiety.[44–51] A woman who has nine mammograms over the decade of her forties has a probability of 55% that she will have at least one false-positive outcome.[52] False positives have their own set of negatives. These include additional anxiety and additional workups, including the possibility of biopsies.[53]

There are negative aspects of screening per se. Inconvenience is one that will depend on individual women and their proximity to the mammography clinic. Cost is also specific to individual women and depends on their insurance, their means of travel, proximity to the clinic, and the like.

A number of "risks" are included as negatives on the benefit side of the ledger[29] and should not be addressed separately as risks. These include radiation-induced breast cancer, false-negative readings, false reassurance from false-negative results (which might lead a woman to eschew breast self-examinations and clinical breast examinations), and using less than optimal treatment when an aggressive tumor happens to be found while it is still small and seemingly not very aggressive.

A risk properly considered as a negative of screening is that screened women are more likely to have cancer diagnosed, and they learn about their cancers sooner than had they not been screened. For example, the 54 women depicted in Figure 17.2 would have learned about their cancers an average of 1.22 years sooner when screened than when not screened. It may seem strange to say that finding cancers early is negative because this is precisely the goal and the virtue of mammography. Finding cancer early is both good and bad. The extent to which it is good is reflected in the estimated 18% reduction in breast cancer mortality. Knowing one has cancer and the process of dealing with it is a price paid for such a reduction. Other things (such as survival) being equal, people are happier without knowing that they have cancer. Therefore, given that the positives are also listed, finding extra cancers is properly viewed as a negative. Extra cancers lead to extra surgery. Surgery may itself be a reasonable price to pay for extending life, but it is still a price, and it should be listed as a negative in weighing against the positive side of screening. The Cochrane Breast Cancer Group found 20% more mastectomies and 30% more mastectomies and lumpectomies in the screened group than in the control group.[4]

An important special case of finding more cancers involves DCIS. In the United States, 25% of screen-detected breast cancers are staged as in situ at the first screening (32% in subsequent screenings),[54] whereas only approximately 4% of breast cancers detected by other means are in situ. Moreover, this was also true before the advent of screening programs.[55] Finding DCIS may be a benefit in that it can be treated before it becomes invasive, and thereby finding it may prolong survival but, again, if finding DCIS as part of screening prolongs survival, this will have contributed to the estimated 18% reduction in mortality from the randomized trials. Therefore, DCIS is properly viewed separately as a risk.

Table 17.3 is a list of benefits and risks. The risks are listed roughly in decreasing order of importance. However, the ordering of importance of identified risks will differ among women. For example, monetary costs may be all-important to some women, whereas preserving one's breasts may be the critical issue for others.

COMMUNICATING BENEFITS AND RISKS

To convey benefits and risks accurately requires quantification, but numeric risks are difficult for many people to understand.[56] Health care providers and health guidelines should provide lists of benefits and risks of screening mammography to the women they serve. Table 17.3 is such a list. However, this table may be of little help to a woman contemplating screening. One reason is that the benefits and risks are given on different scales, with different denominators. For example, the estimated 18% mortality reduction compares with mortality among controls, whereas the 15% reduction in severe pain is in comparison with all women undergoing mammography. It is possible to compare directly the 1.4 days in expected life saved in the first 15 years with the time it takes to obtain mammograms during one's forties. However, it is less than clear how to factor in other risks. One way to combine risks is through utility assessment in which risks and benefits are put onto the same scale (such as days of life). This entails an extensive

TABLE 17.3 Potential Benefits and Risks of Screening Mammography for Women in Their Forties

Benefits	Risks
Estimated mortality reduction of 18% for regular mammograms in one's forties (prolonged life averaged 1.4 days in first 15 years, 5.3 days over lifetime)	Probability (55%) of one or more false-positive results in 9 mammograms, with associated risks (extra clinical visits, extra mammograms, biopsies, added anxiety); increased probability of discovering cancers, living longer with cancer; 30% probability of finding DCIS; 30% added breast surgeries (lumpectomies, mastectomies); mild to severe pain experienced during mammograms; anxiety about having mammograms; inconvenience (time spent traveling to clinic, etc.); costs (mammograms, travel, etc.)

development in which the woman's preferences are compared with standard risks. However, the "benefits" side of the table is not very strong. Most women's assessments of the utilities of the "risks" will surpass that of the benefits by the time they get part way down the list. Therefore, presenting the table with some help in reading it may avoid an extensive assessment of utilities.

Another defect of the lists in Table 17.3 as regards decision making is that it fails to convey the uncertainties involved. Previously in this chapter, I addressed the uncertainty regarding the estimated 18% reduction in breast cancer mortality. Some researchers think it is greater, and some think it is less (and some that it is nonexistent), whereas still others remain open-minded about screening's benefits. Suffice to say that all other numeric estimates in the table are uncertain. Indeed, some of these estimates are controversial. The 18% mortality reduction is subject to much greater uncertainty than are the risks, but all uncertainties should be made clear to a woman who is contemplating screening.

The estimated 18% reduction in breast cancer mortality is a relative benefit: The reference population is unscreened women who developed cancer. A disadvantage of such measures is that they do not account for incidence, so they are of little value in making decisions. The estimated 1.4 days of life saved in the first 15 years is an absolute benefit in that it does account for incidence.

Most people do not like "days of life saved" as a measure of screening effectiveness. They say that saving only 1.4 days of life over 15 years for a regular schedule of mammograms trivializes the benefit of screening. However, if prolonging life by 1.4 days is trivial, the benefits of screening are trivial. This is a case of killing the messenger—or the measure—because of the message. People do not know how to interpret such statistics as 18% reduction in mortality, but they do understand days of life gained.

Communicating benefit is easier if the units are understandable. It is easy to relate to gain in days of life expectancy. One can compare 1.4 days of life lost for failing to get mammograms with that of more familiar risks. For example, one would lose an estimated 1.4 days of life by not wearing a seat belt over 5 years of typical automobile travel in the United States, by riding a bicycle for 4 hours without a helmet (or 15 hours while wearing a helmet), and of gaining half an ounce of body weight (and keeping it on).[56] A commonly used measure of absolute benefit is number of deaths prevented for each 10,000 women screened regularly during their forties—or, what is closely related, the number of mammograms required to save one life. However, neither measure is easy to calculate, and neither can be calculated from the trial results. The number of deaths prevented depends on the time of follow up. If screening prolongs survival but does not effect cures, any advantage in the number of deaths prevented at 15 years may be lost by 20 years. The reported results of the trials allow for calculating these statistics at 15 years after randomization. Combining the results of all eight randomized trials, there were 36 breast cancer deaths per 10,000 women in the control groups and 29 deaths due to breast cancer per 10,000 women assigned to receive mammograms. (The implied reduction is slightly greater than the 18% reduction in breast cancer mortality already discussed because the latter figure refers to reduction in overall hazard rather than in mortality at 15 years; in addition, the latter is based on a Mantel-Haenszel statistic, which is slightly different from simply combining the trials' results.) Women should understand that screening is a lottery. Any winnings are shared by a minority of women—approximately one in 60 or 70—who have breast cancer diagnosed in their forties. The remaining women, who represent the overwhelming majority, experience no benefit. In the lottery analogy, they lose their entry fee; in screening, they ante the time involved, and they take the risks that are associated with screening.

The lottery analogy is appropriate both for individual decision making and for setting national policies. Consider a lottery in which each of 1,000 women antes $1. The total contributed is $1000. A few of the 1000 women win. If the total amount returned to these women is $1000, the lottery is "fair." If the total returned is greater than $1000, the lottery is favorable, and if the total returned is less than $1000, the lottery is unfavorable. In screening, the 1000 women receive an estimated total of 3.8 years, divided among those with diagnosed breast cancer. Whether the screening is favorable and worthy of participation depends on whether the 1000 women contributed more than the equivalent of 3.8 years to the pot, or more than 1.4 days per woman.

Some women have an elevated risk of developing breast cancer. For example, carriers of mutations of BRCA1 have over the decade of their forties a risk of developing breast cancer approximately 15 times that of noncarriers.[57–59] For carriers, an 18% mortality reduction will be potentially 15 times as important as it is for noncarriers. Although there is no evidence that screening reduces mortality in women who carry mutations, any absolute benefit of screening is likely to be magnified in these women.

SCREENING MAMMOGRAPHY ADVICE TO WOMEN IN THEIR FORTIES

Mammography is effective in finding breast cancer, and it finds cancer earlier than do other means of detection. The problem is that finding cancer early may or may not help in treating it. Although some people feel passionately about the question, no one knows for certain whether, or how much, having mammograms before the age of 50 increases life expectancy. Some women die from breast cancer even if their cancers are small when detected by mammography.

Although eight randomized trials have addressed the question of whether mammography reduces the numbers of deaths due to breast cancer, there is still substantial uncertainty about its benefits for women in their forties. Some trials find that it lowers the breast cancer death rate among these women, and others find that it does not. On balance, there seems to be a modest reduction in breast cancer mortality associated with regular screening, but this conclusion may change as more information becomes available.

In the eight randomized trials, assignment of women in their forties to receive or not to receive regular mammograms was accomplished, in effect, by the toss of a coin. For the first 8 years or so after enrolling in the trials, there was little difference in the numbers of deaths in the two groups. However, at 15 years, there were approximately 29 deaths due to breast cancer per 10,000 women assigned to receive mammograms and approximately 36 breast cancer deaths per 10,000 women in the control groups. The reduction of seven deaths per 10,000 women at 15 years is a rough estimate, and it may not apply to women outside the trials. Also, it does not mean that these seven women were cured of their disease. It is possible that finding the cancer early and treating it while it was small extended these women's lives without curing their cancer. Moreover, the reduction of seven deaths per 10,000 women is subject to many types of uncertainties and may be far from what is achieved by programs outside the context of screening trials. For example, there might be no mortality reduction in a particular set of women who are aged 40–49 and undergo regular screening.

At least 59 of 60 women in their forties gain nothing in the mammography lottery. This is because only approximately 1 in 60 women who are screened regularly in their forties receives a diagnosis of breast cancer. The 1 woman in 60 shares any gain she receives from the lottery with the other women who are given diagnoses of breast cancer. An unknown proportion of the women who receive diagnoses of cancer actually gain but, assuming that the figure of 7 of 10,000 accurately reflects reality, the average gain in the first 15 years after they started screening is approximately 3 months of additional life. This equates to prolonging each of the original participants' lives by an average of 1.4 days. This figure should be compared with the cost of playing the lottery. This cost is in terms of the risks associated with mammograms.

The risks of mammography are better understood than are the benefits. All women who obtain mammograms are subject to these risks. Possibly the most important risk is that of false-positive outcomes. A false-positive result occurs when a woman who does not have cancer has an abnormal mammogram reading and requires follow-up procedures. Approximately 55 of 100 women who have nine mammograms between ages 40 and 49 experience at least one false-positive diagnosis. Between 10 and 15 of these 100 women will undergo at least one biopsy: the surgical removal of a small amount of breast tissue that can be checked for cancer by a pathologist. There are side effects and negative aspects to any surgery, but a biopsy is a very low-risk procedure. Women usually experience anxiety as a result of a false-positive mammogram result, and some women's anxiety continues even after they find that they do not have cancer. In addition, approximately 15 of 100 women experience severe pain from mammograms. Finally, as it is good at finding cancer, mammography can find cancers that would never threaten the woman's life; however, we are unable to tell which cancers these are. So women who are screened are more likely to have more extensive surgery—lumpectomy or mastectomy—and chemotherapy.

Some of the women who were screened in the randomized trials had annual mammograms, but for others the time between mammograms was longer. If having five mammograms between ages 40 and 49 is beneficial, having 10 mammograms is probably better. However, there is no evidence from the trials that a yearly schedule is better than biannual mammograms. Most of any benefit of mammograms occurs with having them every other year, and any incremental benefit of yearly mammograms is smaller. Of course, having twice as many mammograms approximately doubles the chances of the risks.

Regular mammograms between ages 40 and 49 probably lengthen some women's lives, but the overall benefit is not great. Some women in their forties choose regular mammography, and some do not; both decisions are rational. Screening may benefit some of those women who choose it, but screening has risks. Each woman should weigh the potential benefits and risks and decide whether screening is appropriate for her.

DISCUSSION AND SUMMARY

Most U.S. medical organizations recommend regular screening for all women in their forties. Such a blanket recommendation is troubling for several reasons. First, whether screening mammography is beneficial for women in their forties is questionable, as I have argued in this chapter. Second, such a recommendation may be viewed by women as promising that screening mammography is a major tool in the fight against breast cancer. Such a promise would be false. In the United States alone, tens of thousands of women die each year from breast cancer detected by screening mammography. There has been a modest (10%–15%) drop in the U.S. breast cancer mortality rate between years 1990 and 2000, and similar drops have been observed in other countries. Some radiologists have argued that this is due to the increased use of screening in the United States, commencing in the early 1980s. This is pure speculation. Although mammography may play a role in lowering mortality, most of and even all the observed benefit can be easily explained by improvements in chemotherapy and—especially—by the widespread use of tamoxifen for patients with estrogen-receptive positive tumors. The benefits of these improvements have been demonstrated in numerous top-quality randomized clinical trials.[7]

Regular screening mammography is not an imperative health measure for women in their forties. According to Horton,[5] who was referring to women of all ages, "At present, there is no reliable evidence from large randomized trials to support screening programmes." Moreover, as I have shown, even if the trial results are taken at face value, the benefits of screening are small for women in their forties. Also, screening has a number of important risks. Taken together, and depending on a woman's preferences, these risks may more than cancel any benefit. Women should be informed of the risks of screening. Those who are most concerned about their health will probably choose regular screening; others will not. Both choices may be rational and reasonable.

Most clinicians and health care providers go along with medical organizations in recommending screening mammography for women in their forties. Such recommendations should be accompanied by the qualification that the scientific community is divided concerning the merits of such screening. Women should understand that there is great uncertainty concerning whether screening can save lives. It is deceptive for a medical professional to promote screening as an essential part of maintaining good health. Women who might otherwise eschew screening will be persuaded to seek a medical intervention that is of uncertain value and that may be harmful. It is wrong for medical professionals to hold out false hopes and to extend potentially empty promises to the people they serve. Doing so leaves the profession open to the charge that it serves only itself.

REFERENCES

1. Fletcher SW. Whither scientific deliberation in health policy recommendations? Alice in the Wonderland of breast-cancer screening. N Engl J Med 1997;336(16):1180–1183.
2. Taubes G. The breast-screening brawl. Science 1997;275(5305):1056–1059.
3. Ransohoff DF, Harris RP. Lessons from the mammography screening controversy: Can we improve the debate? Ann Intern Med 1997;127(11):1029–1034.
4. Olsen O, Gøtzsche PC. Cochrane review on screening for breast cancer with mammography. Lancet 2001;358(9290):1340–1342.
5. Horton R. Screening mammography—an overview revisited. Lancet 2001;358(9290):1284–1285.
6. Behavioral Risk Factor Surveillance System, 1999 survey data, National Center for Chronic Disease Prevention and Health Promotion, Centers for Disease Control and Prevention, U.S. Department of Health and Human Services. URL: *apps.nccd.cdc.gov/brfss/index.asp*
7. Early Breast Cancer Trialists' Collaborative Group. Tamoxifen for early breast cancer: an overview of the randomized trials. Lancet 1998;351(9114):1451–1467.
8. Tabár L, Larsson L-G, Andersson I et al. Breast cancer screening with mammography in women aged 40–49 years: report of the organizing committee and collaborators, Falun Meeting, Sweden, March 21–22, 1996. Int J Cancer 1996;68:693–699.
9. Tabár L, Vitak B, Chen HHT et al. Beyond randomized trials: organized mammographic screening substantially reduces breast carcinoma mortality. Cancer 2001;91(9):1724–1731.
10. Cady B, Michaelson JS. The life-sparing potential of mammographic screening. Cancer 2001; 91(9):1699–1703.
11. Gøtzsche PC, Olsen O. Is screening for breast cancer with mammography justifiable? Lancet 2000;355(9198):129–134.
12. Wald N. Populist instead of professional. J Med Screen 2000;7(1):1.
13. Duffy SW, Tabár L. Screening mammography re-evaluated [letter]. Lancet 2000;355(9205): 747–748.
14. Miller AB, Baines CJ, To T. The Gothenburg breast screening trial: first results on mortality, incidence, and mode of detection for women ages 39–49 years at randomization. Cancer 1998; 83(1):186–190.

15. Miller AB, To T, Baines CJ, Wall C. The Canadian national breast screening study: update on breast cancer mortality. J Natl Cancer Inst Monogr 1997;(22):37–41.

16. Cajdos C, Tartter PI, Bleiweiss IJ et al. Stage 0 to stage III breast cancer in young women. J Am Coll Surg 2000;190(5):509–515.

17. Ezzat A, Raja MA, Zwaan F et al. The lack of age as a significant prognostic factor in non-metastatic breast cancer. Eur J Surg Oncol 1998;24(1):23–27.

18. Winchester DP. Breast cancer in young women. Surg Clin North Am 1996;76(2):279–287.

19. Albain KS, Alfred DC, Clark GM. Breast cancer outcome and predictors of outcome: Are there age differences? J Natl Cancer Inst Monogr 1994;(16):35–42.

20. Chung M, Chang HR, Bland KI, Wanebo. Younger women with breast carcinoma have a poorer prognosis than older women. Cancer 1996;77(1):97–103.

21. Adami H, Malker B, Holmberg L et al. The relation between survival and age at diagnosis in breast cancer. N Engl J Med 1986;315(9):559–563.

22. Alexieva-Figusch J, Van Putten WLJ, Blankenstein MA et al. The prognostic value and relationships of patient characteristics, estrogen and progestin receptors, and site of relapse in primary breast cancer. Cancer 1988;61:758–768.

23. Tabár L, Stephen WD, Bedrich V et al. The natural history of breast carcinoma. Cancer 1999; 86(3):449–462.

24. Mustafa IA, Cole B, Wanebo HJ et al. Prognostic analysis of survival in small breast cancers. J Am Coll Surg 1998;186(5):562–569.

25. Kollias J, Elston CW, Ellis IO et al. Early-onset breast cancer—histopathological and prognostic considerations. Br J Cancer 1997;75(9):1318–1323.

26. Saarenmaa I, Salminen T, Geiger U et al. The effect of age and density of the breast on the sensitivity of breast cancer diagnostic by mammography and ultasonography. Breast Cancer Res Treat 2001;67(2):117–123.

27. Saarenmaa I, Salminen T, Geiger U et al. The visibility of cancer on previous mammograms in retrospective review. Radiology 2001;56(1):40–43.

28. Kerlikowske K, Grady D, Barclay J et al. Effect of age, breast density, and family history on the sensitivity of first screening mammography. JAMA 1996;276(1):33–38.

29. Berry DA. Benefits and risks of screening mammography for women in their forties: a statistical appraisal. J Natl Cancer Inst 1998;90(19):1431–1439.

30. Bjurstam N, Björneld L, Duffy SW et al. The Gothenburg breast screening trial: first results on mortality, incidence, and mode of detection for women ages 39–49 years at randomization. Cancer 1997;80(11):2091–2099.

31. Hendrick RE, Smith RA, Rutledge JH III, Smart CR. Benefit of screening mammography in women aged 40–49: a new meta-analysis of randomized controlled trials. J Natl Cancer Inst Monogr 1997;(22):87–92.

32. Alexander FE, Anderson TJ, Brown HK et al. 14 years of follow-up from the Edinburgh randomised trial of breast-cancer screening. Lancet 1999;353(9168):1903–1908.

33. Stangl DK, Berry DA. Meta-Analysis in Medicine and Health Policy. New York: Marcel Dekker, 2000.

34. Berry DA. Statistics: A Bayesian Perspective. Belmont, CA: Duxbury Press, 1996.

35. Black WC, Nease RF Jr, Tosteson AN. Perceptions of breast cancer risk and screening effectiveness in women younger than 50 years of age. J Natl Cancer Inst 1995;87(10):720–731.

36. Gordis L, Berry DA, Chu SY et al. Breast cancer screening for women ages 40–49. J Natl Cancer Inst 1997;89:1015–1026. [Reprinted in the J Natl Cancer Inst Monogr 1997;(22):7–12.]

37. Fletcher SW. Breast cancer screening among women in their forties: an overview of the issues. J Natl Cancer Inst Monogr 1997;(22):5–9.

38. Feig SA, Hendrick RE. Radiation risk from screening mammography on women aged 40–49 years. J Natl Cancer Inst Monogr 1997;(22):119–124.

39. Rimer BK, Bluman LG. The psychosocial consequences of mammography. J Natl Cancer Inst Monogr 1997;(22):131–138.

40. Harris R. Variation of benefits and harms of breast cancer screening with age. J Natl Cancer Inst Monogr1997;(22):139–143.

41. Kerlikowske K, Barclay J. Outcomes of modern screening mammography. J Natl Cancer Inst Monogr 1997;(22):105–111.

42. Ernster VL, Barclay J. Increases in ductal carcinoma *in situ* (DCIS) of the breast in relation to mammography: a dilemma. J Natl Cancer Inst Monogr 1997;(22):151–156.

43. Elmore JG, Barton MB, Moceri VM et al. Ten-year risk of false positive screening mammograms and clinical breast examinations. N Engl J Med 1998;338(16):1089–1096.

44. Rimer BK, Bluman LG. The psychosocial consequences of mammography. J Natl Cancer Inst Monogr 1997;(22):131–138.

45. Andrews FJ. Pain during mammography: implications for breast screening programmes. Australas Radiol 2001;45(2):113–117.

46. Hafslund B. Mammography and the experience of pain and anxiety. Radiography 2000;6(4): 269–272.

47. Keemers-Gels ME, Groenendijk RP, van den Heuvel JH et al. Pain experienced by women attending breast cancer screening. Breast Cancer Res Treat 2000;60(3):235–240.

48. Aro AR, Absetz-Ylostalo P, Eerola T et al. Pain and discomfort during mammography. Eur J Cancer 1996;32A(10):1674–1679.

49. Dolan NC, Feinglass J, Priyanath A et al. Measuring satisfaction with mammography results reporting. J Gen Intern Med 2001;16(3):157–162.

50. Mainiero MB, Schepps B, Clements NC, Bird CE. Mammography-related anxiety: effect of preprocedural patient education. Womens Health Issues 2001;11(2):110–115.

51. Lampic C, Thurfjell E, Bergh J, Sjoden PO. Short- and long-term anxiety and depression in women recalled after breast cancer screening. Eur J Cancer 2001;37(4):463–469.

52. Christiansen CL, Wang F, Barton MB et al. Predicting the cumulative risk of false-positive mammograms. J Natl Cancer Inst 2000;92:1657–1666.

53. Lidbrink E, Elfving J, Frisell J, Jonsson E. Neglected aspects of false positive findings of mammography in breast cancer screening: analysis of false positive cases from the Stockholm trial. Br Med J 1996;312:273–276.

54. May DS, Lee NC, Richardson LC et al. Mammography and breast cancer detection by race and Hispanic ethnicity: results from a national program (National Breast and Cervical Cancer Early Detection Project, United States). Cancer Causes Control 2000;11(8):697–705.

55. National Cancer Institute. Surveillance, Epidemiology and End Results Program, Cancer Incidence Public-Use Database, 1973–1998. August 2000 update. URL: http://seer.cancer.gov

56. Laudan L. The Book of Risks. New York: John Wiley and Sons, 1994.

57. Ford D, Easton DF, Peto J. Estimates of the gene frequency of BRCA1 and its contribution to breast and ovarian cancer incidence. Am J Hum Genet 1995;57(6):1457–1462.

58. Struewing JP, Abeliovich D, Peretz T et al. The carrier frequency of the BRCA1 185delAG mutation is approximately 1 percent in Ashkenazi Jewish individuals. Nat Genet 1995;11(2):198–200.

59. Berry DA, Parmigiani G, Sanchez J et al. Probability of carrying a mutation of breast-ovarian cancer gene BRCA1 based on family history. J Natl Cancer Inst 1997;89(3):227–238.

60. Shapiro S. Periodic screening for breast cancer: the HIP randomized controlled trial. J Natl Cancer Inst Monogr 1997;(22):27–30.

61. Tabár L, Chen H-H, Fagerberg G et al. Recent results from the Swedish two-county trial: the effects of age, histologic type and mode of detection on the efficacy of breast cancer screening. J Natl Cancer Inst Monogr 1997;(22):43–47.

62. Frisell J, Lidbrink E. The Stockholm mammographic screening trial: risks and benefits in age group 40–49 years. J Natl Cancer Inst Monogr 1997;(22):49–51.

63. Andersson I, Janzon L. Reduced breast cancer mortality in women under age 50: updated results from the Malmö mammographic screening program. J Natl Cancer Inst Monogr 1997;(22):63–67.

Indexes

SUBJECT INDEX

A

B

C

D

E

F

G

H

I

K

L

M

N

O

P

R

S

T

U

V

W

X

INDEX OF TABLES

9 780763 720636

Printed in Dunstable, United Kingdom

87945254R00228